Baillière's

CLINICAL OBSTETRICS AND GYNAECOLOGY

INTERNATIONAL PRACTICE AND RESEARCH

Baillière's

CLINICAL OBSTETRICS AND GYNAECOLOGY

INTERNATIONAL PRACTICE AND RESEARCH

Volume 3/Number 3
September 1989

Laparoscopic Surgery

C. J. G. SUTTON MA, MB, BCh, FRCOG
Guest Editor

Baillière Tindall
London Philadelphia Sydney Tokyo Toronto

This book is printed on acid-free paper. ∞.

Baillière Tindall	24–28 Oval Road,
W.B. Saunders	London NW1 7DX

The Curtis Center, Independence Square West,
Philadelphia, PA 19106–3399, USA

55 Horner Avenue
Toronto, Ontario M8Z 4X6, Canada

Harcourt Brace Jovanovich Group (Australia) Pty Ltd,
30–52 Smidmore Street, Marrickville, NSW 2204, Australia

Exclusive Agent in Japan:
Maruzen Co. Ltd. (Journals Division)
3–10 Nihonbashi 2-chome, Chuo-ku, Tokyo 103, Japan

ISSN 0950–3552

ISBN 0–7020–1386–2 (single copy)

Baillière's Clinical Obstetrics and Gynaecology is published four times each year by Baillière Tindall. Annual subscription prices are:

TERRITORY	ANNUAL SUBSCRIPTION	SINGLE ISSUE
1. UK	£40.00 post free	£18.50 post free
2. Europe	£50.00 post free	£18.50 post free
3. All other countries	Consult your local Harcourt Brace Jovanovich office for dollar price	

The editor of this publication is Margaret Macdonald, Baillière Tindall, 24–28 Oval Road, London NW1 7DX.

Baillière's Clinical Obstetrics and Gynaecology was published from 1983 to 1986 as *Clinics in Obstetrics and Gynaecology*.

Typeset by Phoenix Photosetting, Chatham.
Printed and bound in Great Britain by Mackays of Chatham PLC, Chatham, Kent.

Contributors to this issue

IVO A. BROSENS MD, PhD, University Hospital Gasthuisberg, Herestraat 49 B-3000 Leuven; St. Elizabeth Hospital, 206 De Fré Avenue, B-1180 Brussels, Belgium.

M. A. BRUHAT MA, Department of Obstetrics and Gynaecology, Polyclinique Hotel Dieu, University of Clermont-Ferrand, 13 Boulevard Charles de Gaulle, Clermont-Ferrand, France.

M. CANIS MD, Department of Obstetrics and Gynaecology, Polyclinique Hotel Dieu, University of Clermont-Ferrand, 13 Boulevard Charles de Gaulle, Clermont-Ferrand, France.

JAMES F. DANIELL MD, 2222 State Street, Nashville, TN 37203, USA.

ALAN H. DECHERNEY BS, MD, John Slade Ely Professor of Obstetrics and Gynecology, Yale University School of Medicine, 333 Cedar Street, PO Box 3333, New Haven, CT 06510, USA.

MICHAEL P. DIAMOND BA, MD, Yale University School of Medicine, Division of Reproductive Endocrinology, Department of Obstetrics and Gynecology, 333 Cedar Street, PO Box 3333, New Haven, CT 06510, USA.

JACQUES DONNEZ MD, PhD, Head of Department of Gynecology, Catholic University of Louvain, Cliniques Universaires St. Luc, Avenue Hippocrate 10, B-1200 Brussels, Belgium.

G. MARCUS FILSHIE DM, FRCOG, Reader and Consultant Obstetrician and Gynaecologist, Queen's Medical Center, University Hospital, Nottingham NG7 2UA, UK.

ALAN G. GORDON MB, BCh, FRCS, FRCOG, Consultant Gynaecologist, Princess Royal Hospital, Saltshouse Road, Hull HU8 9HE, UK.

JÖRG KECKSTEIN MD, Scientist, Institute of Laser Technologies, Ulm; Senior Lecturer, Department of Gynaecology and Obstetrics, University of Ulm, Prittwitzstrasse 43, D-79 Ulm, West Germany.

G. MAGE MD, Department of Obstetrics and Gynaecology, Polyclinique Hotel Dieu, University of Clermont-Ferrand, 13 Boulevard Charles de Gaulle, Clermont-Ferrand, France.

ADAM LASZLO MAGOS BSc, MD, MRCOG, Clinical Lecturer/Honorary Senior Registrar, Nuffield Department of Obstetrics and Gynaecology, University of Oxford, John Radcliffe Hospital, Maternity Department, Oxford OX3 9DU, UK.

WILLIAM ROBERT MEYER MD, Postdoctorate Associate, Division of Reproductive Endocrinology, Department of Obstetrics and Gynecology, Yale New Haven Medical School, 333 Cedar Street, PO Box 3333, New Haven, CT 06510, USA.

MICHELLE NISOLLE MD, Catholic University of Louvain, Cliniques Universitaires St. Luc, Avenue Hippocrate 10, B-1200 Brussels, Belgium.

ISEULT O'NEILL-FREYS MD, Department of Obstetrics and Gynaecology, University of Kiel and Michaelis Midwifery School, Michaelisstrasse 16, D-2300 Kiel 1, West Germany.

J. L. POULY MD, Department of Obstetrics and Gynaecology, Polyclinique Hotel Dieu, University of Clermont-Ferrand, 13 Boulevard Charles de Gaulle, Clermont-Ferrand, France.

PATRICK J. PUTTEMANS MD, Department of Obstetrics and Gynaecology, St. Elizabeth Hospital, 206 De Fré Avenue, B-1180 Brussels, Belgium.

HARRY REICH MD, FACOG, SRS, Nesbitt Memorial Hospital, Wyoming Avenue, Kingston, PA 18704, USA.

KURT SEMM MD, MvetD, Professor of Obstetrics and Gynecology, Department of Obstetrics and Gynaecology, University of Kiel and Michaelis-Midwifery School, Michaelisstrasse 16, D-2300 Kiel 1, West Germany.

CHRIS SUTTON MA, MB, BCh, FRCOG, Consultant Obstetrician and Gynaecologist, Royal Surrey County Hospital and St Luke's Hospital, Warren Road, Guildford, Surrey, UK.

KEES WAMSTEKER MD, PhD, Staff Gynaecologist; President, EndoGyn Foundation and Hysteroscopy Training Centre; President, European Society of Hysteroscopy; Spaarne Hospital Haarlem, Department of Gynaecology and Obstetrics, van Heythuijzenweg 1, PO Box 1644, 2003 BR Haarlem, The Netherlands.

A. WATTIEZ MD, Department of Obstetrics and Gynaecology, Polyclinique Hotel Dieu, University of Clermont-Ferrand, 13 Boulevard Charles de Gaulle, Clermont-Ferrand, France.

Table of contents

PREVIOUS ISSUES

March 1987
Fetal Monitoring
M. J. WHITE

June 1987
Gynaecological Surgery
J. M. MONAGHAN

September 1987
Fetal Diagnosis of Genetic Defects
C. H. RODECK

December 1987
Renal Disease in Pregnancy
M. D. LINDHEIMER & J. M. DAVISON

March 1988
Antenatal and Perinatal Causes of Handicap
N. PATEL

June 1988
Gynaecology in the Elderly
S. L. STANTON

September 1988
Anti-hormones in Clinical Gynaecology
D. HEALY

December 1988
Operative Treatment of Cervical Cancer
E. BURGHARDT & J. M. MONAGHAN

March 1989
Operative Treatment of Ovarian Cancer
E. BURGHARDT & J. M. MONAGHAN

June 1989
Dysfunctional Uterine Bleeding and Menorrhagia
J. O. DRIFE

FORTHCOMING ISSUES

December 1989
Psychological Disorders in Obstetrics and Gynaecology
M. OATES

March 1990
Antenatal Care
M. HALL

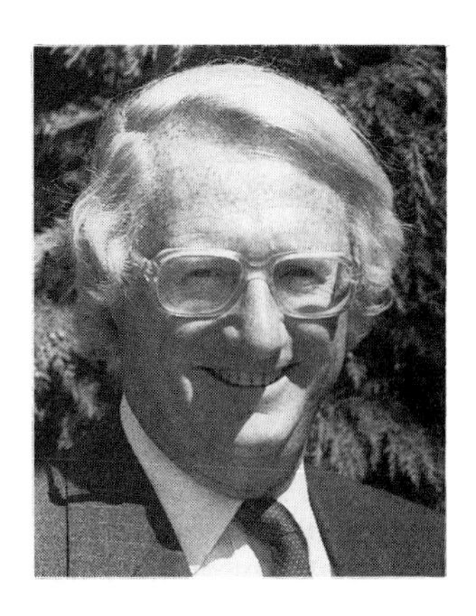

Foreword

The advent of laparoscopy heralded a new era in gynaecology, replacing art with science and taking the guesswork out of the diagnosis of many pelvic and abdominal ailments. Many gynaecologists, proud of their previously unchallenged clinical acumen, were surprised to find that the ovarian cyst their fingers had detected so confidently was in reality distended caecum and the recurrent pelvic infection so stubbornly resistant to antibiotics was, in fact, endometriosis.

The book opens with a fascinating account of the historical aspects involved in the development of endoscopy. It may come as a surprise to discover that the first visual incursions inside the human body date back to 400 BC but these early attempts at endoscopy by Hippocrates and his disciples were 'per vias naturales'. For many centuries the light source was a problem, progressing slowly from the lowly candle to a more sophisticated lantern (originally used by burglars) until eventually Edison invented the light bulb whereupon Man became less afraid of the dark and acquired the ability to peer inside his own bladder. The first laparoscopies using a pneumoperitoneum were performed as long ago as 1910 by Jacobaeus and since then the technique has had its ups and downs in popularity, even being replaced for a while in the 1940s by culdoscopy. It was not until after the Second World War that the development of the cold light source in France and the Hopkins rod lens system in England enabled the safe transmission of light and optimal visualization that is a prerequisite for laparoscopic surgery.

Early attempts at laparoscopic surgery were primarily directed at simplified methods of female sterilization, pioneered mainly in Continental Europe by Fragenheim and Palmer who are generally hailed as the fathers of modern laparoscopy. The original electrodiathermy instruments produced an unacceptable number of complications leading Kurt Semm at Kiel to invent the safer alternative of endocoagulation. The excellent haemostasis provided by this instrument and the development of a whole range of endoscopic operating instruments, endoloops and sutures allowed Semm and his team to enormously expand the number of operations that could be performed through the laparoscope. A further refinement was introduced by Bruhat and his gifted team at Clermont–Ferrand, who first used the unique properties of laser energy to perform delicate fertility surgery through the laparoscope. In this book we are indeed fortunate to have contributions from both of these pioneers in their fields of conventional operative laparoscopy and of laser laparoscopy.

In this volume I have tried to cover the whole spectrum of operative laparoscopy as it exists at the present time, and have gathered together an international team of experts from both sides of the Atlantic. I have struggled hard to resist my obvious bias towards the use of lasers but inevitably they feature prominently in this volume with chapters from the leading pioneers in both Europe and the USA. While editing this book I have been intrigued how many of us have developed laser laparoscopic techniques working completely independently and, certainly in the early days, unaware of each others existence and yet the results obtained are surprisingly similar. In Guildford we have achieved exactly the same viability rate for infertility patients with endometriosis as Professor Donnez working in Brussels and our results for the relief of dysmenorrhoea are virtually identical to those of Joe Feste and Jim Daniell in the USA, yet none of us were aware of the practical details such as the laser power densities used by the others.

It is important to realize that it is not necessary to have access to expensive lasers to perform most of the operations described in this book. Polycystic ovarian syndrome, unruptured ectopic pregnancy and ovarian cystectomy can all be treated by sophisticated electrodiathermy as long as the necessary ancillary instruments and the skill to use them are available. In the final chapter of this book, Harry Reich takes laparoscopic surgery to its very limits and yet many of the advanced techniques such as pelvic lymphadenectomy and laparoscopic hysterectomy can be performed without the use of lasers. Apart from the technical skill needed, the main requirement is patience and the ability to allow considerable time; some of these 'foreveroscopies', as they are called in the USA, can last up to six hours and would create havoc on a busy welfare operating list in the UK. Although some may scoff at the rationale for such procedures as laparoscopic hysterectomies, further developments in anastomotic clip technology may considerably shorten the operating time and increase the feasibility of these operations—unless those other endoscopic surgeons, the hysteroscopists, relegate traditional hysterectomy to oblivion by the simple technique of endometrial ablation.

There is inevitably some repetition in certain chapters but since this usually concerns safety precautions I have deliberately allowed them to remain in the text. At this stage in the development of laparoscopic surgery we are quite correctly obsessed with safety and I was genuinely concerned that a novice might read one chapter and then feel qualified to embark on the endoscopic operation described therein. Many of the techniques detailed here require great skill, manual dexterity and excellent hand–eye co-ordination. They are not for everyone and, indeed, may only have a place in a few specialized centres. If anyone is interested in acquiring these skills I beg of you that you do not tread the path alone but rather attend the relevant courses and workshops and then acquire some individual tuition on a one-to-one basis with an acknowledged expert. That is the only way that operative laparoscopy will maintain the excellent safety record that it has achieved over the past two decades.

Diagnostic laparoscopy came to us from Continental Europe and had already been well established there for a number of years by the time the late Patrick Steptoe wrote the first monograph on the subject in the English language in 1967. Although most modern gynaecologists were keen to learn the new technique and recognize its value there were others who for many years stood resolute, like Canute before the waves, refusing to accept the importance of this diagnostic aid in patient management. A similar situation now exists with regard to operative laparoscopy and this volume is a timely reminder to our colleagues in gynaecology, and also in general surgery, that they should not merely be content to gaze at the wondrous view afforded by the laparoscope but should see it as a method of performing a variety of operations ranging from ovarian cystectomy and ectopic pregnancy to appendicectomy and even cholecystectomy. Although these endoscopic procedures require great technical virtuosity and are often more time consuming than conventional surgery the benefit to the patient is enormous and throughout this volume this message is repeated time and again. Most of these endoscopic operations can be performed on a day case basis, avoiding a long hospital stay and the unsightly scar associated with a laparotomy and allowing an earlier return to social, domestic and working life. The savings to the health services and the economy are huge and it behoves us all to rethink the old methods and teaching and, for the sake of our patients, try to acquire the necessary skills to perform laparoscopic surgery. If this book contributes in some small way to this end then the effort expended in its production will have been worthwhile.

CHRIS SUTTON

1

The development of laparoscopic surgery

A. G. GORDON
A. L. MAGOS

'An eye in the pelvis is worth more than a thousand pelvic examinations' (Soderstrom, 1978). For centuries gynaecologists have been concerned by the elusive nature of pelvic pathology and women have undergone unnecessary surgery for medically treatable conditions or have been observed for too long before appropriate treatment was instituted. In the past two decades diagnostic laparoscopy has opened new doorways to the management of infertility and pelvic pain, and in more recent years operative laparoscopy has enabled gynaecologists to treat a large number of women with pelvic disease without subjecting them to the added problems of open surgery.

HISTORY OF LAPAROSCOPY

Early endoscopy (400 BC–1900 AD)

Endoscopy (400 BC–500 AD)

The first description of endoscopy came from the Kos school led by Hippocrates (460–375 BC) who described the use of a rectal speculum, and the first primitive instruments for gynaecological endoscopy date from the same period. A three-bladed vaginal speculum was recovered from the ruins of Pompei, destroyed in 70 AD, and similar instruments, some of tubular shape, have been described by physicians from Rome between 95 and 117 AD (Semm, 1975). The Babylonian Talmud (500 AD), written after many centuries of work in Mesopotamia, refers to a 'siphopherot', a tube made of lead, through which the vagina and cervix could be observed.

Light sources (1000–1870 AD)

Although the earliest light sources used to illuminate the body cavities were mirrors, probably introduced by the Arabs before 1000 AD, the real impetus to endoscopy came with the use of more sophisticated light sources in the middle ages. In 1587 Aranzi described the use of the 'camera obscura' for medical purposes, an invention attributed by Leonardo da Vinci in 1519 to a Benedictine Monk, Don Panuce. Aranzi used the sun's rays shining through a hole in a window-shutter into a spherical glass flask filled with water to focus the beam into the nasal cavity. In the 17th century the concave mirror was introduced by Peter Borell of Castres, but it was not until the following century that a small lantern used by burglars was adapted by Arnaud to illuminate an endoscope.

It is generally accepted that it was Bozzini in 1806 (Frangenheim, 1988) who gave the first impetus to modern endoscopy. He developed a complex system which conveyed light from a lamp through a tube into the vagina to illuminate it and allow observation of the cervix through a second channel. Cystoscopes without lenses but using light from a candle reflected through a tube were developed by Segal in 1826 and Desormeaux (1865). Gynaecological endoscopy prior to 1890 was restricted to attempts, most of them futile, to inspect the interior of the uterine cavity but otherwise little practical progress was made during this period.

Lens systems (1890–1900)

The development of telescopes with lenses began in the late nineteenth century when Nitze (1897) working with Reinecke, a Berlin optician, and Leiter, a Viennese instrument maker, produced the forerunner of modern optical instruments. Originally their light source was an overheated, water-cooled platinum wire, but after the invention of the electric light bulb by Edison the latter was combined with the cystoscope in the early 1900s. Developments over the next few years included mounting the electric bulb at the distal end of the cystoscope, incorporating an operating channel, and designing an instrument with the lens separate from the operating channel. The modern endoscope was born.

Modern laparoscopy

Laparoscopy (1900–1940)

In the early years of the twentieth century the main impetus for endoscopy moved away from gynaecology towards the inspection of the bladder, rectum, larynx and oesophagus. However, von Ott (1901) from Peterburg reported the first 'ventroscopy', the equivalent of the modern open laparoscopy. One year later Kelling (1902) from Germany suggested that by filling the abdominal cavity with air a better view of the intra-abdominal organs would be obtained. His first observations using 'coelioscopy' were on laboratory animals but in 1910 Jacobeus reported performing 17 laparoscopies on patients with ascites (Jacobeus, 1912). Kelling disputed this claim but nonetheless these three should be considered the 'fathers' of modern laparoscopy.

Subsequently, a number of reports of laparoscopy were documented and further developments took place including the use of the Trendelenburg position and the invention of the laparoscope with trocar by Nordentoeft (1912) in Copenhagen, the production of a new type of insufflating needle by Goetze (1918), the use of carbon dioxide to insufflate the peritoneum by

Zollikofer (1925) in Switzerland, and the introduction of the insufflating needle in present-day use by Veress (1938) of Budapest. The further development of laparoscopy in this period was enhanced by the publication of articles and textbooks on the subject by Unverrichte (1923) in Germany, Stone (1924) in the USA, Short (1925) in England and Korbsch (1927) also in Germany.

Laparoscopy in the 1930s was largely performed by general surgeons and internists for the diagnosis of hepatic disease. The first reported operative laparoscopy was by Fervers (1933), a general surgeon, who performed adhesiolysis. Hope (1937) from the USA was the first to describe the use of a laparoscope for the diagnosis of extrauterine pregnancy. During this period other gynaecologists were also performing laparoscopy, and Bosch (1936) in Switzerland and Anderson (1937) in the USA suggested the use of coagulation or fulguration to perform tubal sterilization. It is not clear whether they actually performed the operation and it may be that the first tubal sterilization by laparoscopy was in the USA by Power and Barnes (1941). Techniques were developing in parallel in several countries at this time, but due to difficulties in communication because of distance and language and also the political constraints on free exchange of scientific information, it is difficult to be certain of the exact sequence of events.

Culdoscopy (1939–1966)

The advance of laparoscopy was limited by deficiencies in light sources and optical systems so there was little further advance in the technique in the 1940's. Instead, many physicians turned to culdoscopy, introduced in the USA by Te Linde who reported 10 years experience in 1948. A detailed view of the pelvic organs by this route was poor until Decker (1946) described the knee–shoulder position. Following this, culdoscopy remained the preferred procedure in the USA until the late 1960s. There were few exponents in Europe apart from Palmer (1950), Thomsen (1951), Clyman (1966), and Scott JS and Hancock (1988).

Post-war developments

After the Second World War, the trend towards gynaecological endoscopy was renewed by Palmer in Paris and Frangenheim in Konstanz. The dual developments of cold light illumination by Fourestiere et al (1943) in Paris, and improved lens systems introduced by Hopkins (1953) of Reading revolutionized the operation. In the early 1950s Frangenheim modified and designed instruments for laparoscopic surgery and also made the first prototype for the modern carbon dioxide insufflation apparatus thereby not only introducing a new form of surgical treatment but also improving the safety of the pneumoperitoneum (Frangenheim, 1988).

Modern trends (1970 onwards)

Development of techniques

Monopolar electrocoagulation had been introduced in the early 1950s for tubal sterilization and this was the method most commonly used for almost 30 years. Complications resulting from electrical burns led to the development of bipolar coagulation by Frangenheim (1972) in Germany and Rioux and Cloutier (1974) in Canada, and thermocoagulation by Semm (see Chapter 2) in Germany, and indeed laparoscopic surgery was initially limited to tubal sterilization by these means. More recently mechanical methods of tubal occlusion by means of rings (Yoon and King, 1975) and clips (Hulka et al, 1975; Lieberman et al, 1977; Filshie et al, 1981) have largely replaced these electrical procedures.

Laser, which in the field of gynaecology had already been used for the treatment of cervical lesions (Kaplan et al, 1973) and for some open abdominal surgery, was introduced to laparoscopic surgery by Bruhat et al (1979) in France, Tadir et al (1981) in Israel and Daniell and Brown (1982) in the USA. This technique allowed for more complicated laparoscopic operations, particularly extensive adhesiolysis and the destruction of endometriotic foci.

As the scope of laparoscopic procedures has increased, so modifications in attitudes and techniques have become necessary. Prolonged surgery has led to the problems of fatigue and discomfort which have been overcome by repositioning the patient, the use of body platforms for support, and finally video monitoring instead of through-the-lens viewing. The latter innovation has the added advantages of improving the co-ordination between the surgeon and assistants, magnifying the operative field, maintaining interest of theatre staff as well as being useful for teaching.

The most recent development in this field has been the introduction of 'double-optic' laparoscopy by Brosens et al (1987), initially for salpingoscopy and subsequently to perform microlaparoscopy in early peritoneal endometriosis (Brosens and Gordon, 1989) and ovarioscopy and intraovarian surgery in cases of ovarian endometriosis (Brosens, 1988).

Education

Teaching endoscopic techniques was promoted by the first gynaecological textbooks on laparoscopy by Palmer (1950), Frangenheim (1959), Albano and Cittadini (1962), Steptoe (1967), Cognat (1973) and Phillips (1976). More recent works include those of Semm (1975, 1987), Gomel et al (1986) and Gordon and Lewis (1988). To Jordan Phillips must go much of the credit for the international spread of laparoscopy by the formation of the American Association of Gynecological Laparoscopists (AAGL) and by initiating national surveys of complications. In later years he also organized international teaching teams who introduced laparoscopy to China and the Third World. Other national and international societies have been formed to develop gynaecological endoscopy which now accounts for some 20% of all gynaecological operations.

INSTRUMENTS FOR OPERATIVE LAPAROSCOPY

The main advances in the last 25 years in laparoscopic instrumentation have been the development of automated instruments for the safe distension of the abdomen with gas, fibreoptic cables for transmission of light from a source outside the body, and telescopes with the rod lens system which allows for a clearer, undistorted view of the pelvic organs. Safer methods for the control of bleeding and for incising tissues combined with newly developed forceps for effective and gentle tissue handling have also increased the scope of laparoscopic surgery.

Pneumoperitoneum

The first requirement for laparoscopy is the safe provision of a pneumoperitoneum. The modern electronic insufflation apparatus maintains adequate abdominal distension at a safe preset pressure. This is especially important in operative laparoscopy where multiple punctures with frequent changes of instruments lead to loss of gas which cannot readily be replaced by manually operated instruments. Pneumoperitoneum with carbon dioxide is safer than nitrous oxide, but with either gas, pulse and blood pressure should be monitored throughout the procedure which should be performed with endotracheal intubation and controlled positive pressure ventilation.

Light source

Illumination to the laparoscope should be provided by a minimum of 150 watt cold-light source via a fibreoptic or liquid cable. More powerful light sources are required if closed circuit television (CCTV) is used or if photographs are to be taken. The modern laparoscopist should be trained to use CCTV which allows him to operate while watching the image on the screen instead of through the eye piece. The modern chip camera with its light weight and improved definition has been one of the major factors in the development of laparoscopic surgery by allowing the assistant to manipulate tissues more accurately and making supervision of trainees safer as well as permitting prolonged surgery.

Laparoscope

The development of the rod lens by Professor Hopkins (1953) has improved the performance of laparoscopes giving a brighter image with better definition. Whilst 5 mm telescopes are satisfactory for simple inspection, a 10 mm instrument is required for surgery to give adequate illumination and wide enough field of vision. Some prefer an operating laparoscope which has a channel for instruments, but any advantage is outweighed by the narrower field of view through the relatively smaller lens. Magnification by a factor of two to three can be obtained by the addition of a lens to the laparoscope cap thus allowing for laparoscopic 'microsurgery'.

In the new development of 'double-optic' laparoscopy a second fine telescope is passed along the operating channel of a 10 mm operating laparoscope into the tubal lumen to examine the mucosa or into the cavity of endometriotic and other ovarian cysts for the purposes of inspection or coagulation of vessels at the ovarian hilum.

Electro- and thermal coagulation

The control of intraperitoneal bleeding is an essential prerequisite for any form of surgery and in the case of laparoscopy can usually be achieved by mono- or bipolar electrocoagulation or by thermal coagulation. The classic instrument for electrocoagulation was the Palmer biopsy forceps with a monopolar current, originally used for tubal coagulation. Unfortunately, its use was responsible for a number of complications related to accidental burns. Excessive heat can be produced with danger of damage to adjacent tissues such as bowel, bladder and ureter. The pathway along which the current returns to the dispersive electrode is also unpredictable so burns outside the surgeon's visual field can occasionally occur when the current 'jumps' from one surface to another within the peritoneal cavity. However, careful use of better designed instruments, particularly microdiathermy, has virtually eliminated these complications which were frequent in the early 1970s, and monopolar current can be recommended where cutting is necessary as in adhesiolysis and salpingostomy.

Bipolar coagulation is safer than monopolar but is not suitable for cutting. With this, the current flows between the electrodes which are usually the blades of tissue forceps. As before, unintentional tissue damage by direct transmission of heat can still take place. Serious complications can also occur when two different electrical generators, one for bipolar the other for monopolar, are connected to the patient simultaneously; here, the current generated by the bipolar instrument may be attracted to the dispersive plate of the latter and cause inadvertent burns to structures distant from the operation site.

The third method of haemostasis is thermal coagulation, where coagulating forceps are heated to 100–120°C for a preset time of 20–40 seconds. This produces coagulation of protein, a response similar to boiling an egg, an effect which is slower but safer than electrocautery as the risk of remote tissue damage is eliminated.

Laser

Laser has become a popular surgical tool during the past 20 years as it allows precise tissue destruction with instruments that are highly predictable. The type, power and delivery system depend on the tissue reaction required, be it vaporization or coagulation.

Carbon dioxide laser, currently the most widely utilised in laparoscopy, must at present be transmitted through a rigid lens system although flexible fibres are at an advanced stage of development. A back stop must be used to limit penetration of the laser and consequent damage to structures lying deep to the target tissue, and a suction system is required to clear the associated smoke.

Argon, neodymium–yttrium aluminium garnet (Nd-YAG) and potassium titanyl phosphate (KTP) lasers, on the other hand, can be transmitted along fibreoptic cables thereby increasing their versatility. Vaporization occurs only in the vicinity of the fibre tip and coagulation in a zone surrounding this. When used in the non-contact mode, increasing the distance between the fibre tip and the target is associated with a decrease in the thermal effect so the risk of inadvertent damage by transmitted heat is less than with electro-cautery.

There is no doubt that laser has added an important dimension to laparoscopic surgery particularly for the performance of adhesiolysis and the vaporization of endometriotic deposits. Unfortunately, at an approximate cost of £1000 per watt with 20–50 watts being generally required, the initial cost of the equipment is expensive, although running costs are relatively cheap. Sharing with other specialties is a practical possibility.

Sutures

Sutures are useful to control or prevent arterial haemorrhage in radical procedures such as salpingectomy or salpingo-oophorectomy and to reconstruct organs such as the ovary. A slip knot based on the Roeder* loop (Ethicon) can be applied to a cut pedicle. The loop is passed down a suture applicator via a 5.5 mm cannula, the proximal end of the ligature applicator snapped off and the knot pushed downwards until it is tight around the bleeding pedicle. These sutures, made of catgut, are also available with a needle but without a knot. This suture is inserted around or through the pedicle and brought out of the abdomen through the cannula before tying the knot. The loop can then be tightened as before by pulling on the proximal end of the applicator until it is tight and haemostasis has been achieved. A third type of suture that must be tied internally is also available but its use requires a greater degree of manual dexterity.

The limitations of laparoscopic suturing must be appreciated in that the finest suture material available is 3/0 which has to be attached to a strong enough needle to be used with laparoscopic needle holders. Equally important is the working distance between the surgeon's hand and the tissue, usually 35 cm or more, with resultant limit on delicate procedures. Repair of ovaries after cyst enucleation and peritoneal defects can be achieved with fibrin glue, so sutures other than for haemostasis will probably be replaced by tissue welding techniques such as those currently used to evert a salpingostomy. Nonetheless, the ability to suture in the pelvis is an essential prerequisite for safe laparoscopic surgery.

Forceps and scissors

A range of forceps is available to allow the surgeon to operate through two or three separate channels, additional cannulae being inserted on either side of the midline above the symphysis pubis. Instruments include flat forceps for holding adhesions during dissection, grasping forceps for stabilizing ovaries while enucleating cysts, atraumatic grasping forceps for manipulating bowel or the fallopian tubes, and large forceps for holding fibroids and cysts during myomectomy or cyst resection.

Most dissection can be performed with 5 mm scissors but finer micro-

* H. Roeder (1866–1918) first described a special loop used in tonsillectomy in children.

scissors should be used when operating close to the fallopian tube or bowel. Alternatively, when excising large ovarian cysts or performing myomectomy, 11 mm scissors are useful. Occasionally cysts and fibroids are too large to deliver through an 11 mm cannula so must be morcellated with a tissue punch.

Irrigation

It is important to be able to remove blood and debris during laparoscopic surgery. Lavage solutions such as normal saline or heparinized Ringer's lactate solution should be kept at 37°C as lower temperatures lead to hypothermia. The solution may be pumped through an irrigation channel using an Aquapurator (Semm, 1979) or more cheaply, a 500 ml bag can be pressurized with a cuff. When laser is used, particularly CO_2, the smoke plume must be removed by intermittent or continuous aspiration.

CONTRAINDICATIONS AND COMPLICATIONS OF LAPAROSCOPIC SURGERY

Contraindications

As for all surgical procedures, there are well defined absolute and relative contra-indications to laparoscopy (Table 1).

Table 1. Contraindications to laparoscopy.

Absolute
Mechanical and paralytic ileus
Large abdominal mass
Generalized peritonitis
Irreducible external hernia
Cardiac failure
Recent myocardial infarction
Cardiac conduction defects
Respiratory failure
Severe obstructive airways disease
Shock
Relative
Multiple abdominal incisions
Abdominal wall sepsis
Gross obesity
Hiatus hernia
Ischaemic heart disease
Blood dyscrasias and coagulopathies

Absolute

Abdominal distension secondary to bowel obstruction is an absolute contraindication to laparoscopy because of the dangers of bowel trauma and perforation. Similarly, the presence of a large intra-abdominal mass (larger than the equivalent of a 14 week pregnancy) increases the risk of trauma during the insertion of trocars and cannulae; lesions larger than 6 cm are anyway difficult to deal with laparoscopically with the sole exception of benign ovarian cysts which can be deflated prior to their excision. Generalized and even upper abdominal acute peritonitis should also be managed by laparotomy, but laparoscopy can be a useful diagnostic as well as therapeutic tool with localized peritonitis such as with pelvic abscesses (Mecke and Semm, 1988). (This new and potentially useful technique is described in detail in Chapter 10.) With an irreducible external hernia there is the danger of ischaemic damage to its contents following the creation of the pneumoperitoneum. Similarly, the cardiovascular and respiratory effects of the gases used to distend the abdomen can only aggravate the anaesthetic risks posed by severe cardiorespiratory disease because of effects on acid–base balance, myocardial contractility, venous return and blood pressure. Shock of any origin is also an absolute contraindication.

Relative

Previous abdominal surgery is not in itself an absolute contraindication to laparoscopic surgery, but instruments should ideally be inserted away from scars where bowel and other adhesions may be potential dangers; Semm (1988) has recently described sight-controlled peritoneal puncture which should improve the safety of laparoscopy under these conditions. Likewise, the abdomen should not be entered through infected areas. While gross obesity is associated with obvious technical problems and complications, it should be remembered that in the mid-line, in the umbilicus and along the linea alba, there is little fat tissue between the skin and rectus sheath, and provided the correct safety measures are adhered to, peritoneal insufflation should be without added hazard (Semm, 1987). Alternatively, insufflation can be carried out via the posterior vaginal fornix. Insufflation in the presence of a large hiatus hernia may result in a pneumomediastinum but provided the Trendelenburg tilt is limited to 15° and the intra-abdominal pressure is not allowed to exceed 10 mmHg, laparoscopy is safe; indeed, direct laparoscope trocar insertion without prior pneumoperiteum may be safer in this situation (Dingfelder, 1978). Ischaemic heart disease in the absence of heart failure should not deter from laparoscopy but procedures should be kept as short as possible. Severe bleeding disorders must be corrected prior to laparoscopy just as before any major surgery.

Complications

Laparoscopy is essentially a safe surgical procedure and complications are relatively rare. Several surveys have reported on the morbidity and mortality associated with basic gynaecological laparoscopy, generally carried out for diagnosis or sterilization, but data concerning more advanced surgical laparoscopy is scanty. Furthermore, all surveys suffer from fundamental differences in sample characteristics and definitions which makes attempts at objective comparison almost impossible.

Table 2. Overall morbidity and mortality associated with laparoscopy from different surveys. Figures expressed as the rate per 1000 laparoscopies.

	Number of procedures in different surveys		
	UK 1976–77 50 247	USA 1977 87 275	GDR 1978–82 292 462
Diagnostic laparoscopy			
Minor complications	29.9	NA	NA
Major complications	6.6	4.6	0.9
Laparoscopic sterilization			
Minor complications	40.6	NA	NA
Major complications	12.1	3.7	2.3
Operative laparoscopy			
Minor complications	—	—	NA
Major complications	—	—	3.8
Overall mortality	0.08	0.05	0.05

NA, Not available

As examples, three surveys from different populations are briefly summarized in Table 2. The 1978 RCOG Confidential Enquiry into Gynaecological Laparoscopy from the UK, focusing mainly on diagnostic and sterilizing laparoscopies, revealed an overall complication rate of 34/1000 with a mortality rate of 0.08/1000 (Chamberlain and Brown, 1978). The most recent AAGL report from the USA with sufficient detail for comparison produced superior figures but this is probably explained by the voluntary nature of the data collection and the seniority of the respondents (Phillips et al, 1979). A much larger survey from West Germany, reporting operative laparoscopies as well (e.g. adhesiolysis, tubal surgery, coagulation of endometriosis, etc.) highlights the relative safety of all types of laparoscopy in the hands of experienced operators (Riedel et al, 1986). While the incidence of major complications (defined as the need for laparotomy or re-laparoscopy) was approximately four times greater with operative laparoscopy compared with diagnostic procedures, the rate was still only 3.8/1000 with an overall mortality for all procedures of only 0.05/1000.

Risk factors

Although relatively uncommon and usually minor, the complications associated with laparoscopic surgery have been well defined (Table 3), and shown to depend on the experience and technique of the operator, the pathology being dealt with, the procedure being carried out, as well as the age and overall condition of the patient. Other risk factors relate to the contraindications already mentioned such as previous surgery and obesity, to which must be added ascites – where gas-filled intestinal loops tend to float on the surface and are thus more prone to penetrating injuries.

Gas insufflation

Carbon dioxide insufflation in particular is associated with tachypnoea, a fall in arterial pH, pO_2 and serum Cl^- and a rise in pCO_2 (El-Miawi et al, 1981). There is a small but definite risk of cardiac arrhythmias even after deflation (Carmichael, 1970), but heart failure and arrest are very rare (e.g. 0.2/1000 in the RCOG study) and may occur particularly in the presence of pre-existing ischaemic heart disease combined with inadequate ventilation. Typically arterial and venous blood pressure rises with the use of CO_2, but if the intra-abdominal pressure is allowed to exceed 20 mmHg, both blood pressure and cardiac output start to fall (Motew et al, 1973). Although nitrous oxide causes fewer adverse metabolic and cardiac changes (Scott DB, 1972; El-Miawi et al, 1981) and is more comfortable for the patient (Sharp et al, 1982), it is a combustible gas and so is not safe with diathermy or laser.

Gas embolism was responsible for one of the four deaths in the 1978 RCOG survey; it was fatal because of right ventricular outflow obstruction. This complication was more of a risk when air was used for insufflating the abdomen, but carbon dioxide and to a lesser extent nitrous oxide are highly

Table 3. Complications recorded by the RCOG Confidential Enquiry into Gynaecological Laparoscopy (1978). Figures expressed as the rate per 1000 laparoscopies.

Anaesthetic complications	
Anaesthetist	0.8
Cardiac arrest	0.2
Cardiac arrhythmias	0.4
Failed procedures	
Failed laparoscopy	7.5
Failed abdominal insufflation	3.5
Burns	
Bowel	0.5
Skin	0.3
Other	0.2
Direct trauma	
Bowel	1.8
Urinary tract	0.2
Pelvic organs	3.4
Haemorrhage	
Abdominal wall	2.5
Pelvic blood vessels and tubal mesentery	2.7
Pelvic side-wall and ovarian vessels	0.9
Bowel mesentery	1.1
Infection	
Abdominal wound	0.5
Pelvic infection	0.5
Chest infection	0.2
Urinary tract	0.5
Other complications	
Chest pain	0.3
Lost foreign body	0.6
Damage to pelvic organs not due to laparoscopy procedures	2.6
Pulmonary embolism	0.2
Deep vein thrombosis	0.2
Other	3.1
Late complications	0.8
Deaths	0.1

soluble such that more than one litre of CO_2 would have to be injected before any noticeable cardiovascular effects occurred (Graff et al, 1959). Interestingly, gas embolism is not necessarily the result of direct vascular injury but may occur following uterine trauma or even in the absence of any obvious injury (Yacoub et al, 1982). Pneumothorax and mediastinal emphysema are well recognized but extremely infrequent complications.

Burns

Burn injuries represent an important area of potential trauma during laparoscopy, laparotomy being almost always mandatory when bowel is affected. There is no doubt that high-frequency electrocoagulation, particularly monopolar diathermy, is the most dangerous in this respect whereas endocoagulation as described by Semm (1976) is arguably the safer but slower technique. Although the 1978 RCOG survey suggested that sterilization by cautery was associated with fewer non-fatal complications than by rings or bands, this finding is probably explained by the inexperience with physical methods at that time rather than the relative safety of diathermy, and indeed one of the four deaths during this survey followed an unrecognized bowel perforation during sterilization by electrocoagulation (Chamberlain and Brown, 1978). Experience has shown, and this has been confirmed by the German survey of Reidel et al (1986), that monopolar diathermy in particular should be used with extreme care. It should also be appreciated that diathermy injury may not become apparent for a number of days (Esposito, 1976).

Direct trauma

Penetrative trauma to hollow organs such as bowel and bladder, and vascular injuries may occur but usually relate to poor technique. The most dangerous times are when the Veress needle and the first trocar and cannula are being introduced blindly, or during surgical manipulation; certainly, once the laparoscope is in place all subsequent trocars must be inserted under direct vision. Various techniques have been described to minimize the risks of creating a pneumoperitoneum, the most rigorous of which are the seven steps described by Semm (1987). With increasing resort to operative laparoscopy and particularly adhesiolysis, intraoperative haemorrhage will no doubt become commoner, but bleeding can usually be controlled by coagulation or suturing. As with diathermy injuries, major direct trauma may require laparotomy.

Infection

Superficial wound infections are surprisingly uncommon bearing in mind the bacterial flora of the umbilicus and the inherent difficulties in sterilizing this important laparoscopic landmark. A thorough cleansing procedure is not unreasonable when one considers that necrotizing fasciitis has been recorded as a complication of laparoscopy (Sortel et al, 1983). There seems little more we can do to reduce the risks of urinary tract infections as catheterization prior to laparoscopy is essential to protect against trauma to the bladder.

Miscellaneous

Pulmonary aspiration of gastric contents is one of the commonest lung complications, and neither starvation nor intubation totally protect against its occurrence (Berci and Cuschieri, 1986). Other complications that have been associated with laparoscopy include surgical emphysema (subcutaneous, preperitoneal, omental or affecting bowel mesentery), omental hernia if the abdomen is not deflated sufficiently prior to removal of all instruments, and leakage of ascitic fluid if the incisions are not sutured carefully. Postoperative shoulder pain, sometimes severe and prolonged, is almost universal despite the use of CO_2 or N_2O for insufflation (Sharp et al, 1982); whereas all methods of deflation are equally inefficient (Chamberlain, 1984), the use of a peritoneal drain inserted via the umbilical incision for 6 hours postoperatively has been claimed to reduce this symptom (Alexander and Hull, 1987). Deep vein thrombosis and pulmonary embolism are such rare events following laparoscopy that routine preventive measures are not indicated.

THE SCOPE OF LAPAROSCOPIC SURGERY

The therapeutic options open to the laparoscopic surgeon are many and varied, from simple adhesiolysis to the resection of dense endometriotic

Table 4. Classification of operative laparoscopy procedures (adapted from Martin and Diamond, 1986).

Basic operative laparoscopy
Tubal sterilization
Biopsies
Coagulation of mild endometriosis
Aspiration of small ovarian cysts
Intermediate operative laparoscopy
Lysis of mild to moderate adhesions
Coagulation of moderate endometriosis
Exploration of small ovarian cysts
Uterine suspension
Salpingectomy
Salpingectomy for ectopic pregnancy
Extensive operative laparoscopy
Cuff salpingostomy
Salpingotomy for ectopic pregnancy
Lysis of extensive adhesions
Excision of moderate to severe endometriosis
Enucleation of ovarian cysts (endometriosis, dermoids)
Oophorectomy
Myomectomy
Tubal anastomosis
Appendectomy

tissues and the removal of relatively large benign tumours such as fibroids. Semm (1987), considered the father of operative laparoscopy by many, catalogues over 50 indications for this mode of surgery in his classic manual. Martin and Diamond (1986) have recently suggested a useful classification of procedures based on their complexity (Table 4). Whatever the procedure, however, both the surgeon and patient must be prepared for failure and the need for laparotomy, either because the desired operation cannot be carried out safely laparoscopically or because of some intervening complication. Operative laparoscopy should therefore build on experience gained with conventional surgery, and above all a thorough understanding of intra-abdominal anatomy.

A multiple puncture approach should be used for all but the simplest of interventions as it provides superior depth of field and manipulation possibilities. The correct instruments are also essential as a standard diagnostic laparoscopy set contains few of the necessary tools. However, there are no 'best buys' in terms of instrumentation: an instrument is only as good as the surgeon using it and it is better to operate with something you are familiar with rather than trying to follow the latest fashion.

Adhesiolysis

For any surgery to be successful and safe there must be an unimpeded view of the operative field. For this reason, particularly after previous surgery, adhesiolysis is often the first and at the same time essential preface to more extensive procedures. While the lysis of adhesions can be the simplest of maneouvres, it can potentially be the most difficult and is fraught with the danger of trauma to surrounding tissues and organs. Thus, filmy adhesions are easily and safely divided by blunt dissection using grasping forceps or scissors. More vascular adhesions, such as those attached to omentum, can be divided with or without prior thermal haemostasis or suturing but care has to be taken to keep clear of bowel. The principles of conventional surgery should be adhered to and tissues kept under tension to identify lines of cleavage. In rare instances the laparoscope can initially be placed suprapubically to allow for the lysis of periumbilical adhesions before resiting the optic at its conventional position. The laser has been an exciting new development in laparoscopic adhesiolysis procedures and is described in more detail in Chapters 5 and 6.

Tubal sterilization

In most units sterilization is by far the commonest indication for therapeutic laparoscopy. Various methods are available from mono- and bipolar diathermy to endocoagulation and laser, from occlusive devices (clips and rings) to laparoscopic salpingectomy. There is little doubt that the various clips are comparable to other methods in terms of efficacy while giving the greatest chance of successful reversal (Hulka et al, 1975; Lieberman et al, 1977; Filshie et al, 1981). Not only are these techniques safer but, as is evident from Table 5, failure and ectopic pregnancies occured more

Table 5. Failure and ectopic rates after different methods of laparoscopic sterilization (after Riedel et al, 1986).

	n	Pregnancy rate per 1000	Ectopic rate per 1000
Monopolar diathermy	13966	1.8	0.6
Bipolar diathermy	53522	3.9	1.4
Endocoagulation	42425	1.1	0.3
Occlusive devices	18202	3.0	1.9

frequently after high frequency sterilization (Riedel et al, 1986). The techniques themselves are familiar to many gynaecologists and are discussed further in Chapter 11.

Ovarian biopsy

Although ovarian biopsy has been claimed to be the oldest endoscopic surgical procedure in gynaecology, the indications are now few if any (Sutton, 1974). Sampling should be from the less vascular antihilar region of the ovary using either Palmer's biopsy forceps, or alternatively toothed biopsy forceps with a bevelled cannula acting as a tissue punch. Bleeding can be controlled by coagulation, Semm (1987) recommending endocoagulation as in his experience electrocautery affects the neurovascular supply of the ovaries with resultant permanent dysfunction.

Ovarian cyst resection

Ovarian cysts should only be dealt with laparoscopically if the appearances are consistent with a benign histology, typically meaning a unilateral, unilocular, translucent, freely mobile cyst with a smooth capsule and normal looking vascular pattern, and absence of papillae or ascites. To this usually functional type of cyst can be added endometriotic and dermoid cysts, which however require more complex surgery. It goes without saying that ultrasound scanning is a mandatory part of the preoperative assessment.

Three procedures have been described: puncture, fenestration and excision. While aspiration is simple, it is an unsatisfactory approach as the nature of the lesion can only be confirmed by histology and not cytology, and recurrences are not uncommon (Frangenheim, 1972). Fenestration, that is the cutting of a window in the cyst wall, not only provides a histological specimen but also allows for the laparoscopic inspection of the inner aspect of the cyst to check for any suspicion of malignancy and ensures continuing drainage (Kleppinger, 1978). Recurrence following this procedure is relatively uncommon, the combined series of Kleppinger (1978) and Larsen et al (1986) quoting 1 out of 71 procedures. Ovarian endometriomas or dermoid cysts are unsuitable for this approach.

Total excision of an ovarian cyst is the most radical procedure of the three and theoretically suitable for any benign cyst provided its size does not prevent safe instrumentation. The technique involves partial deflation of the cyst, splitting of the tunica albuginea with scissors (or laser), extraction of the cyst wall by traction with grasping or biopsy forceps, and resection of redundant ovarian cortex in the case of larger cysts. In contrast to ovarian surgery at laparotomy there is usually minimal bleeding following this procedure and coagulation of the base of the cyst is generally sufficient. Suturing of the ovarian edges as advocated by Semm (1987) can be an extra haemostatic measure but is rarely essential; while concern has been expressed about adhesion formation secondary to the insertion of catgut sutures into the ovary, evidence is lacking and this fear may be more theoretical than real. Alternatively, the ovary can be reconstituted with fibrin glue or salpingo-oophorectomy can be performed. The newer approach of ovarian cystoscopy using double-optic laser laparoscopy with the argon laser is described in detail in Chapter 9.

Endometriosis

Endometriosis has become the laparoscopic diagnosis par excellence, and the same approach offers exciting therapeutic possibilities for both superficial and deep disease. Thus, adhesions may be divided and endometriomas resected, and above all endometriotic implants can be excised, coagulated or vaporized with a laser. High frequency current diathermy is associated with all the dangers of burn injuries and so must be used only with extreme care although a recent controlled study has attested to both its safety and efficacy (Seiler et al, 1986) Thermocoagulation and above all laser must nonetheless be the modalities of choice, particularly as the latter allows for the dissection of endometriosis off bowel. Carbon dioxide (Davis, 1986), Nd-YAG (Lomano, 1987) and argon lasers (Keye and Dixon, 1983) have all been tested and conception rates when the treatment is for infertility as well as pain are encouraging (Nezhat et al, 1986). The role of the different lasers in the laparoscopic treatment of endometriosis is discussed in Chapter 4.

Uterine ventrosuspension

Few reports in the literature have detailed this technique, and indeed there is no mention of it by Semm (1987). Steptoe, the father of British laparoscopy, was the first to describe laparoscopic ventrosuspension (Steptoe, 1967), and a later series from the USA discussed the possible complications (Mann and Stenger, 1978). The technique basically involves lysing adhesions and destroying any endometriosis, pulling the mid-portion of the round ligaments on either side through the internal ring with surgical forceps, shortening them and securing them to the external oblique aponeurosis with absorbable sutures. Problems noted by Mann and Stenger (1978) included incisional pains (20/20 cases), avulsion of the round ligament (2/20 cases), haematoma (1/20 cases) and an eventual failure rate of 5%.

Ectopic pregnancy

The laparoscopic removal of a tubal pregnancy was first reported by Shapiro and Adler (1973), and currently the largest published series includes 321 cases (Pouly et al, 1986). Both conservative (linear salpingotomy) and radical (segmental resection or salpingectomy) procedures are possible. Tubal aspiration is associated with a relatively high failure rate because of persistent bleeding and should be reserved for those cases where spontaneous tubal abortion seems imminent (Bruhat et al, 1980). Although Semm (1987) advocates suturing the serosal defect following a salpingotomy, the majority view holds that this is unnecessary (Pouly et al, 1986; DeCherney and Diamond, 1987). Prior injection of 20 ml of a dilute solution of vasopressin into the mesosalpinx reduces the operative blood loss from the tubal incision but care must be taken to ensure that complete haemostasis has been achieved.

Salpingectomy itself can be very neatly carried out using Semm's triple loop technique, but is also possible by thermocoagulation and transection at the isthmus (Dubuisson et al, 1987). The use of laser has also been described (Johns and Hardie, 1986) and the advantages over conventional haemostatic methods are described in Chapters 6 and 8. Tubal rupture is not in itself a contraindication to laparoscopic management provided the patient is haemodynamically stable (Magos et al, 1988). Finally, a recent study has confirmed that the laparoscopic treatment of ectopic pregnancy is associated with less operating time, reduced postoperative pain, and shorter hospital stay and convalescence than laparotomy (Brumsted et al, 1988). In addition the conservative management of ectopic prgnancy by laparoscopy is associated with results at least as good as those obtained at laparotomy (Timoner and Nieminen, 1967) and the subsequent ectopic rate is lower.

TRAINING IN LAPAROSCOPIC SURGERY

Laparoscopic surgery demands a higher degree of skill than that required for diagnostic laparoscopy and simple procedures such as sterilization. Surgeons must learn new techniques, the use of unfamiliar instruments, and also develop a comprehension and clinical judgement of the limits of operative laparoscopy. For these reasons, the operator should be an experienced laparoscopist preferably with a background of microsurgical techniques. Initial training should be with the use of inert models such as the pelvitrainer and watching practical demonstrations and video recordings of procedures. 'Hands on' training with an experienced surgeon is, however, essential. The development of technical skills should commence with simple procedures such as the division of fine adhesions before proceeding to more extensive adhesiolysis, resection of ovarian cysts, salpingectomy, surgery for pelvic endometriosis and laparoscopic tubal reconstructive surgery.

THE FUTURE

At present relatively few surgeons in Europe and North America are performing operative laparoscopy and are demonstrating its potential value. Although DeCherney (1985) feels that these techniques should replace conventional laparotomy, they need to be adopted by more surgeons and their value proved in general use. Compared to laparotomy, there is an average reduction of 49% in overall hospital costs and an 80% reduction in laparotomy for tubal and ovarian disease has been achieved by Semm (see Chapter 2). To this must be added the benefits of a quicker return to normal activities and the consequent savings to the community.

The full potential of gynaecological endoscopic surgery remains to be exploited. The day is sure to come when operative laparoscopy will replace most laparotomies and operative hysteroscopy most hysterectomies. It is up to us to ensure that that day is not too far in the future.

SUMMARY

For centuries people have been trying to look inside the abdomen but it is only relatively recently that the technology has been available to make this a meaningful possibility. Major milestones have included safe peritoneal insufflation, cold-light illumination, laparoscopes with the rod lens system, instruments for the safe manipulation of pelvic organs, techniques to ensure haemostasis, laser, video monitoring and most recently double-optic laparoscopy. As a result, the indications for gynaecological laparoscopy have been greatly extended from its initial use as a diagnostic aid or a means of female sterilization, and procedures such as adhesiolysis, ovarian cystectomy, tubal surgery for infertility or ectopic pregnancy, excision of endometriosis and even myomectomy are now possible without open surgery. Well-defined safety guidelines must of course be adhered to and proper training is essential in the various techniques, but the medical, financial and social advantages are such that we owe it to our patients to exploit the full potential of this new mode of management.

REFERENCES

Albano V & Cittadini E (1962) *La Celioscopia in Ginecologia*. Palermo: Denaro.

Alexander JI & Hull MGR (1987) Abdominal pain after laparoscopy: the value of a gas drain. *British Journal of Obstetrics and Gynaecology* **94:** 267–269.

Anderson ET (1937) Peritoneoscopy. *American Journal of Surgery* **35:** 136–139.

Berci G & Cushieri A (1986) *Practical Laparoscopy*. London: Bailliere Tindall.

Bosch PF (1936) Laparoskopische sterilization. *Schweizerische Zeitschrift fur Krankenhaus und Anstaltswesen.*

Brosens IA (1988) *Ovarioscopy*. Presented at the International Symposium on Gynaecological Endoscopy, Oxford.

Brosens IA & Gordon AG (1989) *Tubal Infertility*. Philadelphia: JB Lippencott, *in press*.

Brosens IA, Boeckx W, Delatin PH et al (1987) Salpingoscopy: a new pre-operative diagnostic tool in tubal infertility. *British Journal of Obstetrics and Gynaecology* **94:** 768–773.

Bruhat MA, Mage G, Manhes M (1979) Use of the CO_2 laser by laparoscopy. In Kaplan I (ed.) *Laser Surgery III. Proceedings of the Third International Congress on Laser Surgery*, pp 275. Tel Aviv: Jerusalem Press.

Bruhat MA, Manhes H, Mage G & Pouly JL (1980) Treatment of ectopic pregnancy by means of laparoscopy. *Fertility and Sterility* **33:** 411–414.

Brumsted J, Kessler C, Gibson C et al (1988) A comparison of laparoscopy and laparotomy for the treatment of ectopic pregnancy. *Obstetrics and Gynecology* **71:** 889–892.
Carmichael DE (1970) Laparoscopy: cardiac considerations. *Fertility and Sterility* **22:** 69–70.
Chamberlain G (1984) The recovery of gases insufflated at laparoscopy. *British Journal of Obstetrics and Gynaecology* **91:** 367–370.
Chamberlain G & Brown JC (1978) *Gynaecological laparoscopy. The Report of the Working Party of the Confidential Enquiry into Gynaecological Laparoscopy.* London: Royal College of Obstetricians and Gynaecologists.
Clyman MJ (1966) Importance of culdoscopy in fertility Studies. *New York Medical Journal* **66:** 1867.
Cognat MA (1973) *Coelioscopie Gynecologique.* Villeurbanne: Simep.
Daniell JF & Brown DH (1982) Carbon dioxide laser laparoscopy: initial experience in experimental animals and humans. *Obstetrics & Gynecology* **59:** 761–764.
Davis GD (1986) Management of endometriosis and its associated adhesions with the CO_2 laser laparoscope. *Obstetrics & Gynecology* **68:** 422–425.
DeCherney AH (1985) The leader of the band is tired. *Fertility and Sterility* **44:** 299–302.
DeCherney AH & Diamond MP (1987) Laparoscopic salpingostomy for ectopic pregnancy. *Obstetrics & Gynecology* **70:** 948–950.
Decker A (1949) Culdoscopy: its diagnostic value in pelvic disease. *Journal of the American Medical Association* **140:** 378–385.
Desormeaux A-J (1865) *De l'endoscope et de ses applications au diagnostic et au traitement des affectations de l'uretre et de la vessie.* Paris: Bailliere.
Dingfelder JR (1978) Direct laparoscope trocar insertion without prior pneumoperitoneum. *Journal of Reproductive Medicine* **21:** 45–47.
Dubuisson JB, Aubriot FX & Cardone V (1987) Laparoscopic salpingectomy for tubal pregnancy. *Fertility and Sterility* **47:** 225–228.
El-Miawi MF, Wahbli O, El-Bagouri IS et al (1981) Physiologic changes during CO_2 and N_2O pneumoperitoneum in diagnostic laparoscopy. *Journal of Reproductive Medicine* **26:** 338–346.
Esposito JM (1976) The laparoscopist and electrosurgery. *American Journal of Obstetrics and Gynecology* **126:** 633–637.
Fervers C (1933) Die Laparoskopie mit dem Cystoskope. Ein Beitrag zur Vereinfachung der Technik und zur endoskopischen Strangdurchtrennung in der Bauchole. *Medizinische Klinik* **29:** 1042–1045.
Filshie GM, Casey D, Pogmore JL et al (1981) The tetaneum silicone rubber clip for female sterilization. *British Journal of Obstetrics and Gynaecology* **88:** 655–662.
Fourestiere M, Gladu A & Vulmiere J (1943) La peritoneoscopie. *Presse Médicale* **5:** 46–47.
Frangenheim H (1959) *Die Laparoskopie und die Kuldoskopie in der Gynakologie.* Stuttgart: Thieme.
Frangenheim H (1972) *Laparoscopy and Culdoscopy in Gynecology.* London: Butterworth.
Frangenheim (1988) History of endoscopy. In Gordon AG & Lewis BV (eds) *Gynaecological Endoscopy*, pp 1.1–5. London: Chapman and Hall.
Goetze O (1918) Die Rontgendiagnostik bei gasgefullter Bauchohle eine neue Methode. *Munch Med Wschr* **65:** 1275–1280.
Gomel V, Taylor PJ, Rioux et al (1986) *Laparoscopy and Hysteroscopy.* Chicago: Year Book.
Gordon AG & Lewis BV (1988). In Gordon AG & Lewis BV (eds) *Gynaecological Endoscopy.* London: Chapman and Hall.
Graff TD, Arbgast NR, Phillips OC et al (1959) Gas embolism. A comparative study of air and carbon dioxide as embolic agents in the systemic venous system. *American Journal of Obstetrics and Gynecology* **78:** 259–65.
Hope R (1937) The differential diagnosis of ectopic pregnancy by peritoneoscopy. *Surgery, Gynecology and Obstetrics* **64:** 229–234.
Hopkins HH (1953) On the diffraction theory of optical images. *Proceedings of the Royal Society* **A217:** 408.
Hulka JF, Omran K, Phillips JM et al (1975) Sterilization by spring clip. *Fertility and Sterility* **26:** 1122–1131.
Jacobeus H (1912) Uber Laparo- und Thoracoskopie. *Beitrage zur Klinik Tuberk* **25:** 183–254.
Johns DA & Hardie RP (1986) Management of unruptured ectopic pregnancy with laparoscopic carbon dioxide laser. *Fertility and Sterility* **46:** 703–705.

Kaplan I, Goldman JM & Ger R (1973) The treatment of erosions of the uterine cervix by CO_2 laser. *Obstetrics & Gynecology* **41:** 795–796.

Kelling G (1902) Uber Oesophagoskopie, Gastroskopie und Cölioskopie. *Munchener Wochenschrift* **49:** 21–24.

Keye WR Jr & Dixon J (1983) Photocoagulation of endometriosis by the argon laser through the laparoscope. *Obstetrics & Gynecology* **62:** 383–386.

Kleppinger RK (1978) Ovarian cyst fenestration via laparoscopy. *Journal of Reproductive Medicine* **21:** 16–19.

Korbsch R (1927) *Lehrbuch und Atlas des Laparo- und Thorakoskopie.* Munchen: Lehmen.

Larsen JF, Pedersen OD & Gregerson E (1986) Ovarian cyst fenestration via the laparoscope. A laparoscopic method for the treatment of non-neoplastic ovarian cysts. *Acta Obstetrica et Gynecologica Scandinavica* **65:** 539–545.

Lieberman BA, Gordon AG, Bostock JF et al (1977) Laparoscopic sterilisation with spring loaded clips: a double puncture technique. *Journal of Reproductive Medicine* **18:** 241–245.

Lomano JM (1987) Nd : YAG laser ablation of early pelvic endometriosis: a report of 61 cases. *Lasers in Surgery and Medicine* **7:** 56–60.

Magos AL, Baumann R & Turnbull AC (1988) Laparoscopic management of ectopic pregnancies. *Lancet* **ii:** 694.

Mann WJ & Stenger VG (1978) Uterine suspension through the laparoscope. *Obstetrics & Gynecology* **51:** 563–566.

Martin DC & Diamond MP (1986) Operative laparoscopy: the role of the CO_2 laser. In *Intra-Abdominal Laser Surgery*. Memphis: Resurge Press.

Mecke H & Semm K (1988) Pelviscopic treatment of abscess-forming inflammation in the true pelvis. *Geburtshilfe Frauenheilkdunde* **48:** 479–482.

Motew M, Ivancovich A, Bieniac J et al (1973) Cardiovascular effects and acid–base and blood gases during laparoscopy. *American Journal of Obstetrics and Gynecology* **115:** 1002–1012.

Nezhat C, Crowgey SR & Garrison CP (1986) Surgical treatment of endometriosis via laser laparoscopy. *Fertility and Sterility* **45:** 778–783.

Nitze M (1879) Beobachtung – und Untersuchungsmethode fur Harnrohre, Harnblase und Rectum. *Weiner Med Wochenschrift* **29:** 649–652.

Nordentoeft S (1912) Uber Endoskopie geschlossener Kavitaten mittels meines Trokar-Endoskopes. *Verhandlungen der Deutchen Gesellschaft fur Gynakologie* **41:** 78–81.

von Ott D (1901) Die direkte Beleuchtung der Bauchhohle, der Harnblase, des Dickdarms und des Uterus zu diagnostischen Zwecken. *Rev Med Tcheque* (Prague) **2:** 27.

Palmer R (1950) *La sterilite involuntaire*. Paris: Masson.

Phillips JM (1976) *Laparoscopy*. Los Angeles: Williams & Wilkins.

Phillips JM, Hulka J, Hulka B, Keith DM & Keith L (1979) American Association of Gynecologic Laparoscopists 1977 Membership Survey. *Journal of Reproductive Medicine* **23:** 61–64.

Pouly JL, Manhes H, Mage G, Canis M & Bruhat MA (1986) Conservative laparoscopic treatment of 321 ectopic pregnancies. *Fertility and Sterility* **46:** 1093–1097.

Power FH & Barnes AC (1941) Sterilization by means of peritoneoscopic fulguration: a preliminary report. *American Journal of Obstetrics and Gynecology* **41:** 1038–1043.

Riedel H-H, Lehmann-Willenbrock E, Conrad P & Semm K (1986) German pelviscopic statistics for the years 1978–1982. *Endoscopy* **18:** 219–222.

Rioux JE & Cloutier D (1974) Bipolar cautery for sterilization by laparoscopy. *Journal of Reproductive Medicine* **13:** 6–10.

Scott DB (1972) Cardiac arrhythmias during laparoscopy. *British Medical Journal* **ii:** 49–50.

Scott JS & Hancock KW (1988) Culdoscopy. In Gordon AG & Lewis BV (eds) *Gynaecological Endoscopy*, pp 11.1–10. London: Chapman and Hall.

Seiler JC, Gidwani G & Ballard L (1986) Laparoscopic cauterization of endometriosis for infertility: a controlled study. *Fertility and Sterility* **46:** 1098–1100.

Semm K (1975) *Atlas of Gynecologic Laparoscopy and Hysteroscopy*, pp 3–14. Philadelphia: WB Saunders.

Semm K (1976) Endocoagulation: a new field of endoscopic surgery. *Journal of Reproductive Medicine* **16:** 195–203.

Semm K (1979) Gynecological surgical interventions with the laparoscope. In Phillips JM (ed.) *Endoscopy in Gynecology*, pp 514–521. Downey: AAGL.

Semm K (1987) *Operative manual for endoscopic abdominal surgery*. Chicago: Year Book.

Semm K (1988) Sight controlled peritoneum puncture for surgical pelviscopy. *Geburtshilfe Frauenheilkunde* **48:** 436–439.
Shapiro HI & Adler DH (1973) Excision of an ectopic pregnancy through the laparoscope. *American Journal of Obstetrics and Gynecology* **117:** 290–291.
Sharp JR, Pierson WP, Brady III CE (1982) Comparison of CO_2- and N_2O-induced discomfort during peritoneoscopy under local anaesthesia. *Gastroenterology* **82:** 453–456.
Short R (1925) The uses of coelioscopy. *British Medical Journal* **ii:** 254–255.
Soderstrom RM (1978) Foreword. In Phillips JM (ed.) *Endoscopy in gynaecology. Proceedings of the 3rd International Congress on Gynecologic Endoscopy*, pp viii-ix. Downey: AAGL.
Sortel G, Hirsch E & Edelin K (1983) Necrotizing fasciitis following diagnostic laparoscopy. *Obstetrics & Gynecology* **62** (supplement): 67–69.
Steptoe PC (1967) *Laparoscopy and Gynaecology*. London: Livingstone.
Stone WE (1924) Intra-abdominal examination by aid of the peritoneoscope. *Journal of the Kansas Medical Society* **24:** 63–64.
Sutton C (1974) Limitations of laparoscopic ovarian biopsy. *British Journal of Obstetrics and Gynaecology* **81:** 317.
Tadir Y, Ovadia J, Zuckerman Z et al (1981) Laparoscopic applications of the CO_2 laser. In Atsumi K & Nimsakul N (eds) *Proceedings of the 4th Congress of the International Society for Laser Surgery*, pp 25–26. Tokyo: Japanese Society for Laser Medicine.
Thomsen K (1951) Erfahrungen und Fortschritte bei der Douglasskopie. *Geburtshilfe und Fraunheilkunde* **11:** 587–601.
Timonen S & Nieminen U (1967) Tubal Pregnancy, choice of operative method of treatment. *Acta Obstetricia et Gynecologica Scandinavica* **46:** 327.
Unverrichte W (1923) Die Thorakoskopie und Laparoskopie. *Berliner Kliniche Wschr* **2:** 502–503.
Veress J (1938) Ein neues Instrument zur Ausfuhrung von Brust – oder Bauchpunktionen und Pneumothoraxbehandlung. *Deutsche Medizinische Wachenschrift* **64:** 1480–1481.
Yacoub OF, Cardona I, Coveler LA et al (1982) Carbon dioxide embolism during laparoscopy. *Anesthesiology* **57:** 533–535.
Yoon IB & King TM (1975) A preliminary and intermediate report of a new laparoscopic ring procedure. *Journal of Reproductive Medicine* **15:** 54–56.
Zollikofer R (1924) Zur Laparoskopie. *Schwizerische Medizinische Wochenschrift* **5:** 264–265.

2

Conventional operative laparoscopy (pelviscopy)

KURT SEMM
ISEULT O'NEILL-FREYS

The recent technical advances in endoscopic equipment, coupled with man's never-ending quest to improve and simplify has led to the possible replacement of over 75% of gynaecological laparotomies by operative pelviscopic surgery. The concept of 'minimally invasive surgery' has been realized. This chapter discusses the instrumentation, techniques, and role of advanced pelviscopic surgery in gynaecology.

With the advent of endocoagulation in 1972, the controversial and often destructive use of mono- or bipolar, high-frequency current became obsolete in endoscopic surgery. Endocoagulation, in conjunction with the development of the endosuture in 1977, established a thorough and reliable method of haemostasis which ultimately led to even newer operative instruments and techniques. The triple-loop ligation technique as well as the extracorporeal and intracorporeal knotting techniques have played a pivotal role in the migration from classical gynaecological laparotomy towards operative pelviscopic surgery.

The range of operative procedures performed by pelviscopy is large. Classical gynaecological operations such as adnexectomy, myoma enucleation, repair of uterine perforation, ovariolysis and salpingolysis, ovarian biopsy and cyst enucleation, and endocoagulation of endometriosis, are now routinely performed. Microsurgical operations, for example, in the conservative treatment of ectopic pregnancy, through longitudinal salpingotomy, and salpingostomy with tubal eversion have demonstrated results superior to those obtained through classic laparotomy. Operative pelviscopy also reaches effectively into the domain of classical abdominal surgery, e.g. visceral and parietal peritoneum adhesiolysis, bowel-omental adhesiolysis, and appendicectomy. Pelviscopic surgery also has an increasing role in the diagnosis and follow-up of the (sometimes debilitated) patient suffering from malignant disease.

This chapter will try with the help of illustrations to make the advanced principles and techniques of this method clear.

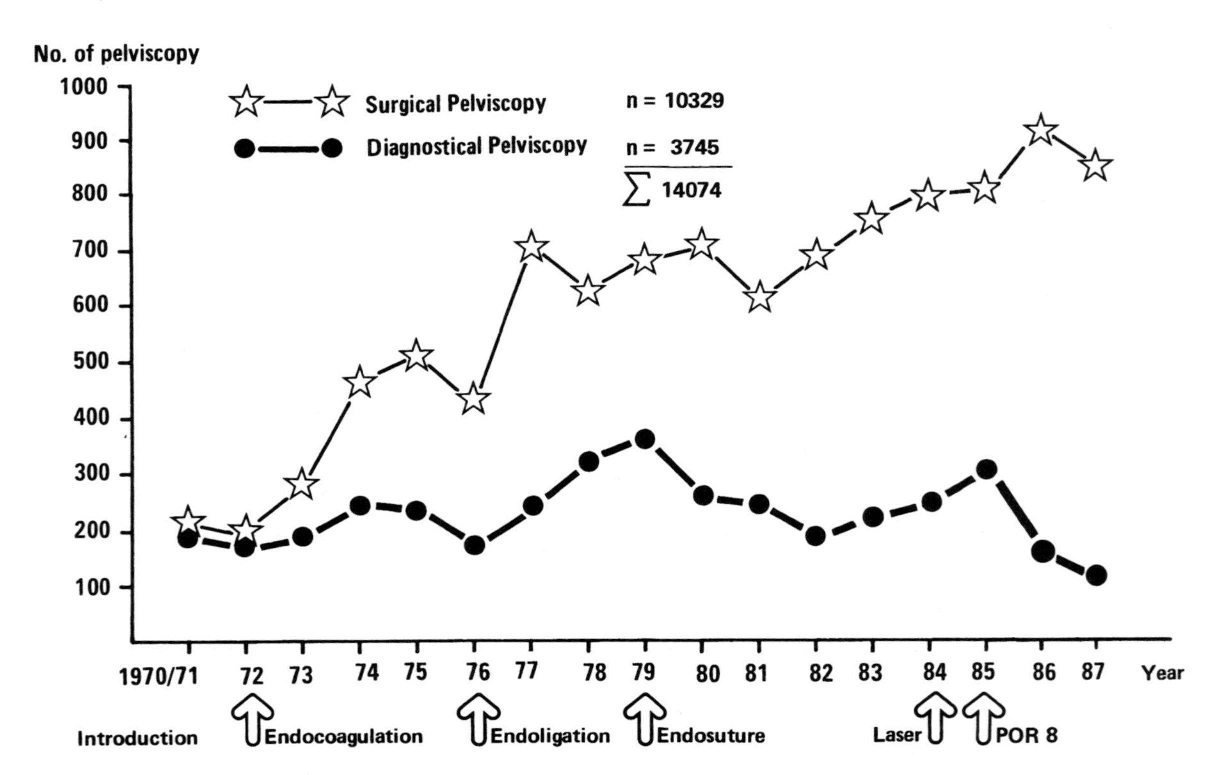

Figure 1. Increase of surgical pelviscopy at the Department of Gynecology, Kiel (1971–1987).

INSTRUMENTATION AND EQUIPMENT FOR OPERATIVE PELVISCOPY

The clinical and operative experience at the Department of Obstetrics and Gynaecology at the University Womens' Clinic of Kiel/Western Germany, where over 15 000 operative pelviscopies have been performed since 1971, has set a standard for endoscopic operations (Figure 1) (Riedel et al, 1986a, b, 1989; Semm, 1987a, b). Constant advances in techniques and equipment have established an operative system which provides the greatest efficacy for the surgeon and at the same time the greatest safety to the patient.

Operative pelviscopy requires the following equipment:

1. *Semm's electronic* 'OP-PNEU' *insufflator*. A pneumoperitoneum of constant pressure and volume is mandatory for operative pelviscopy. The exchange of instruments, pelvic irrigation and suction, all disturb the equilibrium of the conventionally established penumoperitoneum. The electronically controlled insufflator designed by Semm (Figure 2) provides, via the Monofilar Bivalent System (MBS, see Figure 3) a constant delivery of 7 litres of CO_2 per minute even in the presence of intraperitoneal pressures of up to 12 mmHg.

2. *Pelviscope and light source*. To perform operative pelviscopy we recommend the use of the pelvic 'Circum-Vision Optics Set' designed by Semm (Figure 4). The set consists of a 5 mm diameter, 30° angled pelviscope, a 10 mm diameter, 30° angled pelviscope, and a straight pelviscope. An optimal light transmission is provided by a fluid light cable. The light source

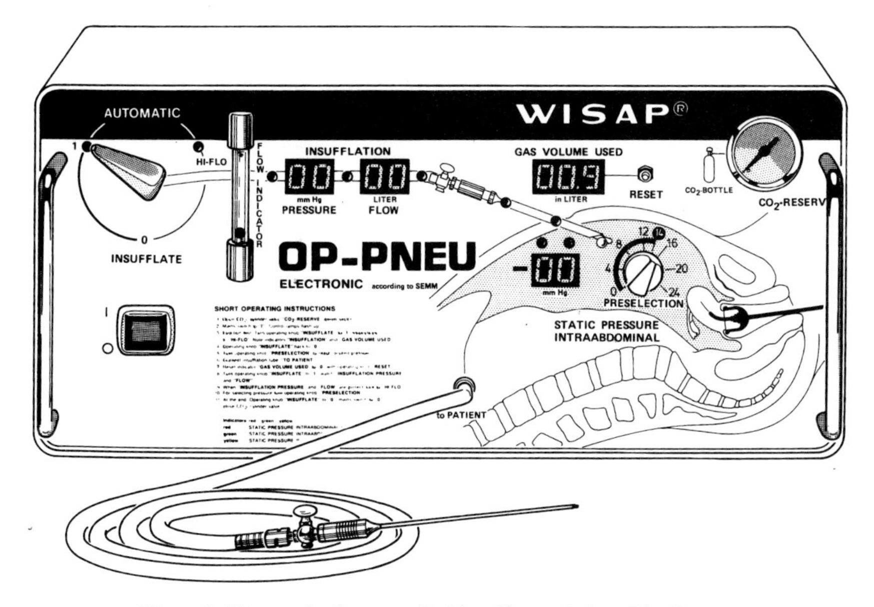

Figure 2. Electronically controlled insufflator designed by Semm.

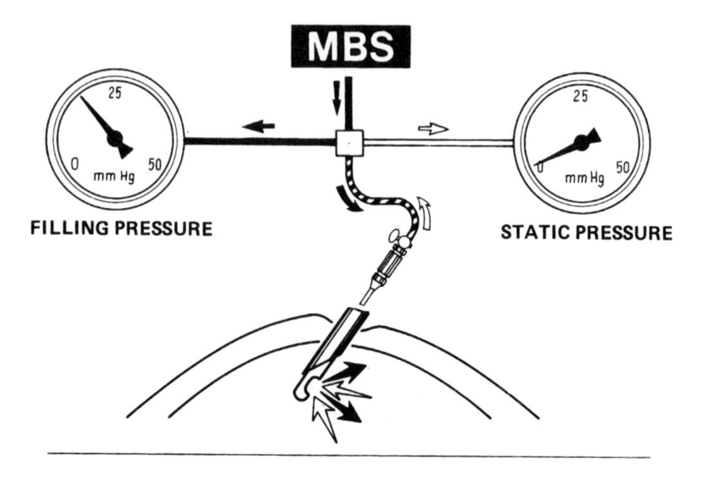

Figure 3. Monofilar Bivalent System (MBS).

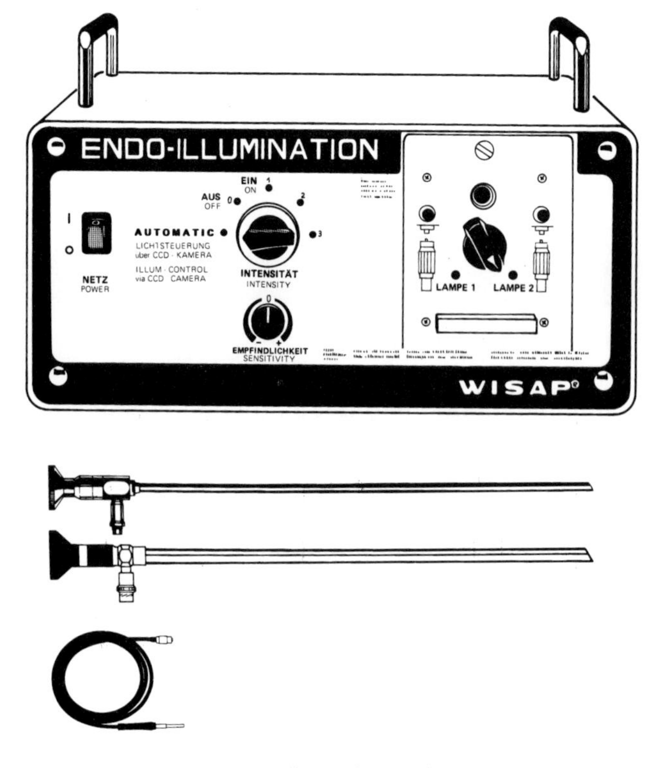

Figure 4. Circum-Vision Optics set.

must generate 150 W and is adequately provided by the Endo-Illumination Apparatus (Figure 4).

3. *Endocoagulator*. The advent of destructive heat at a temperature of only 100C as an effective method of haemostasis has become an integral part of operative pelviscopy. For this reason the endocoagulator together with its attachments (Figure 5), the crocodile forceps, the point coagulator, and the myoma enucleator are mandatory. Endocoagulation prevents the risk of uncontrollable burning which can occur with the application of monopolar or bipolar high-frequency current.

4. *Suture and suture materials*. With the advent of endosuture (Figure 6), endoloop (Figure 7), and endoligature (Figure 8) and the intra- and extracorporeal operative knotting techniques (Figure 9.1–6) in 1977, classical methods used at laparotomy were introduced into endoscopic surgery and have become a mainstay.

5. *Instruments*. A full range of instruments (Figure 10a–c) allowing the surgeon to perform the operative steps are necessary. Included are instruments for perforation, dilatation, grasping, cutting, aspiration, instillation, morcellation, haemostasis, drainage, and emergencies.

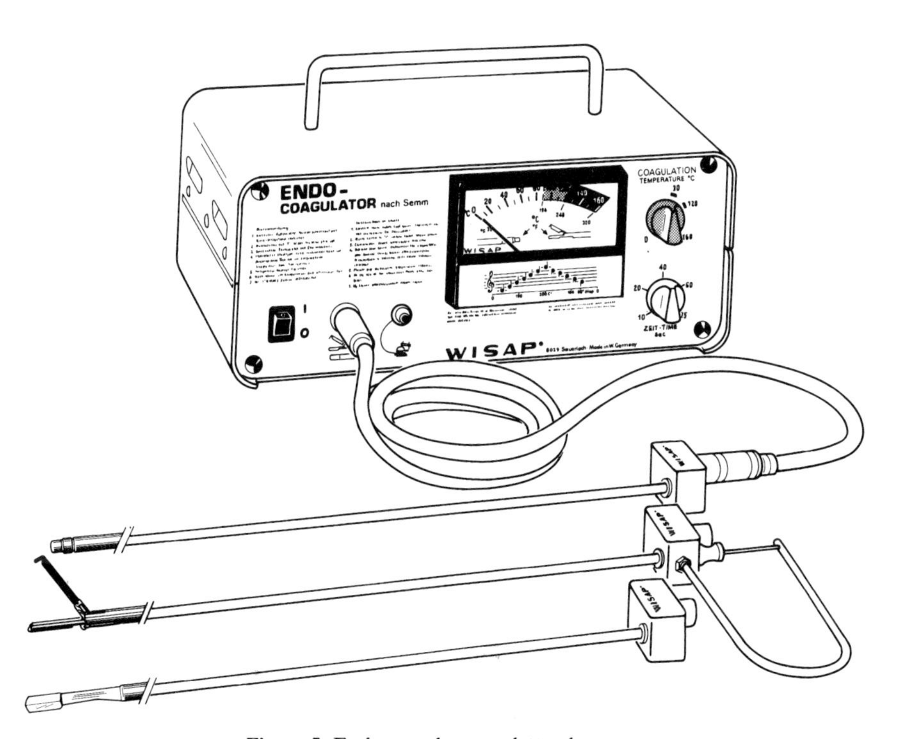

Figure 5. Endocoagulator and attachments.

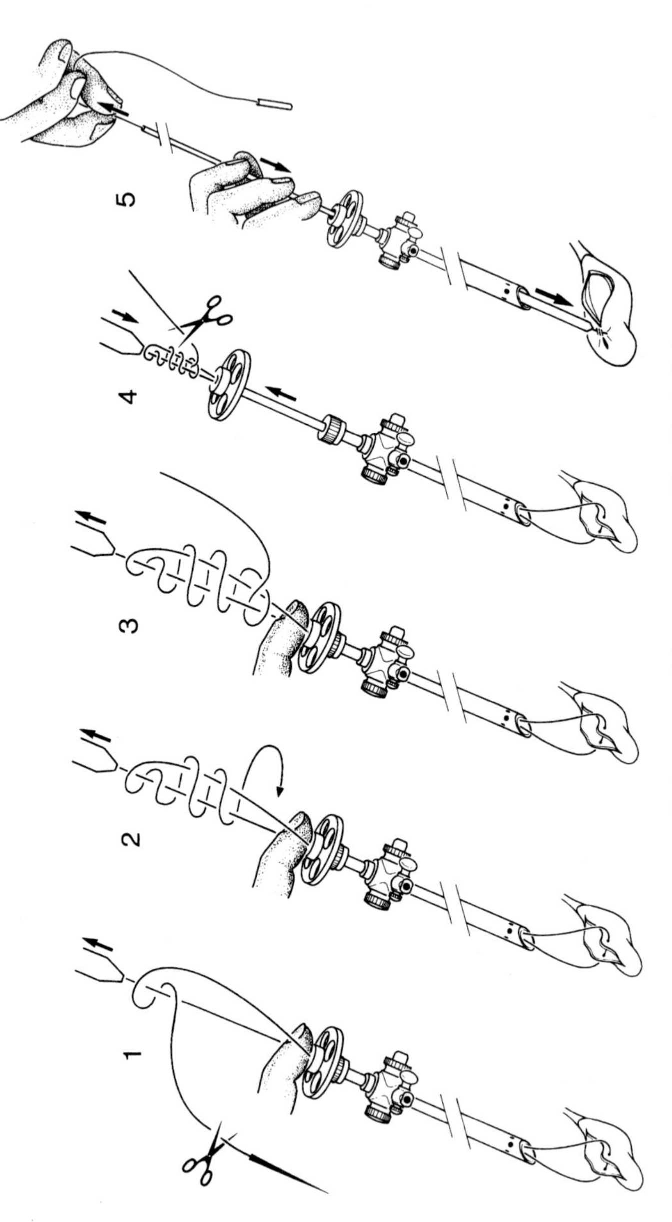

Figure 6. Endosuture and the extracorporeal knotting technique.

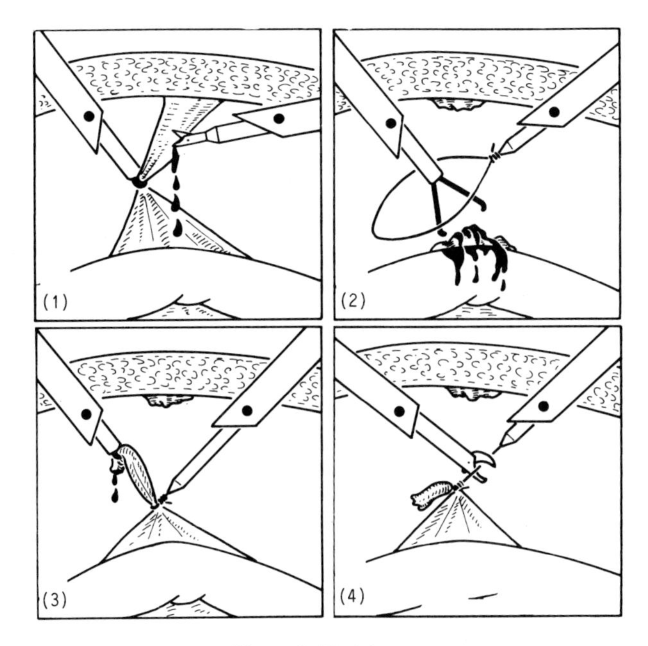

Figure 7. Endoloop.

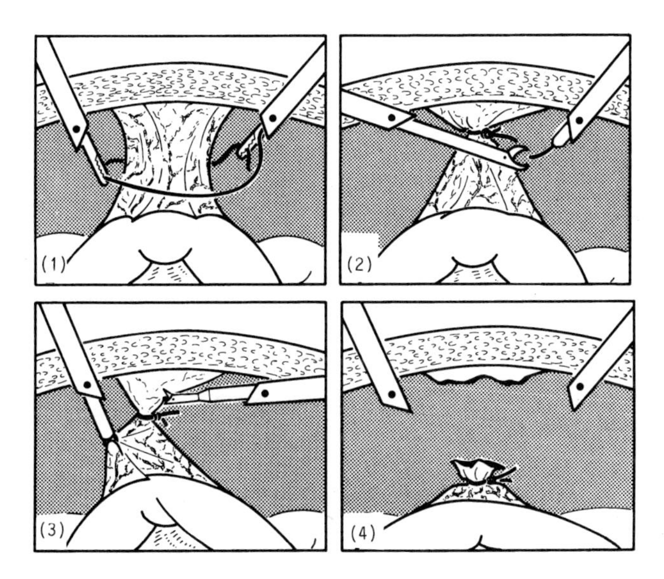

Figure 8. Endoligature.

6. *Aquapurator*. In order to maintain a clear view of the operative field pelvic irrigation and lavage is necessary. This is adequately provided by the monofilar-bivalent irrigational system, the Aquapurator or the CO_2 Aqua Purator with its attachments (Figure 11). This system allows for effortless instillation and aspiration of physiological saline at 37°C. During the operation 2–4 litres of normal saline solution are kept in a warm water bath set at 37°C; a second bath set at 50°C is used for cleaning and prevention of fogging of the pelviscope.

7. *Pertubation apparatus*. Endoscopic tubal diagnosis and surgery requires an initial controlled pertubation using either CO_2 gas or a blue dye solution (methylene blue) (Figure 12). This is performed using the pertubation apparatus which is connected to a cervical vacuum adaptor which also allows for easy manipulation of the uterus during the procedure.

8. *Aids for the surgeon*. The surgeon must work in a relaxed and comfortable position. An optic holder with a flexible arm attachment, an operative stool, and a shoulder rest are obligatory (Figure 13).

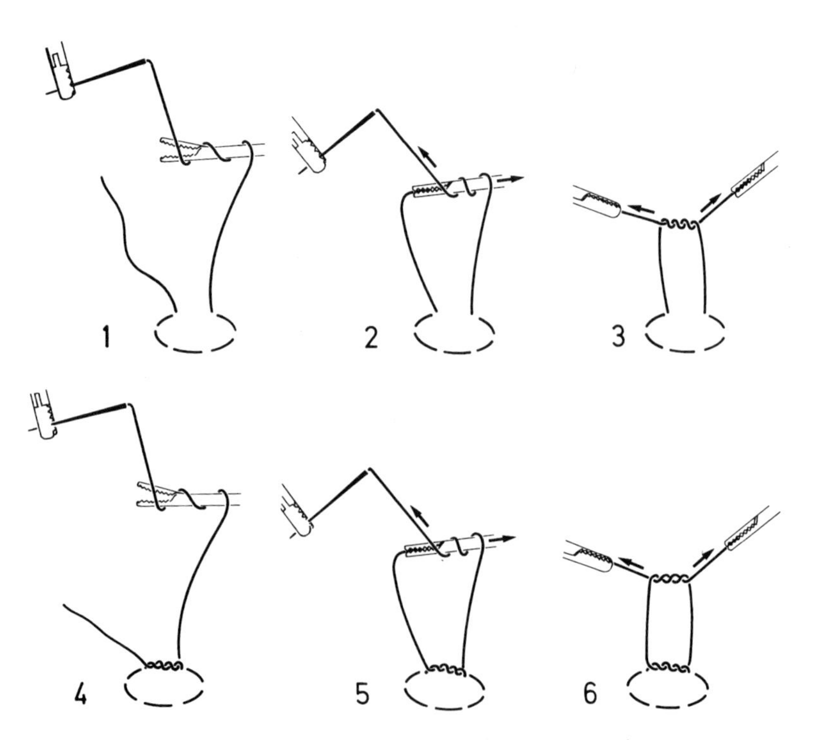

Figure 9. Intra- and extracorporeal operative knotting techniques.

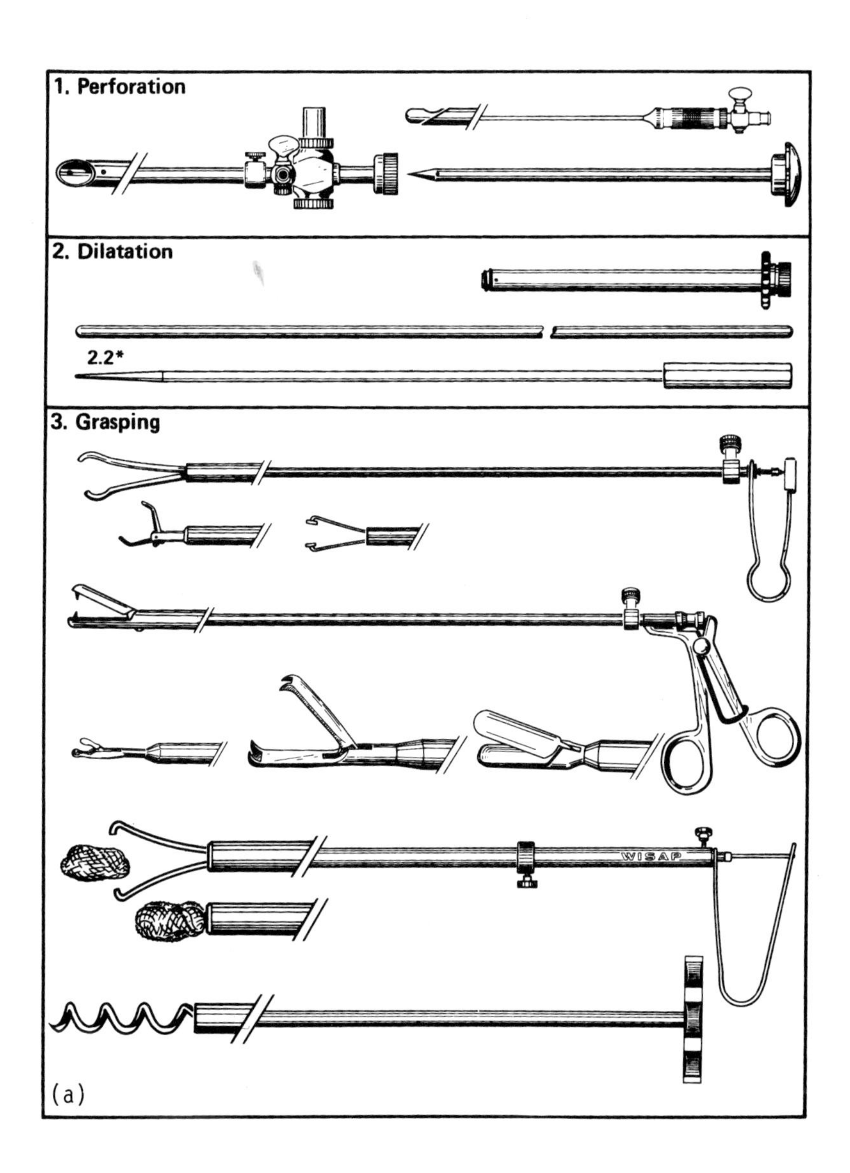
1. Perforation
2. Dilatation
2.2*
3. Grasping
WISAP
(a)

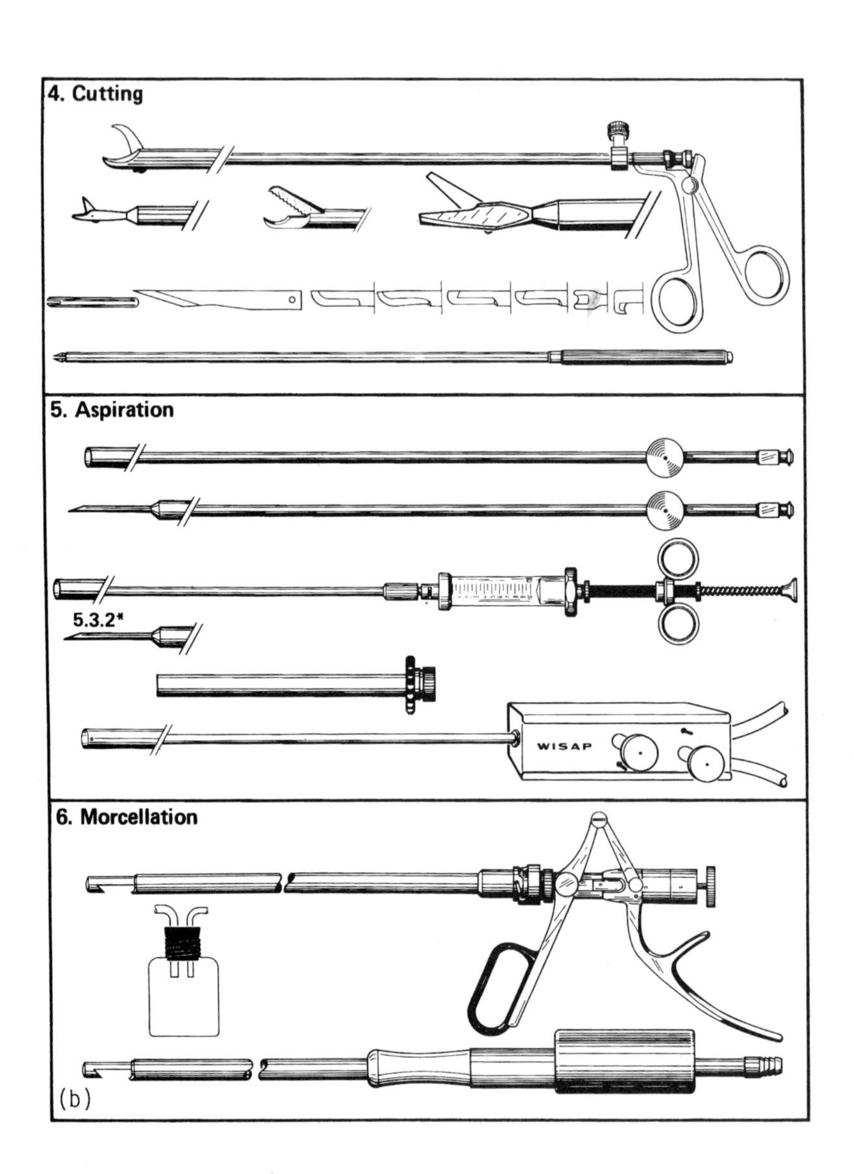
4. Cutting
5. Aspiration
5.3.2*
WISAP
6. Morcellation
(b)

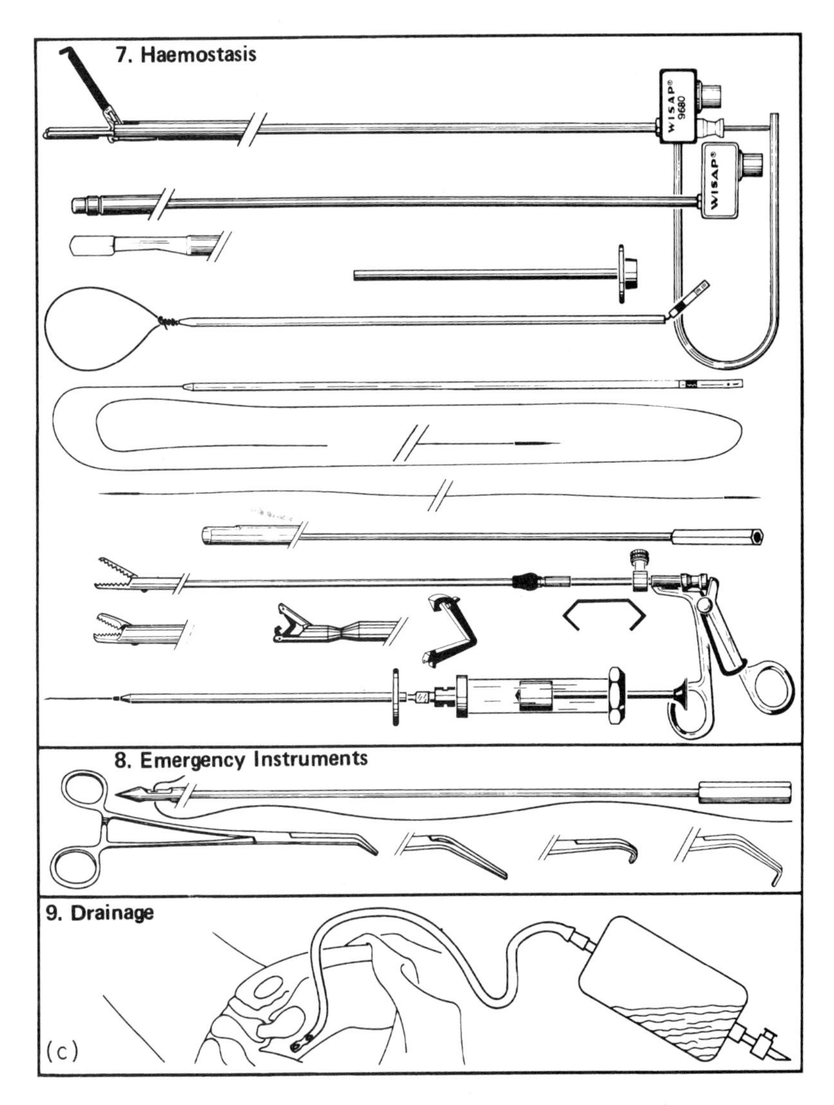

Figure 10. The full range of instruments for operative pelviscopy.

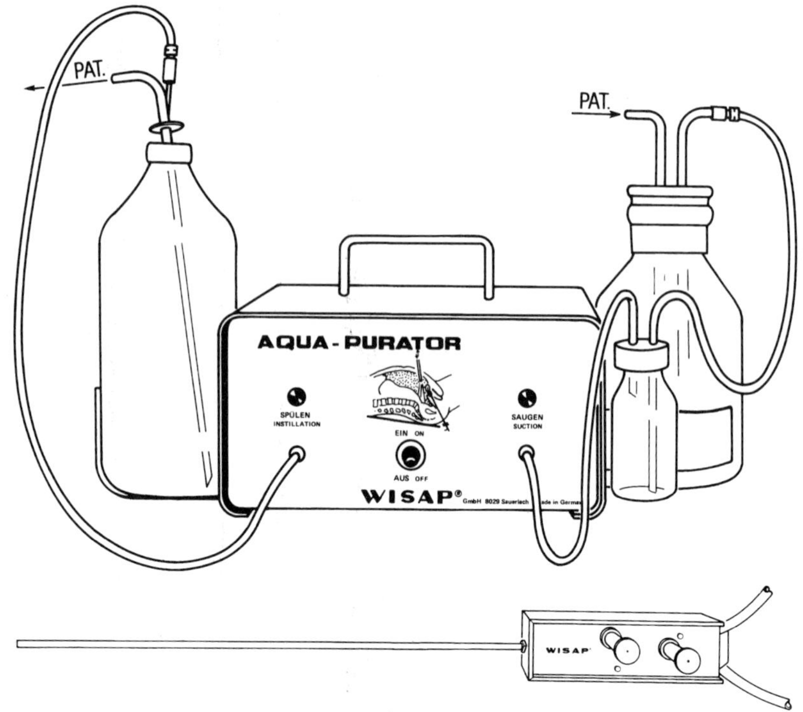

Figure 11. The Aquapurator.

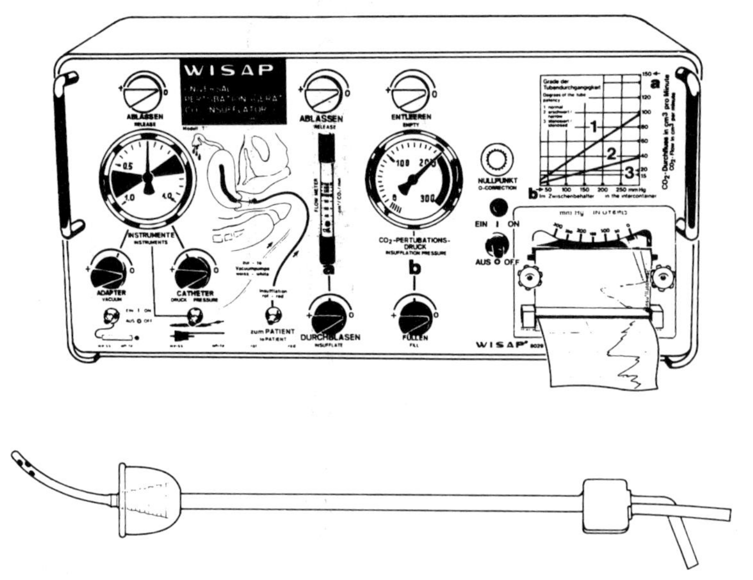

Figure 12. Pertubation apparatus (designed by Fikentscher and Semm) and Semm's cervical vacuum adapter.

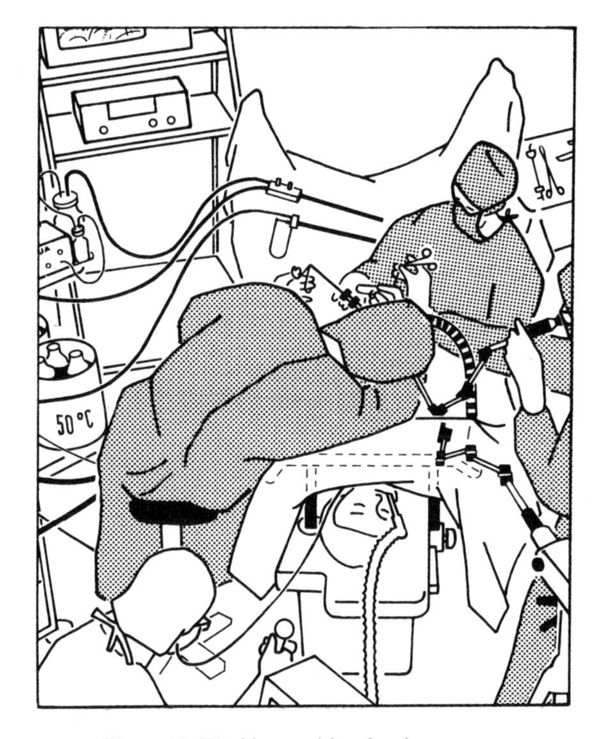

Figure 13. Working position for the surgeon.

DISADVANTAGES OF HIGH FREQUENCY CURRENT

High frequency current is not recommended in pelviscopic abdominal surgery (Semm, 1983). It is routinely used in general surgery for haemostasis and coagulation; these effects are principally provided through the production of a destructive heat which ranges from 100°C to 500°C. The 'skin effect' of high frequency current allows it to flow over the surface of the human body and it can therefore be used without any risk to the patient. This phenomenon is described in figure 14. Faraday's law states that the flux of current causes a clockwise magnetic field around the electric conductor. Lenz (see Figure 14) described a negative feedback whereby the effect tends to oppose its source. This change in magnetic field generates AD currents. These AD currents are thus rotating against the direction of the current. This forces the electrical current to migrate out of the conductor onto its surface as the frequency increases (Figure 15). Thus, high frequency current is not dangerous to patients so long as it flows over the surface of the conductor, as in open laparotomy. If, however, we force the current to flow through the human body (i.e. at pelviscopy) it takes the path of least resistance and flows now through the second-order conductors, i.e. electrolytes conduct the current. The current now flows in tissues having the highest

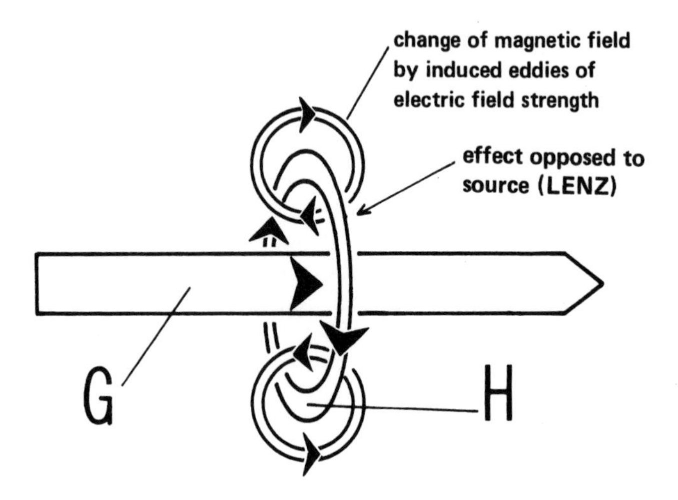

Figure 14. Faraday's Law.

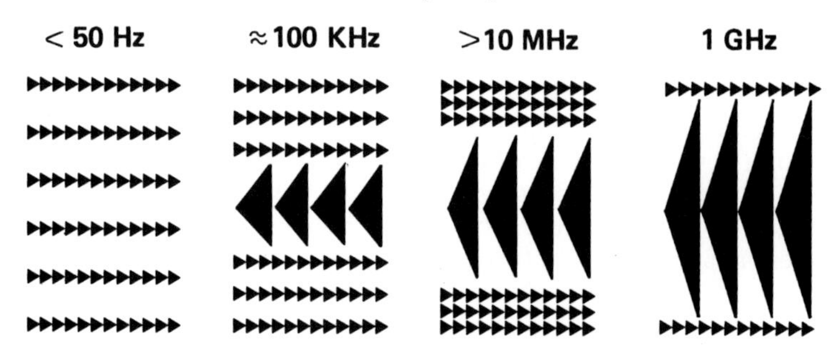

Figure 15. The skin effect.

electrolyte content, for example nerves, blood vessels, intestines; the skin effect causes the current to flow always on the surface of these tissues. High frequency current therefore reaches the return electrode through many indeterminable pathways, and is capable of leaving the body wherever there is an earth, including the nose, eyes and ears of the surgeon, if he is earthed; all could sustain damage (Figure 16). Another variable, which demonstrates how uncontrollable high frequency current may be, is that current can alter the electrolyte content of the tissues through which it passes, thus causing the pathways of current to fluctuate constantly.

The widespread use of high frequency current for sterilization procedures in the 1970s in the USA and Europe, was associated with many unforeseen injuries to bowel, ureter, and abdominal wall. It is important, therefore, to measure the amount of energy applied objectively, not for example by determination of the discolouration of the tissue, which commences at over 94°C. At this temperature biological death (starting at 57°C) has occurred and the thermolabile enzymes are destroyed, leading to thermal necrosis (Stalsand, 1978). This necrotic process occuring in the mesovarium in procedures such as fallopian tube sterilization upsets the vital blood and nerve supply to the ovary and leads to disturbed exocrine and endocrine ovarian function (Riedel et al, 1983). Bipolar high frequency current tends to damage a smaller area of the mesovarium but nonetheless damage to the mesovarium still occurs (Figure 17 b and c).

As high frequency current is so uncontrollable with respect to the region

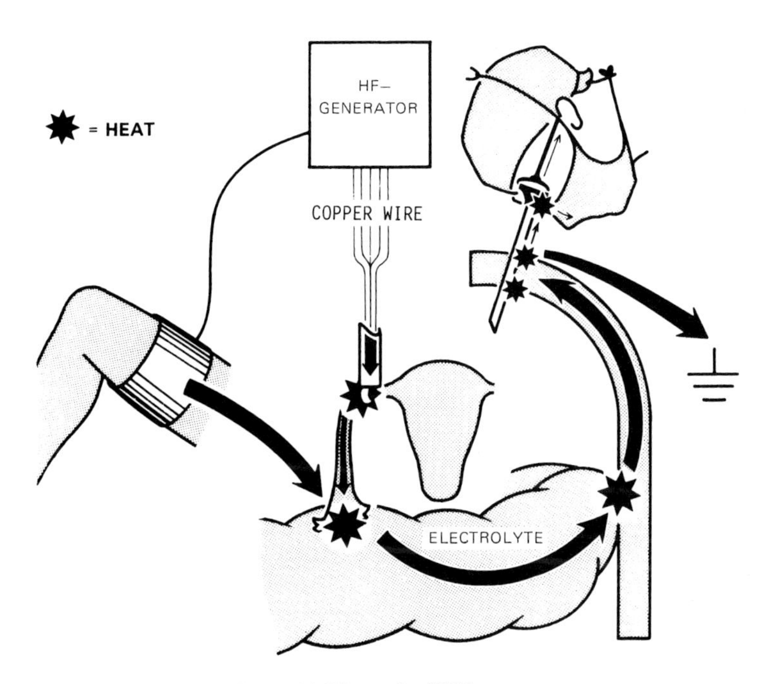

Figure 16. The path of HF current.

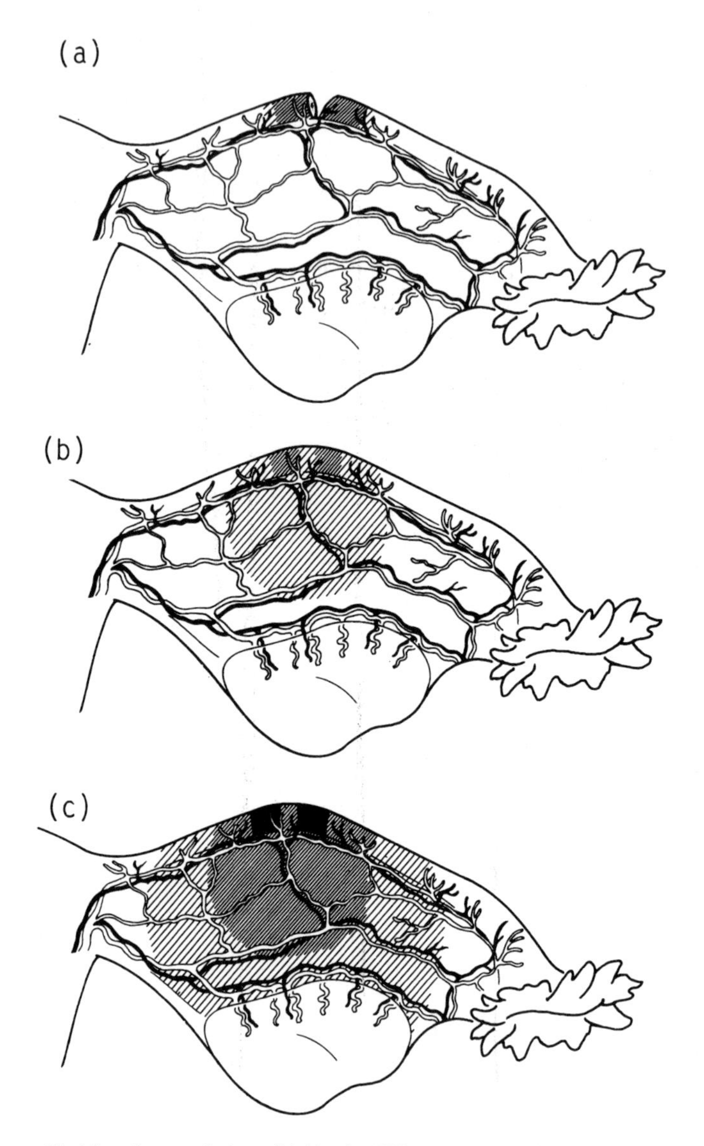

Figure 17. (a) endocoagulation; (b) bipolar HF coagulation; (c) HF coagulation.

of the body that it affects, it is completely unsuitable for endoscopic use. We therefore advocate its replacement by a safe and electronically-directed destructive heat—that of endocoagulation (Brackebusch and Semm, 1976).

ENDOCOAGULATION AND ITS ADVANTAGES IN ENDOSCOPIC SURGERY

With endocoagulation, destructive heat is produced in the abdomen without endangering the patient. The endocoagulator designed by Semm has three principal attachments (see Figure 5) (Semm 1966): the point coagulator for use in haemostasis and destruction of endometriotic implants; the myoma enucleator for removal of myomas and adhesioloysis; the crocodile forceps necessary for bowel adhesiolysis and fallopian tube sterilization. Their use will be described later in the description of the operation techniques.

These instruments are fully insulated and heated with approximately 5 V of direct current, and they heat only the tissue with which they come in contact. Heat is convected only for a diamater of 2–3 mm around their active surface, thus they can be used in many operative procedures such as adhesiolysis. As the endocoagulator delivers an exact heat dose it was possible to determine the thermic load capacity for a certain tissue depth. The on–off function is controlled via a pneumatic foot switch. The desired coagulation temperature may be preselected having a range from 80–140°C. The coagulation time is coupled with an acoustic signal; this may also be preselected. This acoustic signal increases and decreases according to the temperature, and shuts off when the tip of the applied instrument cools down to 60°C. This allows the surgeon to devote his entire attention to the operative field as he does not have to look at the machine at the same time.

Tissues accidently touched with the instrument when in the off position are in little danger of burning as the instrument is too small to release much heat to the tissue via convection. The low voltage required and the fact that endocoagulation is confined to a small area are both very positive factors but we must examine the biophysical changes in the tissue after application of this method of tissue destruction by heat.

When animal tissue is heated at greater than 120°C the protein becomes glue-like; a further rise in temperature causes charring as we see with high frequency current. This tissue is sloughed off after a few days and the open wound produces a fibrinous exudate; histiocytes and fibroblasts migrate to the area, and a perfect site for the formation of intra-abdominal adhesions is produced. However, with endocoagulation the temperature is maintained at that of boiling water; no tissue sloughs off—the dead cells remain—no cell migration occurs and no exudation of fibrin takes place as there is no open wound. As there is no tissue defect the regeneration process is stimulated and a protein coat (the sloughed off dead cells) is laid like a film over the wound, preventing the formation of adhesions. This is one of the major benefits of the endocoagulation process (Riedel et al, 1986a, b).

In a study done on 1260 sterilization cases we performed fallopian tube sterilization by application of endocoagulation followed by haemostatic transection of the tube. The success rate was 99.9% with this method (Riedel and Semm, 1982). We have demonstrated electron-microscopically (Semm and Phillip, 1979, 1980) that an inadequate separation or transection of the fallopian tube can lead to recanalization; this of course indicates that a proper transection of the tube is mandatory. The advantages of endo-coagulation are:

1. that it is accurately controllable,
2. that it prevents the formation of later adhesions, and
3. that the amount of heat energy applied to tissues of the human body may be correctly measured, therefore avoiding method-related burns and ovarian dysfunction (see Figure 17a) (Riedel et al, 1983).

TECHNIQUES INVOLVED IN ADVANCED OPERATIVE PELVISCOPY

Here we describe briefly the major haemostatic techniques used in operative pelviscopy. These are incorporated in many of the detailed descriptions of the procedures which follow (Semm , 1986, 1987a, b, 1988a).

Loop ligation (see Figure 7)

Loop ligation is performed using the endoloop or Roeder loop which is a prepackaged, pretied, slip knot described by Roeder in the late 1890s for paediatric tonsillectomy. Incorporated now within the realm of pelviscopic surgery it is safe and easy to use. It is used as an adjuvant to haemostasis and as a classic ligature, e.g. in the case of salpingo-oophorectomy or oophorectomy. When ligating the loop is applied on three consecutive occasions; this procedure is therefore known as the pelviscopic 'triple loop technique' (see Figure 22).

Endosuture (see Figure 6) and endoligature (see Figure 8) with subsequent extracorporeal knotting technique

In all cases where it is technically impossible to pull bleeding tissue through an endoloop, either endosuture or endoligature is required. The suture or ligature material used is sterile catgut approximately 80 cm long with one end attached through a plastic push rod. Once the suture or ligature has been set a slip knot as described by Roeder is tied extracorporeally (see Figure 6). The knot tied extracorporeally is now reintroduced into the abdomen, pulled tight, and the suture material is resected.

Intracorporeal knotting technique

The intracorporeal knotting technique is required for all microsurgical procedures in the case of tubal surgery, intestinal serosal defects, or fine ovarian sutures. The suture material used is 4-0 or 6-0 PDS. The suture is

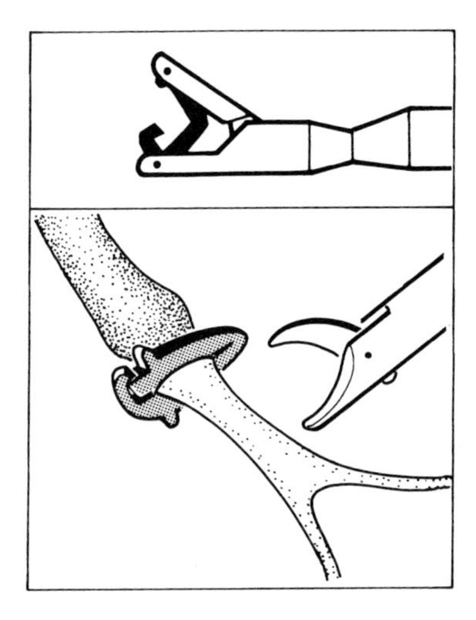

Figure 18. The Endoclip technique.

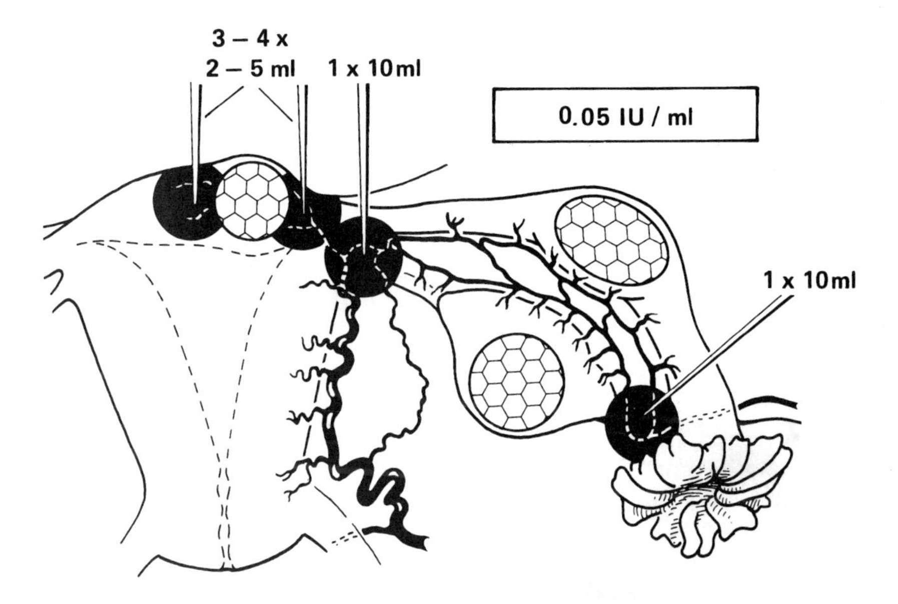

Figure 19. Instillation of POR 8.

laid and tied in the classical surgical fashion (see Figure 9), either without or (easier) with the needle attached.

Endoclip techique

For smaller tissue bundles requiring ligation the endoclip may be applied. The clip is made of PDS material and is available in 2 sizes, 5 mm and 10 mm. The clip is applied using the 5 or 10 mm diameter clip applicator (Figure 18).

Instillation of POR 8 (Sandoz)

This is a synthetic Ornipressin and it is used in much of our adnexal and uterine surgery as a haemostatic adjuvant (Semm and Mettler, 1988). We have achieved excellent results using this solution in a concentration of 5 IU per 100 ml of normal saline. Usually, we inject 2–3 boluses each containing 10 ml of solution into the myometrium and mesosalpinx (Figure 19), along specific areas of distribution of branches of the ovarian and uterine arteries.

PELVISCOPIC SURGERY ON THE UTERUS

Repair of uterine perforation

Pelviscopy is of indisputable value in cases of uterine perforation whether caused by sounding probe or operative curette in that it identifies the extent of extrauterine damage and rules out the possibility of internal bleeding. In intrauterine device (IUD)-associated perforation the IUD may be sought and easily removed using the biopsy forceps. When the IUD becomes entangled within the omentum, omental resection of that segment via ligation with an endoloop is required. Where the IUD remains within the uterine wall POR 8 injection is performed followed by point coagulation producing an adequate haemostasis. Biopsy forceps are then used to remove the IUD. Point coagulation suffices to arrest any residual bleeding.

Enucleation of myomata

Both subserosal and intramural myomata may be safely and effectively removed with a minimal loss of blood by pelviscopy.

Subserosal myomata

These myomas are removed practically without blood loss combining the haemostatic techniques of POR 8 instillation and endocoagulation. The tissue surrounding the base of the myoma is instilled with two to three depots of POR 8 (Figure 20.1a). Endocoagulation using the myoma enucleator is then performed. The myoma itself is held with the grasping forceps or the myoma screw and its pedicle is rotated with the myoma enucleator until the myoma is completely severed (Figure 20.1b). The remaining uterine wound

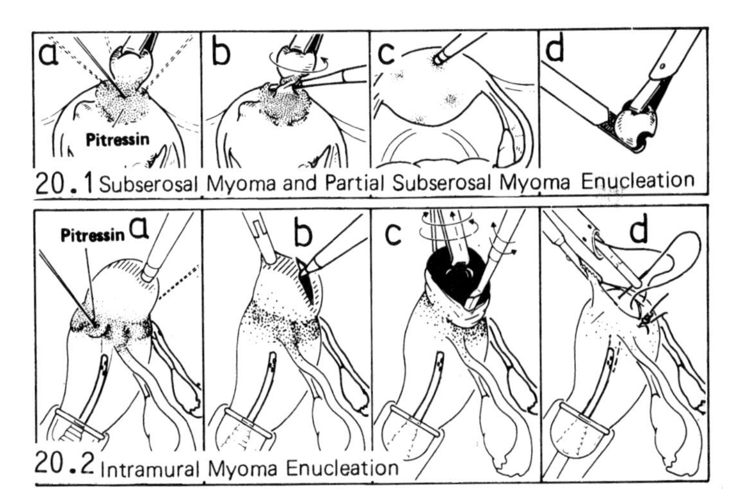

Figure 20. Enucleation of myomata.

is coagulated using the point coagulator (see Figure 20.1c). The myoma is then morcellated using the hand or automatic morcellator (Figures 10.9 and 20.1d).

Intramural myomata

After POR 8 instillation (Figure 20.2a) an additional haemostasis of the myoma capsule is established using endocoagulation along the intended incisional site. The incision is made using the microscissors which dissect the uterine muscle until the capsule of the fibroid is exposed (Figure 20.2b). The wound edges are now splayed open using biopsy forceps (it is important to use the bidentate forceps to ensure a firm grip on the wound margins). The fibroid itself is grasped with the claw forceps. Using the myoma enucleator set at 120°C the myoma may be completely disencapsulated (Figure 20.2c). A slow progression is recommended so that the vessels split by the myoma enucleator may recoil back into the uterine wall. When thick veins are observed a loop ligation or endoligation is recommended. If the pedicle is very large pedicle ligation is first performed using an endoligature.

Once the myoma has been enucleated it is left resting in the pouch of Douglas. We recommend that the surgeon closes the uterine wound first using endosuture with extracorporeal knotting (Figure 20.2d). Wound closure prior to morcellation is performed so that the surgeon has enough time to observe whether or not the haemostasis established by the suturing has been adequate. The myoma is then morcellated.

Obligatory to the myoma enucleation procedure is the placing of a Robinson drain at the end of the procedure (see Figure 10.9). This has a dual purpose: to recognize immediately postoperative bleeding and to drain developing exudate—the drain remains in situ for 24–48 hours (Semm and Popp, 1989).

OPERATIONS ON THE ADNEXA—CONSERVATIVE

Ovariolysis

It must be mentioned that adhesiolysis of all types, whether on the adnexa, bowel or anterior abdominal wall, are most effectively performed by pelviscopy because of the very small extent of disturbance to the peritoneum.

Ovariolysis may either be performed with the microscissors (Figure 21.1), or through the application of endocoagulation using the myoma enucleator (see Figure 10.6). As already discussed, the application of endocoagulation has the advantage that the generated protein film produced by the destructive heat helps to prevent the redevelopment of adhesions.

Ovarian biopsy

The bidentate, long-jawed biopsy forceps are used for this procedure. The

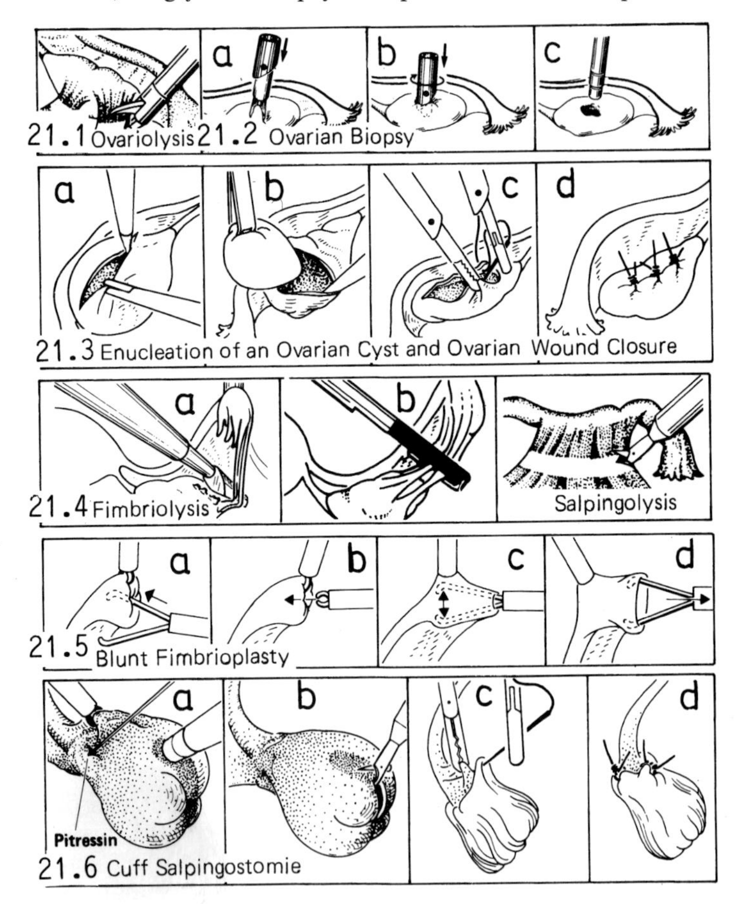

Figure 21. Conservative operations on the adnexa.

chosen site for ovarian biopsy is grasped using the forceps. This is in principle a punch biopsy that is performed by pressing the elliptical trocar sheath down to meet the tissue which has been grasped by the biopsy forceps: then, using a twisting motion the biopsy is taken. Haemostasis is achieved using the point coagulator (Figure 21.2).

Ovarian cyst enucleation

Ovarian cysts suspected of being malignant must be excluded from treatment by pelviscopic surgery. This is made possible by means of pre-operative vaginal sonography, whereby one can determine whether a cyst is simple, multiloculated, or if papillomatous protrusions are present.

Pelviscopic ovarian cyst enucleation requires proper haemostasis. Instillation of 10 ml of POR 8 solution into the mesovarium (see Figure 19) forming two to three wheals coupled with the application of endocoagulation along the intended incision site using the point coagulator provides adequate haemostasis.

The next step is to split the tunica albuginea using the microscissors until the capsule of the ovarian cyst is exposed. The wound is then splayed open using two biopsy forceps, and the ovarian cyst itself is enucleated (Figure 21.3a). Grasping the ovarian cyst using the claw forceps or the large spoon forceps allows for a complete enucleation of the cyst (Figure 21.3b). Where the cyst has been ruptured and it is difficult to remove the entire cyst wall, biopsy forceps are employed. Using the so-called 'hair curler technique', the cyst wall is wrapped around the biopsy forceps in a ravelling motion and is thus more easily and completely excised. The bed of the ovarian wound is now re-inspected to ensure that the entire cyst wall has been removed. Using the point coagulator the ovarian wound bed is coagulated ensuring complete haemostasis. Finally, the ovarian wound itself is closed by endosuture with extracorporeal knotting (Figure 21.3c). We recommend the use of interrupted sutures or a Z-suture. A Robinson drain is placed in all cases of ovarian surgery (see Figure 10.9).

Fimbriolysis

Fimbriolysis (Figure 21.4) is effectively and haemostatically performed using the myoma enucleator set at 100°C. Where a sharp transection of adhesions is required application of the crocodile forceps to the adhesional strands prior to resection is extremely effective.

Fimbrioplasty

A prerequisite for this procedure is the application of a vacuum intrauterine cannula suctioned onto the cervical ostium which, via a reservoir containing chromopertubation fluid (methylene blue), is attached in series to a universal pertubation apparatus (as designed by Fikentscher and Semm, see Figure 12). Ascending chromopertubation using pressures of up to

250 mmHg demonstrates stenoses of the fallopian tube fimbria. Manual insufflation is not adequate.

For blunt fimbrioplasty, the fimbrial end of the tube is held with atraumatic grasping or bowel forceps (Figure 21.5a). A second atraumatic grasping forceps now in the closed position is then passed into the ampulla (Figure 21.5b), opened approximately 2–3 cm (Figure 21.5c), and then in this open position removed from the tube (Figure 21.5d). Through this procedure the ampullary end of the tube is atraumatically, i.e. bluntly dilated. We recommend repetition of this procedure two or three times.

Salpingostomy

Here again, a prerequisite for salpingostomy is ascending chromopertubation whereby the course of the tube and the ampulla itself may be visually and effectively demonstrated. Optimal haemostasis is provided by injecting the mesosalpinx with POR 8 solution (5 IU/100 ml of normal saline). Multiple depots of the solution are injected into the mesosalpinx each containing 2–5 ml of solution (see Figure 16); following this, sometimes, a small streak like area at the site of the old ampullary opening is coagulated using the point coagulator (Figure 21.6a). Haemostasis is now assured.

The ampullary end of the tube is now opened using the microscissors (Figure 21.6b); free flow of the blue dye solution follows and allows the inner wall of the hydrosalpinx to be inspected to assess the possibility for future fertility. A cuff is now formed in this area using either two atraumatic grasping forceps, two bowel forceps, or two needle holders (Figure 21.6c). This cuff or everted ampulla is fixed by suturing the fimbrial edge to the ampullary serosa (Figure 21.6c and d) 4-0 or 6-0 PDS sutures with intracorporeal knotting technique are used for this purpose. Three suprapubic incisions 5 mm in diameter are recommended for this procedure.

Continuous ascending chromopertubation and subsequent fallopian tube pertubation using CO_2 gas is used to demonstrate the patency of reconstituted fallopian tube.

NON-ORGAN PRESERVING OPERATIONS ON THE ADNEXA

Oophorectomy

Oophorectomy is performed using the 'triple loop technique'. For this procedure 3 suprapubic incisions are necessary, two 5 mm in diameter on the left and right, and one 11 mm in diameter lying between the two, directly in the mid-line. The ovary is grasped with the big-claw forceps which is carried in the medially-lying 11 mm diameter trocar. The Roeder loop is introduced on the ipsilateral side to the oophorectomy being performed. The claw forceps passes first through the Roeder loop and then grasps the ovary to be ligated (Figure 22.1a). Correct setting of the Roeder loop over the meso-

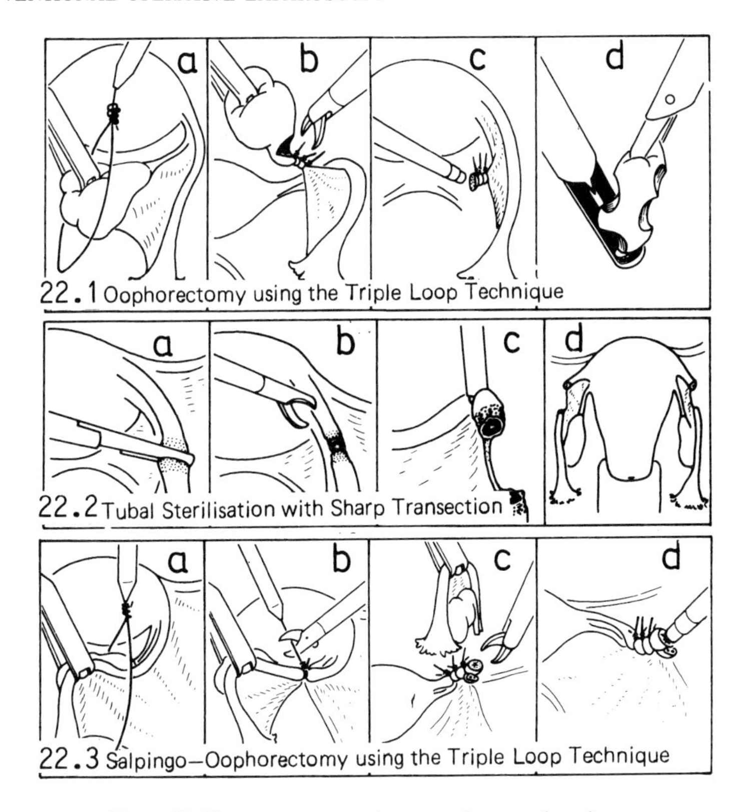

Figure 22. Non-organ preserving operations on the adnexa.

varium is guided by an atraumatic grasping forceps being held in the remaining 5 mm diameter trocar.

Three Roeder loops are set, each one being placed behind the previous one in order to establish a full and secure pedicle. After the three Roeder loops have been set ovarian resection is performed using the hooked scissors (Figure 22.1b). The hooked scissors should be inserted on the same side as the resection as this ensures the necessary 90° cutting angle. This approach prohibits the accidental cutting of the set ligatures.

The resected ovary is now removed with the claw forceps through the 11 mm diameter trocar. Sometimes, it is necessary to morcellate the ovary; this is easily done using the morcellator (Figure 22.1d). Finally, the amputation stump is coagulated using the point coagulator in order to avoid the formation of adhesions later (Figure 22.1c).

Fallopian tube sterilization with sharp transection

As previously mentioned it is extremely important, when performing tubal sterilization, not to damage ovarian function by destruction of the blood supply to the rete ovarii contained within the mesovarium. The best method, we believe, is therefore endocoagulation of the tube with transection of the coagulation site (Figure 22.2). This form of sterilization is also ideally suited to subsequent tubal reversion surgery as it lends itself well to end-to-end anastomosis; it has also statistically the highest rate of success (Riedel and Semm, 1982). The tube is first grasped using the crocodile forceps attachment of the endocoagulator; the endocoagulator is set at 110°C (Figure 22.2a).

Following endocoagulation, the tube is transected using the hooked scissors (Figure 22.2b). It is extremely important to perform a complete transection. To ensure this the transected ends are splayed apart and examined so as to properly identify the tubal lumina on both sides (Figure 22.2c). The later peritonealization of these tubal stumps ensures tubal occlusion (Figure 22.2d).

Salpingo-oophorectomy

This procedure is also performed using the triple loop technique. The larger mass of tissue, consisting of ovary and tube, makes this procedure technically easier than oophorectomy alone since the ligation is simpler. Again three suprapubic incisions are necessary. Following introduction of a Roeder loop on the ipsilateral side the claw forceps grasps the adnexa and pulls it through the loop (Figure 22.3a). The tissue mass is pulled taut using the claw forceps and the Roeder loop is pushed with the aid of an atraumatic forceps deep into the mesosalpinx close to the tubal interstitium at the level of the pelvic infundibular ligament; subsequent ligation is then carried out.

Two further loops are then set. Once three Roeder loops have been positioned and tied (Figure 22.3b) the adnexal pedicle is resected at an angle of 90° using the hooked scissors (Figure 22.3c). It is important to leave a sufficiently large stump in order to guard against inadvertent slipping of ligatures. The tissue stump is coagulated using the point coagulator in order to prevent later adhesion formation (Figure 22.3d). Again each subsequent Roeder loop is placed behind the previous one. However, it may happen that occasionally the Roeder loops slip; in this case the bleeding ascending vessels of the uterine artery (tubal branch), and the ovarian artery must be seperately ligated using Roeder loops.

As with all ovarian procedures a Robinson drain is inserted and left in for 24–48 hours. It is important to stress that in cases of previous adnexal surgery where a patient requires a pelviscopic intervention it is imperative to observe and identify accurately the course of the ureter.

Ectopic pregnancy

The treatment of ectopic pregnancy no longer necessarily requires laparotomy (Semm, 1989).

Radical therapy of ectopic pregnancy

Using the triple loop technique salpingectomy is easily and quickly per-

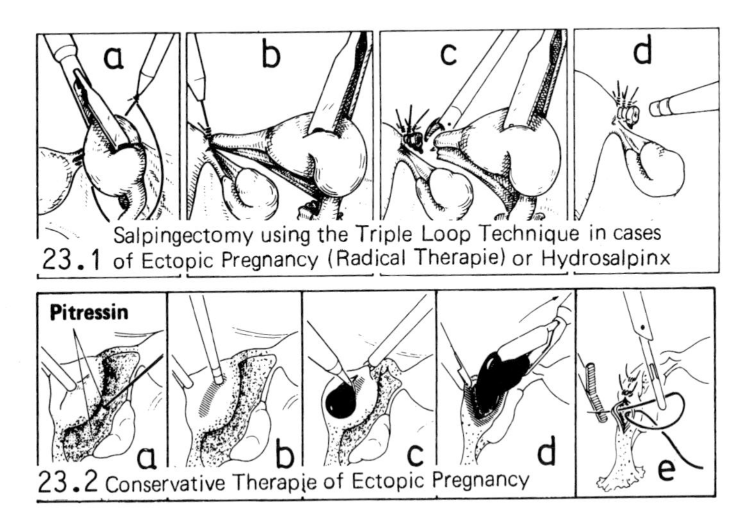

Figure 23. Radical and conservative therapy of ectopic pregnancy.

formed: Following a thorough pelvic irrigation using the aquapurator (see Figure 11) the ectopic pregnancy is located. Using the claw forceps the tube is then, together with the products of conception, pulled through a Roeder loop and subsequently ligated. If the loop is too small for the tissue bundle an endoligature may be used. This step must be approached from the same side as the tubectomy, thus ensuring a perpendicular endoligation (Figure 23.1b). As little tubal tissue as is possible should be resected in order to ensure maintenance of the ovarian blood supply.

After setting three Roeder loops the tube is transected, the scissors having been introduced on the ipsilateral side to the salpingectomy (Figure 23.1c). The stump is now coagulated using the endocoagulator (Figure 23.1d). Finally a meticulous pelvic lavage using the aquapurator is performed to prevent the later formation of adhesions. Here, once again, the insertion of a Robinson drain for 24–48 h is obligatory.

Conservative surgery of ectopic pregnancy

Following the aspiration of blood from the lower pelvis using the aquapurator, the pregnancy nidation site is located. In cases of ampullary implantation, the products of conception may be either suctioned from the ampulla or mechanically removed using the big spoon or biopsy forceps. In cases of isthmic or interstitial implantation, a longitudinal salpingotomy with subsequent wound closure is necessary.

Prior to salpingotomy extensive ischaemia along the course of the tube is provided through instillation of POR 8 solution (5 IU/100 ml of normal saline) forming two to three wheals each containing 10 ml of solution (Figure 23.2a); then, on the convex anti-mesosalpinx side of the tube (Figure 23.2b) a coagulation streak is made using the point coagulator in order to prevent bleeding from the serosal vessels. The layers of the tubal wall are then individually dissected using the microscissors until the ectopic tissue becomes visible (Figure 23.2c).

After splaying the tubal walls open using two atraumatic forceps or two needle holders the products of conception may be slowly removed as a complete unit using the large spoon or biopsy forceps (Figure 23.2d). Finally, a thorough washout of the nidation bed is performed with the aquapurator.

Once all the products of conception have been removed the salpingotomy wound (Figure 23.2e) is closed by approximation of the tubal serosa using only 4-0 or 6-0 PDS endosuture with subsequent intracorporeal knotting; only the serosal layer is closed in order to prevent tubal stricture. A careful and well-sealed closure prevents later tubal fistula formation.

We recommend that tubal insufflation is performed for several weeks postoperatively either through pelviscopy (a rather aggressive procedure) or through tubal pertubation using CO_2 gas with vaginal ultrasound control.

PELVISCOPIC OPERATIVE PROCEDURES FOR ENDOMETRIOSIS

A visual diagnosis of endometriosis may be obtained by employing the 'Thermo-colour test', as described by Semm, which is diagnostically accurate in 85% of cases. Once the diagnosis has been made surgical removal of the endometriotic implants may be performed during the same operative session either by endocoagulation or excision.

Endometriotic implants may be best detected in the last third of the menstrual cycle owing to the typical blue discolouration of the peritoneum at this time. These implants are biologically destroyed through the application of endocoagulation via the point coagulator at 120°C.

The thermo-colour test is best applied at the beginning of the cycle. Here, healthy peritoneum becomes white at 100°C whereas pale red endometriotic implants become dark brown, almost black, owing to their haemosiderin content. Endometriotic implants in the area of the utero-sacral ligaments are located either superificially or deeper in the form of nodules.

With the superficial implants endocoagulation using the point coagulator for removal suffices (Figure 24.2), however, with the deeper nodular form the nodule and its overlying peritoneum must first be split either using the point coagulator or microscissors; the endometriotic nodule is then subsequently coagulated while carefully observing the course of the ureter. Large

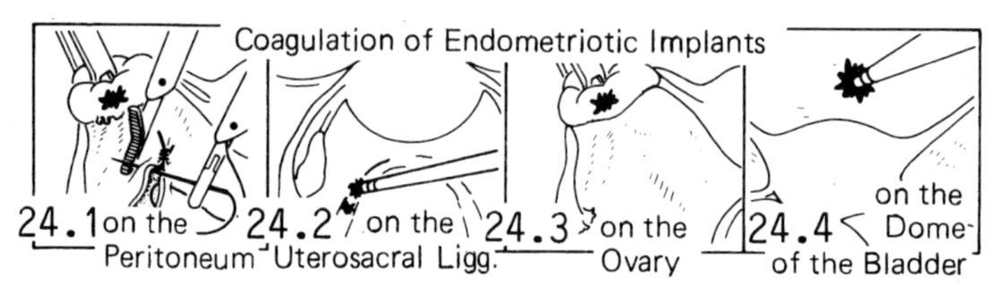

Figure 24. Coagulation of endometriotic implants.

peritoneal defects are closed via endosuture with extracorporeal knotting technique (Figure 24.1). Twenty per cent of all endometriotic implants lie behind the ovary (Figure 24.3). Therefore, in diagnostic pelviscopy, a second and third suprapubic incision are always necessary in order to adequately expose this aspect of the ovary. Removal of the implants is performed using either the point coagulator or through ovarian biopsy.

PELVISCOPIC OPERATIONS ON THE BOWEL

Intra-abdominal adhesiolysis

Owing to the very limited amount of peritoneal damage at pelviscopy this method is ideal for intra-abdominal adhesiolysis. When describing intra-abdominal adhesiolysis per pelviscopy we must differentiate between 'bloody' and 'non-bloody' adhesiolysis.

'Bloody' adhesiolysis

Firstly, the adhesion is pulled taut with an atraumatic grasping forceps (Figure 25.1a), then, using scissors the adhesion is resected (Figure 25.1b). If the pedicle then bleeds it is grasped with an atraumatic grasping forceps which has been passed through a Roeder loop and is then ligated (Figure 25.1c and d). Once ligation is complete the parietal adhesion site (normally the anterior abdominal wall) is coagulated using the point coagulator in order to prevent the later formation of adhesions.

'Non-bloody' adhesiolysis

This procedure is normally performed for mid-abdominal adhesions which are in most cases highly vascularized. Firstly an endoligature is introduced into the abdomen using the 3 mm diameter needle holder (Figure 25.2a). The endoligature is placed around the vascularized adhesion using the 5 mm

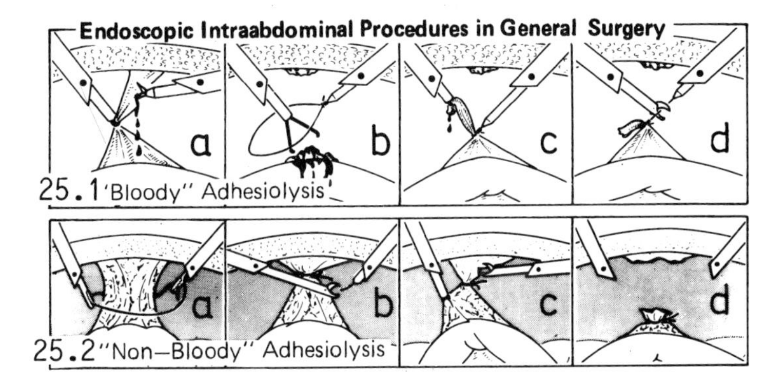

Figure 25. Endoscopic intra-abdominal procedures in general gynaecological surgery.

diameter needle holder; this needle holder then represents the endoligature to the 3 mm in diameter needle holder which withdraws the endoligature from the abdomen whereby the extracorporeal Roeder slip knot may be tied (Figure 25.2b). The Roeder slip knot is then reintroduced into the abdomen and pulled taut. Once ligation is complete sharp dissection of the adhesion using the hooked scissors is performed (Figure 25.2c). The parietal adhesion site may be coagulated using the point coagulator and the previously ligated stump may be additionally secured with a Roeder loop if necessary (Figure 25.2d).

Adhesiolysis involving the bowel

Parietal peritoneum

Adhesions involving one or more loops of bowel and the anterior abdominal wall are primarily of postoperative aetiology. The intimate relationship between the parietal peritoneum (which in cases of dehiscence shows invasion of the abdominal fascia) and the visceral fascia, requires a sharp dissection using microscissors (Figure 26.1a).

This procedure is made easier by pulling the bowel taut; this is performed atraumatically using a small swab set in the swab holder (Figure 26.1a). If during intestinal adhesiolysis the bowel serosa is damaged repair is carried out using the intracorporeal knotting technique with 4-0 PDS suture (Figure 26.1b and c). In case of bowel perforation the wound is closed in two layers following classical surgical protocol. Through the use of bowel forceps intestinal injury is avoided.

Visceral peritoneum

In case of fused adhesions, i.e. visceral peritoneum of one organ adherent to that of another, for example bowel adherent to bowel, there is an increased risk of intestinal hernia, subsequent ileus, and ultimately bowel obstruction. Ligation of vascular adhesions is mandatory following a careful dissection (Figure 26.2a).

The adhesion is first endoligated (Figure 26.2a and b) using a 3 mm diameter needle holder. With larger adhesions the insertion of a suture ligature may be required. In both cases the Roeder extracorporeal slip knot is performed as the final step. Once tied the slip knot is reintroduced into the abdomen and set in an area that is not too close to the bowel serosa (Figure 26.2b). Upon completion of a double ligation (Figure 26.2c) the vascular adhesion is transected without blood loss using the hooked scissors (Figure 26.2d). Recurrence of adhesions is thus almost completely avoided.

Appendicectomy

Appendicectomy whether in the orthograde or retrograde position may be performed per pelviscopiam according to the classical surgical rules set forth by McBurney and Sprengel (Grewe and Kramer, 1977).

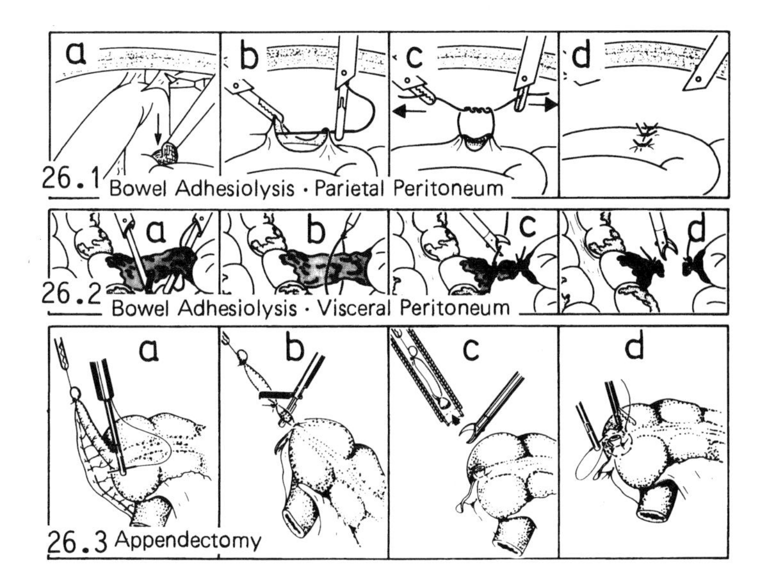

Figure 26. Adhesiolysis involving the bowel and appendectomy.

The appendix is first fixed using a Roeder loop which acts as a stay suture, then the appendicular artery is suture ligated (Figure 26.3a). Skeletelization of the appendix follows, prior to ligation of its base using a Roeder loop (Figure 26.3b). Faeces are expressed using the crocodile forceps which simultaneously destroys bacteria at 90°C (Figure 26.3b). The hooked scissors then transects the appendix (Figure 26.3c) which subsequently is pulled into the appendix extractor without contamination. After iodinization of the appendicular stump a purse string suture (Figure 26.3d) is inserted in the classical manner bringing about subsequent stump invagination. At the end of the operation the classical Z-suture is performed (Figure 26.3d).

It is important to mention that we have also had extremely good results in leaving the stump bare, e.g. the final surgical step is as depicted in Figure 26.3c. If the appendix is too thick for the 11 mm in diameter extractor the stab incision is atraumatically dilated up to fit a 15 mm in diameter extractor.

PELVISCOPIC SURGERY AS AN AID TO INTRA-ABDOMINAL CANCER DIAGNOSIS

In using the above mentioned techniques histologic confirmation of tumour tissue is achieved through biopsy, ligation and subsequent resection of tissue, and aspiration of ascites. In some cases, for example early tumour recurrences, tumour cytoreduction is possible. For tumour staging, especially in the case of retroperitoneal lymph nodes, underwater pelviscopy is a method of choice.

ROBINSON DRAIN

A Robinson drain is routinely inserted at the end of the following pelviscopic procedures: salpingostomy, conservative surgical treatment of an ectopic pregnancy, extensive pelvic adhesiolysis, lysis of adhesions involving omentum and bowel, ovarian cyst enucleation, enucleation of myomata (Robinson and Brown, 1950; Oberhammer, 1979). The drain has two purposes:

1. To absorb developing exudate, and, thus, promote wound healing.
2. To immediately recognize postoperative bleeding.

The Robinson drain is a closed system gravity drain and is inserted via an suprapubic 5 mm in diameter trocar. It is left in situ from 24–48 hours (Figure 27).

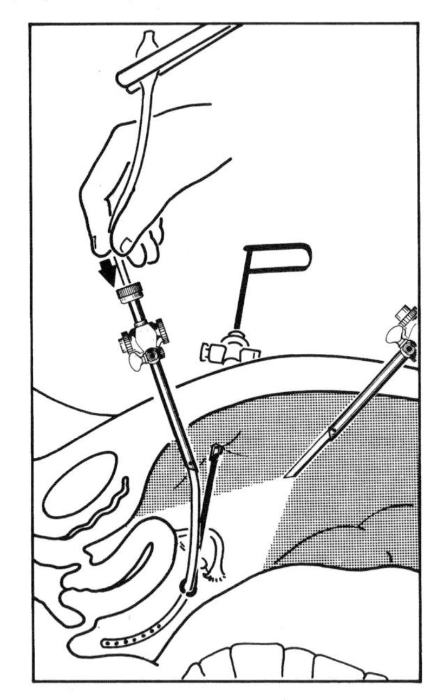

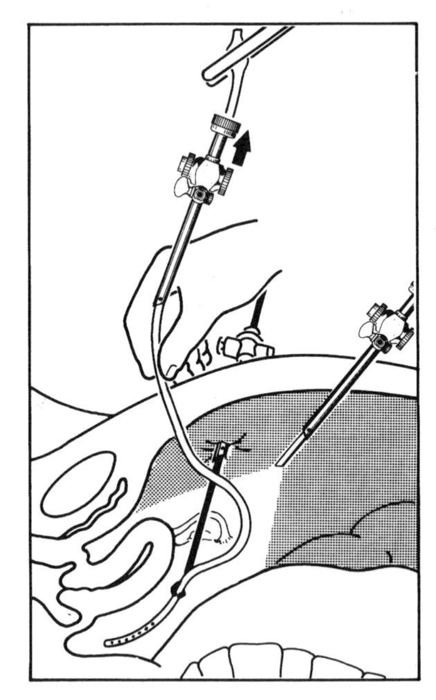

Figure 27. The Robinson drain.

SECOND-LOOK PELVISCOPY

Following pelviscopic operative procedures such as conservative treatment of ectopic pregnancy, conservative operations on the adnexa, enucleation of endometriomas, and in particular extensive lysis of adhesions involving omentum and bowel, we recommend performing a second-look pelviscopy on the third postoperative day.

The above mentioned procedures are all associated with the production of pelvic adhesions. The purpose of a second-look pelviscopy is to lyse new

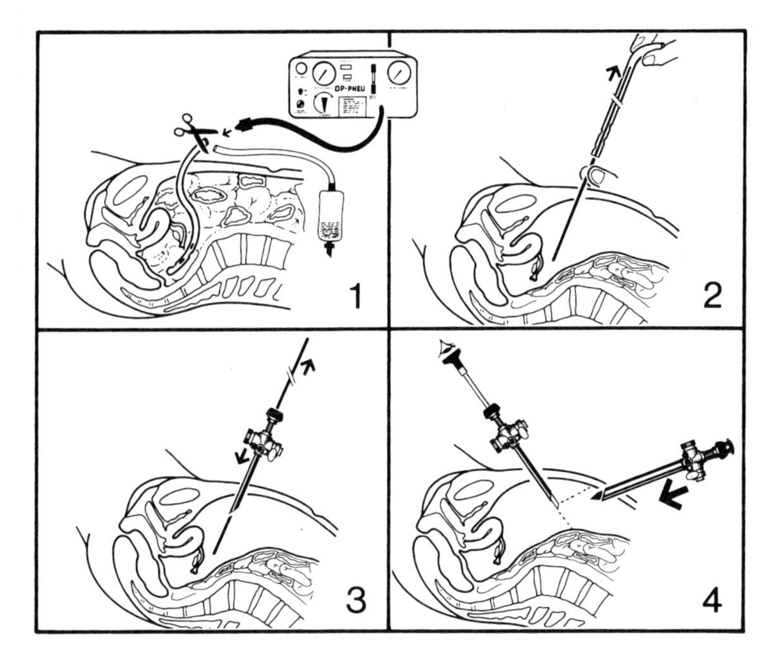

Figure 28. Second-look pelviscopy.

adhesions in the initial stages of their formation.

As a Robinson drain is inserted as part of the protocol in these procedures, the pneumoperitoneum is established via this drain (Figure 28.1). A 3 mm diameter guide rod is then introduced through the drain, and the drain is then removed (Figure 28.2), and a 5 mm diameter trocar is introduced over the guide rod (Figure 28.3). Introduction of further trocars, i.e. the 11 mm umbilical trocar, is now safely performed under visual control (Figure 28.4).

VISUALLY CONTROLLED PERITONEAL PERFORATION

In patients who have undergone multiple laparotomies and those suspected of having massive abdominal adhesions. We recommend performing a visually controlled peritoneal perforation. The bevelled trocar is inserted under visual control following the classic Z-puncture technique (Semm, 1988b):

1. The 5 mm diameter trocar or elliptic shaped sheath is inserted via the z-puncture technique through the umbilicus, carrying its conical end to the depth of the muscle layer.
2. The conical trocar is now replaced by the 5 mm diameter pelviscope, and the trocar sheath is then under visual control advanced (Figure 29a) through the musculature to the peritoneum.

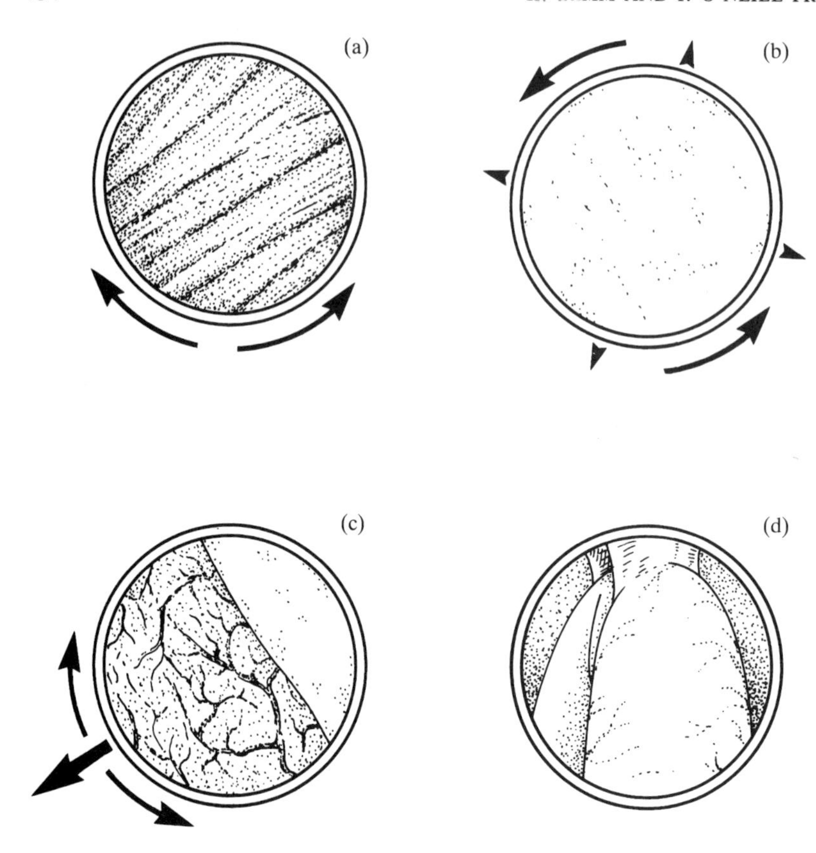

Figure 29. Visually controlled peritoneal perforation.

3. Where peritoneal adhesions (omentum or bowel adherent to the peritoneum) are present a dull white surface is seen as the endoscopic light is totally reflected (Figure 29b).
4. The bevelled trocar is now moved laterally on the rectus fascia and peritoneum revealing a translucent area of peritoneum (Figure 29c).
5. This area may now be perforated under visual control by exerting blunt pressure providing a free view into the abdominal cavity (Figure 29d).

Sometimes the procedure described in (5) may be difficult to perform, for example, in patients with thick layer of fascia. In this situation peritoneal perforation is performed following the Z-puncture technique by exchanging the pelviscope for the conical trocar.

REFERENCES

Brackebusch H-D & Semm K (1976) Die biophysikalischen Prinzipien bei der diagnostischen und therapeutischen Anwendung des elek trischen Stromes in der Endoskopie. *Acta Endosc. et Radiocinematogr.* **VI:** 41–54.

Eisenburg J (1966) Ueber eine Apparatur zur schonenden und kontrollierbaren Gasfuellung der Bauchhoele fuer die Laparoskopie. *Klin. Wschr.* **44:** 593–594.
Grewe HE & Krämer K (1977) Appendektomie nach McBurney und Spregel. In Chirurgische Operationen, Bd II, pp 186–190. Stuttgart: Thieme.
Oberhammer E (1979) Eine neue Drainagegeneration als hygienische Alternative für Bauchraumdrainage. Krkh. Hygiene + Infektionsverhütung **6:** 14.
Riedel H-H & Semm K (1982) An initial comparison of coagulation techniques of sterilization. *Journal of Reproductive Medicine* **27:** 261–267.
Riedel H-H, Cordts-Kleinwordt G & Semm K (1983) Tierexperimentelle, morphologische und endokrinologische Untersuchungen nach Anwendung verschiedener Koagulationstechniken. *Zbl. Gynäk.* **105:** 1568–1584.
Riedel H-H, Semm K & Corts-Kleinwordt G (1986a) Tubal coagulation techniques in animal models with follow-up morphological and endocrinological studies. In Siegler AM *The Fallopian Tube: Basic Studies and Clinical Contributions*, pp 311–318. Mount Kisco, New York: Futura.
Riedel H-H, Lehmann-Willenbrock E, Conradt P & Semm K (1986b) German Pelviscopic statistics for the years 1978–1982. *Endoscopy* **18:** 219–222.
Riedel H-H, Lehmann-Villenbrock E, Mecke H & Semm K (1989) The frequency distribution of various pelviscopic (laparoscopic) operations, including complication rates statistics of the Federal Republic of Germany in the years 1983–1985. *Zentbl. Gynäkol.* **111:** 78–91.
Robinson JO & Brown AA (1950) A new closed drainage system. *British Journal of Surgery* **67:** 229–230.
Semm K (1966) New apparatus for 'cold-coagulation' of benign cervical lesions. *American Journal of Obstetrics and Gynecology* **95:** 963–967.
Semm K (1983) Physical and biological considerations militating against the use of endoscopically applied high frequency current in the abdomen. *Endoscopy* **15:** 51–60.
Semm K (1986) Operative Pelviscopy. *British Medical Bulletin* **42:** 284–295.
Semm K (1987a) Operative Manual for Endoscopic Abdominal Surgery (transl. by Ernst R. Friedrich/St Louis, Missouri) Chicago, London: Year Book Medical Publishers Inc.
Semm K (1987b) Surgical pelviscopy: review of 12 060 pelviscopies 1970–85. In Studd J *Progress in Obstetrics and Gynaecology* Vol. 6, pp 333–345. Edinburgh, London, Melbourne, New York: Churchill Livingstone.
Semm K (1988a) Pelviscopy operative guidelines (translated by Iseult Freys O'Neill). *Department of Obstetrics and Gynecology*, University of Kiel.
Semm K (1988b) Sichtkontrollierte Peritoneumperforation zur operativen Pelviskopie. *Geburtsh. u. Frauenheilk* **48:** 436–439.
Semm K (1989) *Die pelviskopische Therapie der Tubargravidität Speculum* 7, pp 3–13. (Schering).
Semm K & Mettler L (1988) Local Infiltration of Ornithine 8-Vasopresin (POR 8) as a vasoconstrictive agent in surgical pelviscopy (applied to myoma enucleation, salpingotomy in cases of tubal pregnancy and peripheral salpingostomy). *Endoscopy* **20:** 298–304.
Semm K & Philipp E (1979) Eileiterregeneration post Sterilisationem. *Geburtsh. u. Frauenheilk* **39:** 14–19.
Semm K & Philipp E (1980) Vermeidung von Spontanrekanalisation des Eileiters post sterilisationem. *Gynaek. Prax.* **4:** 63–74.
Semm K & Popp L (1989) *Die Drainage der Bauchhöhle nach operativer Pelviskopie.* Ingelheim: Boehringer.
Stalsand B (1978) Treatment of premalignant lesions of the uterine cervix by means of moderate heat thermosurgery using the Semm coagulator. *Ann. Chirurg. et Gynaec.* **67:** 112–116.

3

CO_2 laser laparoscopy

M. A. BRUHAT
A. WATTIEZ
G. MAGE
J. L. POULY
M. CANIS

Lasers have been used via laparoscopy for 10 years now. The first prototype was developed by the Polyclinique team Clermont-Ferrand, France, back in 1979 (Bruhat et al, 1979). Since then techniques have evolved considerably and the indications have become far wider, to the extent that many laparoscopic surgeons now have a decided preference for the laser.

There are a number of different lasers available for endoscopy. At the time of writing, the techniques which have received the most attention are the CO_2 laser, the neodymium-yttrium aluminium garnet (Nd-YAG) laser and the argon laser. The CO_2 laser is by far the most commonly used. It has the advantage of combining three functions: incision, by which it provides a real scalpel effect without opening the abdomen; vaporization, enabling pathological surfaces to be destroyed; and coagulation of the tissues making it possible to 'shape' the surfaces in question. Each of these functions is governed by physical parameters which are for the most part under the operator's control. A knowledge of laser theory and training in the use of these lasers is therefore absolutely essential.

Laser plus laparoscopy is the combination of two efficient, elegant and atraumatic techniques which can provide great practical and economical benefit to our patients.

ELEMENTS OF LASER THEORY

Laser is an acronym for 'light amplification of stimulated emission of radiation', and is a beam of light made up of photons with identical characteristics. Its radiation respects a certain uniformity:

1. Each laser emits a single wavelength of radiation, meaning it is monochromatic.
2. The photons are all emitted in phase.
3. The photons are all emitted in one direction.

In other words the light is composed of photons all having the same energy, the same direction and the same phase of vibration, as compared with ordinary light which is given off in all directions and over a wide range of wavelengths. The laser produces a very pure beam of light, exceptionally easy to manipulate through optical systems, because the single wavelength means it is not subject to diffraction phenomena. Laser radiation can thus be concentrated on infinitessimal surface areas making it possible to reach extremely high temperatures at the point of impact. Whereas ordinary light radiating in all directions gives 2π steradian, a non-focused beam of laser light produces a cone whose angle is approximately 10^{-6} steradian. So for a given power source (e.g. 10 W) the energy received at a given point will be 10 W/2π steradian for ordinary light and 10 W/10^{-1} steradian for laser light; the laser is 6 million times more intense. It is also easier to focus a laser beam than ordinary light, further accentuating its usefulness. The energy produced at the point of impact is measured as a power density, i.e. in W/cm^2; this gives the relationship between the intensity of the laser source and the surface area of the tissue treated.

Lasers differ mainly in their power and wavelength, ranging from the microlaser used for biological measurements which has a power of 1–2 mW to the experimental 'star war' lasers with something like 100 000 W.

There are three types of laser in common use in surgery although others will no doubt join them soon: Nd-YAG, argon and CO_2. Each has a specific wavelength, which for the CO_2 is 10.6 nm (at the far end of the infrared range), for the Nd-YAG 0.636 nm (in the infrared) and for the argon laser 0.437 nm (visible green light). These differences in wavelength confer important characteristics with respect to their use in surgery:

1. The argon and Nd-YAG lasers, but not the CO_2 laser, can be transmitted by flexible optical fibres.
2. CO_2 laser radiation is quickly absorbed by water, but not the argon, and even less so the Nd-YAG.

A laser just coming into use, the potassium titanyl phosphate (KTP) laser, can be transmitted by optical fibres and has characteristics that place it between the Nd-YAG and the CO_2 lasers.

THE BIOLOGICAL EFFECTS OF LASERS

Laser radiation transmits energy in the form of heat to the tissues. The effects of this heat depend on the amount of energy per unit volume of tissue, which is governed by two parameters: the power density transmitted to the tissues and the depth required for complete absorption of the radiation. That is, for a given power, e.g. 10 W, applied to a surface of 0.001 cm^2 (power density 10 000 W/cm^2), the CO_2 laser is absorbed in approximately 0.01 cm, the argon laser in 0.4 cm and the Nd-YAG laser in 3 cm. So the power density per unit volume of tissue is respectively 1 000 000 W/cm^3 for the CO_2 laser, 25 000 W/cm^3 for the argon laser and 3333 W/cm^3 for the Nd-YAG laser. This description is in fact somewhat simplified because absorption obeys geometrical rather than linear rules. Such widely differing energy values have different biological effects, three of which are of particular interest to the laparoscopic surgeon: vaporization, coagulation and thermal stimulation (Beytout et al, 1983).

When the tissues absorb a very high level of energy, *vaporization* (or incision) occurs: the heat causes the intracellular water to boil. As the cells boil and explode, they give off steam and cell debris. This vaporization effect takes place within a very small volume, and can thus be used either to destroy a mass of tissue such as in endometriosis, or to carry out surgical incision of a tissue, for example adhesions or the wall of a hydrosalpinx.

When the tissues absorb sufficient energy to raise temperatures to above 55C but below 100C, *coagulation* takes place. The cells are destroyed by chemical denaturation of their proteins. Coagulation is accompanied by vascular obliteration which helps haemostasis by sealing off vessels up to 0.5 mm with the CO_2 laser.

If the temperature of the tissues rises above 40C but remains below 55C, the effect is of *thermal stimulation*. The cells are not destroyed but may acquire an increased capacity for tissue regeneration, which could in turn be why healing is so rapid after laser treatments (Baggish, 1985).

In practice a laser beam produces all three of these effects simultaneously: tissue is vaporized, heat generated at the impact area is transmitted to produce an area of coagulation and a further area of thermal stimulation. The coagulation layer has a haemostatic effect on small vessels, which is why tissues sectioned with the laser do not bleed unless large vessels are severed. The relative importance of these three effects depends on several factors:

1. *The wavelength*. The CO_2 laser vaporizes far more than it coagulates. The Nd-YAG vaporizes poorly, but coagulates well. The argon laser is a compromise between these two. The effect produced with each laser depends on the power density used. So a CO_2 laser used at a very low power density ($<10\ W/cm^2$) gives surface coagulation (vaporization requiring about 500–1000 W/cm^2) and the Nd-YAG laser can have a cutting effect at very high power densities or if the energy is focused by artificial sapphire tips.

2. *The power density*. How much energy is transmitted per surface unit can be controlled by varying the size of the point of impact. The spot size depends on the focal length of the lens in the apparatus and can be increased by the operator by defocusing the spot.

3. *The exposure time*. This is of paramount importance when considering the damage to tissues around a laser shot. How much peripheral coagulation is caused by the heat generated at the point of impact depends essentially upon how long the shot lasts. This is why laser sections must be carried out quickly, and vaporization achieved by maintaining a sweeping movement of the impact point, not allowing the beam to stand still, rather like shading the inside of an image with a crayon.

All of these biological effects also depend on the nature of the tissue. The

CO_2 laser is rapidly absorbed by water so the more water in the tissue, the less effect it has. The argon laser is not absorbed much by water, but very much so by haemoglobin, thus the coagulation effect is more intense the richer the tissue is in haemoglobin, as in endometriosis (Keye and Dixon, 1983). Mastery of these somewhat complex theoretical elements is essential for correct choice and utilization of a laser.

The CO_2 laser

In practice, the CO_2 laser is the most suitable for gynaecological applications (Bruhat et al, 1979). It cuts well, the peripheral coagulation effect is low but nevertheless sufficient to achieve haemostasis of vessels less than 0.5 mm, and it can be used for surface coagulation. It is thus excellent for tubal surgery but can also be used for tissue vaporization—in endometriosis, for example. There are a number of problems involved using it via laparoscopy, but most of these should be resolved in time.

1. The CO_2 laser cannot be transmitted by optical fibres, but has to travel via an articulated optical arm, in a heavy and awkward apparatus. This system cannot give such a wide range of angles for the laser beam as a fibreoptic system. Recently, however, flexible fibres capable of transmitting the CO_2 laser have been put on the market (Baggish and Elbakry, 1986; Colles J, personal communication).
2. The laser handpiece needs to be leakproof and must accommodate the CO_2 supply required for the pneumoperitoneum, which also keeps the lens free of carbonized debris.
3. Part of the energy is absorbed by the CO_2 of the pneumoperitoneum (Daniell and Brown, 1982).
4. The impact of the laser shots produces smoke which has to be evacuated. There is in fact an automatic pneumoperitoneum ventilation system which comes into operation as soon as the laser is started up, but it is extremely expensive.
5. The red sighting laser (helium–neon laser) is sometimes difficult to see because of the light source of the laparoscope; this is particularly true where defocused shots are concerned.

The route of entry

Which route of entry into the body is the ideal one for the CO_2 laser was the subject of debate during early trials. The suprapubic operative route appeared best for many reasons but did not seem to be safe enough because the operator had no direct visual control over the laser when compared with the coaxial transumbilical route. Comparative tests carried out at that time demonstrated that handling via the suprapubic route was decidedly superior and that the risk of shots going astray had been grossly overestimated. The advent of endoscopic cameras today tips the balance back in favour of the coaxial route because it makes the endoscope–laser assembly easier to manoeuvre. A further advantage for this route is that it frees an introduction route and one hand for the operator.

Lasers and safety

The laser is a light beam of very high energy; its use requires proper training and the strict observance of basic safety rules. The literature contains very few reports of accidents due to use of the laser. Most of these can be explained by the use of an unsuitable wavelength for the desired result and by the surgeon's inexperience.

As the laser completely destroys the tissues, no pathological tests can be carried out when it is used for vaporization. This raises a very real possibility of making mistakes due to incorrect assessment of the severity and extent of the lesion being treated—i.e. vaporization of a malignant tumour (Daniell, 1985).

The main types of damage reported in endoscopy are lesions due to breaching a large vessel and perforation of hollow organs by burns (mainly the urinary and digestive tracts). The main causes for these accidents are stray shots and overshots, or excessively high power. All such accidents can be avoided if extreme diligence is exercised at all times when the laser is used.

INDICATIONS FOR USE OF LASER LAPAROSCOPY

At present the use of the laser is indicated essentially for three pathologies: adhesions, endometriosis and tubal obstruction.

Adhesions

The CO_2 laser is capable of simulating the scalpel with its high precision, and can thus be used to incise adhesions. It has the additional advantages of causing little peripheral tissue damage, and enabling filmy adhesions on the surface of the ovary to be vaporized. Finally, when confronted with very tight, type C adhesions, incisions can be carried out with simultaneous coagulation of small vessels; however with this last application there is a certain danger due to the creation of an artificial cleavage plane which may result in damage to neighbouring structures.

The technique is similar to that of conventional laparoscopic surgery: the adhesion is put under tension and vaporized as close as possible to the least vulnerable organ. That is to say, for a tubo-ovarian adhesion the section should be as close as possible to the ovary, whereas with a tubo-intestinal adhesion, it should be as close as possible to the tube. Stray shots or damage to the organ behind the adhesion can be avoided either by creating a physiological 'backstop' by flooding the cavity with irrigation fluid or by stretching the adhesion over the laparoscopic forceps and cutting it with laser shots.

There have so far been no studies to settle definitively whether laparoscopic laser adhesiolysis and laparoscopic scissor adhesiolysis is the most effective. The laser has certain points in its favour, however: (i) simultaneous haemostasis, (ii) high precision, and (iii) the ability to free very tight adhesions. The disadvantages are the risk of stray shots, and the risk of

Table 1. Results for adhesiolysis via laparoscopy alone.

Reference	Number of cases	Intrauterine pregnancy	Ectopic pregnancy
Madelenat & Palmer (1973)	144	42 (29%)	11 (7.6%)
Mintz	65	24 (37%)	7 (11.0%)
Gomel	92	57 (62%)	5 (5.4%)
Audebert	50	15 (30%)	0
Abeille	19	7 (37%)	3 (16.0%)
Mettler & Semm (1979)	44	13 (29%)	
Fayez (1983)	50	30 (60%)	2 (4.0%)
Henry-Suchet	38	15 (39%)	1 (3.0%)
Bruhat et al (1979)	93	48 (51%)	7 (5.0%)

damage to fragile tissues when freeing a tight adhesion. The results are at least equal to those with conventional laparoscopic adhesiolysis, that is, up to 60% positive results for fertility (Table 1). How efficient adhesiolysis is in reducing pain is more controversial since the exact relationship of adhesions to abdominal pain is still unresolved.

Endometriosis

Endometriosis is a pathology which gives rise to peritoneal implants, adhesions which are often dense, and ovarian cysts. The laser can be used to treat all of these by vaporizing the peritoneal implants, cutting the adhesions free and vaporizing the endometriotic cyst walls when it is not possible to find a cleavage plane for them. Laser vaporization of the peritoneal implants is carried out using a spot diameter of 0.5–2 mm and between 10 and 20 W power in continuous mode. If the implants are close to the ureter or to large retroperitoneal vessels, these can be protected by infiltrating normal saline solution. When vaporization is completed a thorough peritoneal lavage is necessary to eliminate all carbonized debris which might otherwise provoke postoperative adhesions or be taken for a recurrence of endometriosis at a later checkup (Donnez, 1987).

Our team usually treat ovarian endometriomas by intraperitoneal cystectomy, i.e. complete removal of the cyst wall, rather than puncturing, opening and destroying the cyst wall with the CO_2 laser. The cystectomy technique has the advantage of providing a sample for the pathologist to check on the nature and differentiation of the disease. Some authors recommend that the bottom of the ovary be vaporized after removal of the cyst wall to eliminate deep-seated implants of endometriosis. The CO_2 laser is, however, extremely useful for dealing with endometriotic adhesions which are very dense and thick, as they often are.

In a recent study carried out in our department, 91 patients were given surgery using laser laparoscopy. All 91 complained of chronic pain, 20 had stage I endometriosis, nine stage II, 31 stage III and 31 stage IV. Ten patients were lost to follow-up, the remainder being followed up for over 9 months. Whatever the stage, 70% of the patients showed a distinct functional improvement. The stage involved was equally of no influence as regards the

Table 2. Treatment of pain.

Level of pain	Number of patients	Improvement (%)	Cure (%)	Success (%)	Failure (%)
Minimal	20	45.0	35.0	80.0	20.0
Mild	9	55.6	22.2	77.8	22.2
Moderate	31	29.0	48.4	77.4	22.6
Severe	31	29.0	42.0	71.0	29.0
Total	91	35.2	40.7	75.8	24.2

Table 3. Results for infertility (Clermont-Ferrand series).

	Stage (AFS, 1985)					
	I	II	III	IV	IV<70	Total
No.	28	16	33	33	20	110
IVF	0	1	4	4	2	9
Lost	4	1	4	5	1	14
No.	24	14	25	24	17	87
IUP	12 (50.0%)	4 (28.5%)	10 (40%)	9 (37.5%)	9 (52.9%)	35 (40.2%)
EP	2 (8.3%)	1 (7.1%)	2 (8%)	0 (0.0%)	0 (0.0%)	5 (5.7%)

IVF, In vitro fertilization; IUP, Intrauterine pregnancy; EP, Ectopic pregnancy.

Table 4. Results in the literature (all stages together).

Reference	Number of patients	Number of pregnancies
Feste 1985	140	82 (59%)
Daniell 1985	48	34 (54%)
Adamson 1986	65	35 (54%)
Bowman 1986	35	18 (51%)
Davis 1986	64	37 (58%)
Martin 1986	115	54 (47%)
Nezhat 1986	102	62 (61%)
Paulsen 1986	282	150 (53%)
Total	851	472 (55%)

failure rates (Table 2). One hundred and ten patients were treated for infertility, of which 14 were lost to follow-up and nine were included in an in vitro fertilization programme immediately after laparoscopy because they each had a very advanced stage of endometriosis and very extensive adhesions. The results after treatment show that the uncorrected rate of intrauterine pregnancies was 40.3%. The fertility results are given in Table 3, and it should be noted that 26 of these 35 intrauterine pregnancies occurred within 8 months after the operation. Table 4 gives the results according to the literature for laparoscopic laser treatment of endometriosis.

Tuboplasty

Distal tuboplasty via laparoscopy is not a new idea. The technique had been abandoned, then received renewed interest with the appearance of the CO_2 laser (Fayez, 1983; Daniell and Herbert, 1984; Gordts et al, 1984).

The first phase in operating is adhesiolysis. This is of prime importance in preparing the best conditions possible for the tuboplasty, as the adhesiolysis has to restore normal tubo-ovarian mobility. Next a methylene blue test should be carried out, when the tension induced in the blocked tube helps in locating the scar of the former ostium. Then a focused shot at high power density is used to make three or four radial incisions on the tube, enabling it to be opened. Once this is achieved, the new tube fringes are exposed using two forceps, and the incisions completed. After this, the serous surface of these new fringes is subjected to defocused shots of low power density which coagulate the peritoneal surface. The consequent retraction of the tube everts the fringes; this eversion is stable with time and means sutures to the tube fringes can be avoided.

Only distal obstruction of the tube can be considered a good indication. Prior assessment by hysterosalpingogram followed by laparoscopy is essential before starting treatment. It has been demonstrated without a doubt that the prognosis depends essentially on the tube status (Table 5) and degree of

Table 5. Distal tube scoring table (Mage et al, 1986).

Tube permeability	Ampulla mucosa	Tube wall
	Folds present 0	Normal 0
Phimosis 2	Folds diminished 5	Thin 5
Hydrosalpinx 5	No folds or alveolar salpingitis 10	Thickened or sclerotic 10

Stage I, 2–5; stage II, 6–10; stage III, 11–15; stage IV >15.

Table 6. Adhesions scoring table (AFS 85; Buttram, 1985).

		Surface covered by adhesions		
Organs	Type	⅓	⅔	3/3
Ovaries	Filmy	1	2	4
	Thick	4	8	16
Distal tube	Filmy	1	2	4
	Thick	4	8	16

None, 0; mild, 1–10; moderate, 11–16; severe, >16.

adhesions (AFS, Table 6). It would seem at present that results giving approximately 29% intrauterine pregnancies for all stages taken together can be expected (Mage and Bruhat, 1983). When the stage is taken into account, stage I gives good results with 45%, stage II 22%, stage III 7.7% and stage IV 0%; the rate of ectopic pregnancies rises in inverse parallel (Tables 7 and 8). These rates are comparable with those obtained with microsurgery to the tube (Table 9). It is not possible to make any definite statement as to relative efficacy when comparing our series with the

Table 7. Clermont-Ferrand results with laparoscopic salpingoneostomy according to the tubal stage.

	Number of patients (%)	IUP(%)	EP(%)
Stage I	22 (32.35%)	10 (45.5%)	1 (4.5%)
Stage II	27 (39.70%)	6 (22.2%)	4 (14.8%)
Stage III	13 (19.11%)	1 (7.7%)	0 (0.0%)
Stage IV	6 (8.80%)	0 (0.0%)	0 (0.0%)
Total	68	17 (25.0%)	5 (7.4%)

Table 8. Clermont-Ferrand results with laparoscopic salpingoneostomy according to the tubal stage and the adhesions stage (Mage et al, 1987).

	Number of patients	Intrauterine pregnancy	Ectopic pregnancy
Stage I, II, with adhesions O, L, M	42 (61.8%)	15 (35.7%)	4 (9.5%)
Stage III, IV or severe adhesions	26 (38.2%)	2 (7.7%)	1 (3.8%)
Total	68 (100.0%)	17 (25.0%)	5 (7.4%)

Table 9. Clermont-Ferrand results with microsurgery for distal lesions.

Stages	Number of cases	Intrauterine pregnancy	Ectopic pregnancy
Tube score			
Stage I	12	7 (58.3%)	1 (8.3%)
Stage II	30	11 (36.6%)	3 (10.0%)
Stage III	21	2 (9.5%)	3 (14.2%)
Stage IV	13	0 (0.0%)	0 (0.0%)
Total	76	20 (26.3%)	7 (9.2%)
Adhesion score			
Stage O	18	7 (38.8%)	3 (16.6%)
Stage L	25	8 (32.0%)	0 (0.0%)
Stage M	15	4 (26.6%)	1 (6.6%)
Stage S	18	1 (5.5%)	3 (16.6%)
Total	76	20 (26.3%)	7 (9.2%)

literature, because the success rates given in the various articles published range from 26% (Mettler et al, 1979) to 0% (Fayez, 1983), and 13% for Lauritzen et al (1983). Not all these series used the CO_2 laser so no conclusions can be drawn. Nevertheless the progress made with the CO_2 laser and laparoscopic techniques in general give reason to hope that distal tubal obstruction will, in the future, be entirely treated via laparoscopy using the laser.

CONCLUSIONS

The use of the laser via laparoscopy originated in our department in 1979. After slow beginnings it is now being widely developed because it overcomes certain barriers in operative laparoscopy. Laser technology is also undergoing rapid changes and even more impressive progress can be confidently expected. This being said, the laser is not totally indispensable and a large number of techniques can be applied perfectly satisfactorily using conventional instrumentation.

REFERENCES

Baggish M (ed.) (1985) *Basic and Advanced Lasers in Gynecology*, East Norwalk, Connecticut: Appleton-Century-Crofts.

Baggish M & Elbakry MM (1986) A flexible CO_2 laser fiber for operative laparoscopy. *Fertility and Sterility* **46:** 16–20.

Beytout M, Mage G, Marquet C, Pouly JL & Bruhat MA (1983) Etude experimentale de l'influence de puissance sur la vitesse de section et des lésions tissulaires en microchirurgie tubaire avec le laser CO_2. *Laser Medical 81/82*. Masson, Paris: ESI publications.

Bruhat MA, Mage G & Menhes H (1979) Use of the CO_2 laser via laparoscopy. In Kaplan I (ed.) *Laser Surgery III, Proceedings of the 3rd International Society for Laser Surgery*. Tel Aviv: International Society for Laser Surgery.

Buttram VC (1985) Evolution of the revised American Fertility Society classification of endometriosis. *Fertility and Sterility* **43:** 347.

Daniell JF (1985) Basic and advanced laser surgery in gynecology. Treatment of gynecology tumors, 345–356.

Daniell JF & Brown D (1982) CO_2 laser laparoscopy: initial experience in experimental animals and humans. *Obstetrics and Gynecology* **59:** 761.

Daniell JF & Herbert CM (1984) Laparoscopic salpingostomy utilizing the carbon dioxide laser. *Fertility and Sterility* **41:** 558.

Davis GD (1986) Management of endometriosis and its associated adhesions with the CO_2 laser laparoscope. *Obstetrics and Gynecology* **68:** 422.

Donnez J (1987) CO_2 laser laparoscopy in infertile women with endometriosis and women with adnexal adhesions. *Fertility and Sterility* **48:** 390.

Fayez JA (1983) An assessment of the role of operative laparoscopy in tuboplasty. *Fertility and Sterility* **39:** 476.

Fayez JA & Collazo L (1986) Comparison of laparotomy and laparoscopy in the treatment of moderate and severe stages of endometriosis. AFS meeting abstract 317.

Feste JR (1985) Endoscopic laser surgery in gynecology. In Reproductive surgery. Postgraduate Course Syllabus, Chicago: American Fertility Society. 51–69.

Gordts S, Boeckx W & Brossens I (1984) Microsurgery of endometriosis in infertile patients. *Fertility and Sterility* **42:** 520.

Keye WR & Dixon J (1983) Photocoagulation of endometriosis with the argon laser through the laparoscope. *Obstetrics and Gynecology* **62:** 383.

Lauritzen JG, Pagel JD, Vangsted P & Starup J (1983) Result of repeated tuboplasties. *Fertility and Sterility* **40:** 472.

Lomano JM (1984) Photocoagulation of early pelvic endometriosis with the Nd-Yag laser through the laparoscope. *Lasers in Surgery and Medicine* **3:** 328.

Madelenat P & Palmer R (1973) Etude critique des libérations per-coelioscopiques des adhérences péri-annexielles. *Journal de Gynecologie Obstetrique et Biologie de la Reproduction* **8:** 347.

Mage G & Bruhat MA (1983) Pregnancy following salpingostomy: comparison between carbon dioxide laser and electrosurgery procedures. *Fertility and Sterility* **40:** 472.

Mage G, Bruhat MA, Bouquet J et al (1987) Score d'opérabilité tubaire. XXXIIIe Assises Françaises de Gynécologie. Poitiers.

Mage G, Pouly JL, Bouquet de Joliniere J et àl (1986) A preoperative classification to predict the intrauterine and ectopic pregnancy rates after distal tubal microsurgery. *Fertility and Sterility* **46:** 807.
Martin DC (1986) Operative laparoscopy with the carbon dioxide laser for the treatment of endometriosis associated with infertility. *Journal of Reproductive Medicine* **31:** 1089.
Mettler L, Giesel H & Semm K (1979) Treatment of female infertility due to tubal obstruction by operative laparoscopy. *Fertility and Sterility* **32:** 384.
Nezhat C, Crowgey SR & Garrisson CP (1986) Surgical treatment of endometriosis via laser laparoscopy. *Fertility and Sterility* **45:** 778–783.
Olive DL & Martin DC (1987) Treatment of endometriosis-associated infertility with CO_2 laser laparoscopy: the use of one- and two-parameter exponential models. *Fertility and Sterility* **48:** 18.
Palmer R (1980) Le coelioscopie dans le diagnostic et le traitement des adhérences pelviennes. *Contraception Fertilite Sexualite* **7**(11): 797.
Paulsen JD & Asmar P (1986) Analysis of the first 150 pregnancy after laser laparoscopy. Presented at the ASCCP/GLS Meeting Boston.
Pouly JL, Bruhat MA, Mage G & Manhes H (1982) Utilisation du laser CO_2 par coelioscopie: Comparison entre un branchement coaxial et un branchement sur trocard suspubien. *Acta Medica Romana* **20:** 257–260.
Tadir Y, Kaplan I, Zuckerman Z, Edelsein T & Ovadia J (1984) New instrumentation and technique for laparoscopic CO_2 laser operations, a preliminary report. *Obstetrics and Gynecology* **63:** 582.

4

CO_2 laser laparoscopy in the treatment of endometriosis

CHRIS SUTTON

Endometriosis is discovered in up to 20% of all gynaecological laparoscopies and laparotomies (Schneider, 1983) making it the second commonest gynaecological disorder after uterine fibroids (Shaw, 1988). Nevertheless it remains a strange and puzzling disease that is shrouded in mystery. In spite of vast amounts of energy, ingenuity and research we are not a great deal further forward in the understanding of the aetiology or pathogenesis than we were 70 years ago (Meyer, 1919; Sampson, 1927a,b). The clinical presentation bears little relationship to the severity of the disease, the natural history is unpredictable and attempts to provide rational treatment are often based on studies that have been largely uncontrolled and retrospective. Against this background it is not surprising that both patients and doctors often find themselves confused and frustrated. It is important therefore to be certain of establishing an accurate diagnosis before embarking on any plan of patient management.

DIAGNOSIS

Although about a quarter of patients with endometriosis are completely asymptomatic (O'Connor, 1987), most present with one or other of the classic quartet of symptoms—congestive dysmenorrhoea, deep dyspareunia, pelvic pain and infertility. Clinical examination may reveal a fixed uterus with tenderness in the adnexae and sometimes the presence of painful nodules in the cul-de-sac or the utero-sacral ligaments. Sometimes rocking the cervix forwards with the examining finger can result in severe pain that often mimics the discomfort felt at intercourse during deep penetration (Coats, personal communication). A normal pelvic examination does not exclude the diagnosis and the only way to be certain that endometriosis is present is to perform a diagnostic laparoscopy.

Diagnostic laparoscopy

The diagnosis of endometriosis carries significant implications for any woman and it is therefore important that the laparoscopy is performed by an experienced gynaecologist. A thorough and systematic inspection of the entire pelvis and abdomen should be made employing a double portal technique with an aspiration cannula inserted suprapubically to suck out, from the pouch of Douglas, the yellow serous fluid which is so often associated with endometriosis. The entire peritoneal surface and as much bowel serosa as possible should be visualized and the ovary rotated on its axis with a probe or atraumatic grasping forceps so that the ovarian fossa can be inspected for the presence of endometrial implants or adhesions. The assistant should carefully palpate the vagina and rectum for the presence of nodularity and by movements of the examining finger such sites should be marked by laser spots since such areas will require deep eradication if treatment is to be successful.

If an ovarian endometrioma is suspected needle aspiration should be performed to test for the presence of the characteristic thick chocolate fluid sequestered in the ovarian stroma.

It is important to inspect closely the peritoneal surface using the laparoscope as a magnifying instrument and to be aware of the appearances associated with acute endometriosis rather than merely looking for haemosiderin which often represents 'burnt out' or inactive disease and is more often present in the older patient (Redwine, 1987). Jansen and Russell drew attention to a number of characteristic non-pigmented lesions which are associated with endometriosis and which they confirmed by histological inspection of the peritoneal biopsy:

1. White opacified peritoneum (endometriosis in 81% of biopsies).
2. Red flame-like lesions (endometriosis in 81% of biopsies).
3. Glandular lesions resembling endometrium at hysteroscopy (endometriosis in 67% of biopsies).
4. Other appearances such as subovarian adhesions, yellow-brown peritoneal patches and circular peritoneal defects had endometriosis in half of the biopsies.

Any gynaecologist who is seriously involved in the treatment of endometriosis should read the article by Jansen and Russell (1986).

Documentation

All these lesions and vascular appearances should be carefully marked on a rubber stamp diagram of the pelvis supplemented, if the equipment is available, by a polaroid photograph from a still camera or a video printer. Ideally the laparoscopy and any operative procedures performed at laparoscopy should be recorded on videotape since this is the only reliable way to monitor the response to treatment at subsequent second-look procedures. The whole subject of documentation at laparoscopy is reviewed by Kees Wamsteker in Chapter 11.

An attempt should be made to grade the severity of the disease using the Revised American Fertility Scale (American Fertility Society, 1985) which, although by no means perfect, is probably the best available classification at present. Clinicians should be aware that the attainment of a high numerical grade on a scoring system does not necessarily correlate with the degree of pain experienced by the patient. Recent studies have shown that the pain in endometriosis is linked to prostaglandin metabolism, particularly that of prostaglandin F (Vernon et al, 1986). Even small lesions are capable of producing large amounts of prostaglandin F which accounts for the finding that patients with mild or moderate disease on the AFS scale can often have more pain than those with extensive disease sometimes found incidentally at laparotomy for a pelvic mass in an otherwise asymptomatic patient.

PRINCIPLES OF TREATMENT

It is important to individualize the approach to treatment because circumstances and situations vary enormously and will depend on the severity of symptoms, previous treatment, the age of the patient and her fertility expectations. If endometriosis is discovered incidentally, for example at the time of laparoscopic sterilization it might be entirely appropriate to advise no treatment at all, especially if the patient is asymptomatic. In the present medicolegal climate, however, it would be prudent to discuss this with the patient because untreated endometriosis may become more severe and give rise to future problems (Thomas and Cooke, 1987a).

The most exciting development in endometriosis therapy in recent years has been the use of different lasers to destroy ectopic endometrial implants and this approach has the overwhelming advantage that treatment can be performed laparoscopically at the same time as the diagnosis is made.

CARBON DIOXIDE LASER LAPAROSCOPY

The first reports of carbon dioxide (CO_2) laser laparoscopy came from Clermont-Ferrand in the Auvergne in Central France (Bruhat et al, 1979). Although this team pioneered the use of endoscopic lasers in gynaecology they subsequently seemed to turn their back on lasers and developed advanced techniques for dealing with ectopic pregnancy and ovarian cysts using instruments with several channels that could irrigate and suck at high pressure as well as delivering a cutting current with a diathermy needle. Recently they appear to have renewed their interest in laser surgery and a review of the contribution by the Clermont-Ferrand team is given by Wattiez and Bruhat in Chapter 3.

Meanwhile other centres started experimenting with laser laparoscopy and prototype instruments and techniques were developed independently in Israel (Tadhir et al, 1981), United States (Daniell and Brown, 1982; Feste, 1985; Martin, 1985), United Kingdom (Sutton, 1985) and Belgium (Donnez, 1987). Many of the original workers were quite unaware of the instruments and equipment developed by the others and it is interesting to see how they have independently achieved very similar results, especially in endometriosis, in terms of pain relief and pregnancies.

Before the advent of lasers the only method of removing endometrial implants endoscopically was by relatively crude cutting techniques, heating the endometrial implants by endocoagulation (Semm and Mettler, 1980) or destroying them by the passage of an electric current (Sulewski et al, 1980). These techniques inevitably result in bleeding or are so imprecise that there is considerable destruction of surrounding tissue with subsequent fibrosis and scarring.

In contrast the CO_2 laser has the advantage of being able to vaporize abnormal tissue precisely so that, although there is some cellular damage up to 500 μm from the impact point, the zone of thermal necrosis is usually less than 100 μm (Bellina et al, 1984). Since all the tissue debris is evacuated as smoke in the laser plume there is minimal fibrosis or scar tissue formation and laser wounds heal with virtually no contracture or anatomical distortion (Allen et al, 1983). These characteristics make the carbon dioxide laser particularly suitable for the vaporization of endometriosis and its associated adhesions especially in patients who are infertile or who may wish to have children in the future.

In our hospital the operating theatre staff are trained to have all the necessary equipment for laser laparoscopy available at every diagnostic laparoscopy for pelvic pain or infertility. It is important therefore to obtain informed consent from the patient to proceed to laser treatment once the diagnosis of endometriosis or adhesions is made. A few patients object to this and prefer to discuss the therapeutic options open to them after recovery from the anaesthetic. Most patients, however, appear happy to allow us to use the laser to vaporize endometriosis whenever it is discovered at a diagnostic laparoscopy. Since we are one of the few centres in the UK performing this operation on a regular basis almost 50% of our patients are secondary referrals when the diagnosis has already been made and informed consent is therefore easier to obtain.

Practical aspects

Once the initial assessment has been performed the operator should note the sites of the endometriosis and, depending on these and the preference of the individual surgeon, plan the incisions for the laser and the irrigation–retraction probes. He should decide on a single- or double-puncture technique, the delivery system for the laser energy and obtain a rough estimate of the time the procedure is likely to take and the effect this is going to have on his operating schedule for the day. Some laser laparoscopies can take a mere 10 minutes whereas others can last well over an hour (in the United States they can last longer than 3 hours) and certainly in this country where many general and oncological cases can be included in the same operating session it may be entirely appropriate to establish the diagnosis and leave the therapeutic aspect of the laparoscopy to a future occasion when the number of other cases can be reduced accordingly. This is particularly true of ovarian endometriomas and patients with complete obliteration of the cul-de-sac when corrective laparoscopic operations can be very time-consuming and can take far longer than a similar procedure performed at laparotomy. The reward for the patient, however, lies in the short hospital stay and early return to full activity.

Single-puncture technique

The advantage of the single-puncture approach lies in the fact that the path of the laser beam is exactly the same as the operators line of vision through the laparoscope. The laser energy passes down the operating channel of the angled laparoscope and the beam is finely focused by a micromanipulator joystick using the thumb of the right hand (Figures 1 and 2). Unfortunately the laser channel has to be rather large to stop the beam reflecting off the side-walls and this means an inevitable sacrifice in the amount of the cross-sectional area that is available for the passage of the light fibres. Thus, although the operating laser laparoscope is 14 mm in diameter, the visibility is poor compared to a conventional laparoscope. In this kind of surgery this is a grave disadvantage.

The other advantage of the single-puncture technique is that it allows the operator to have a free hand to manipulate irrigators, retractors or back-stops with less need to rely on assistants to perform these tasks. The position of insertion at the umbilicus also makes this an ideal situation for dealing with bowel adhesions in the paracolic gutter or the perihepatic adhesions of the FitzHugh Curtis syndrome, both of which are awkward to access with

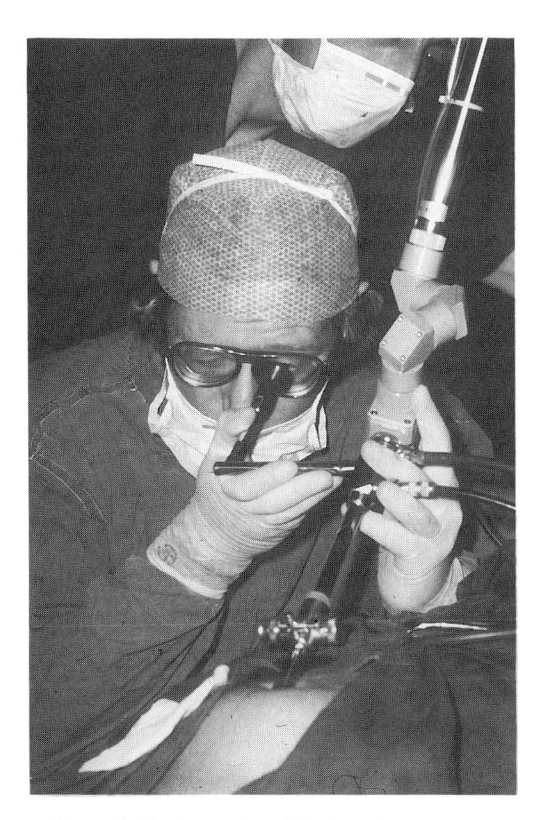

Figure 1. Single-puncture CO_2 laser laparoscope.

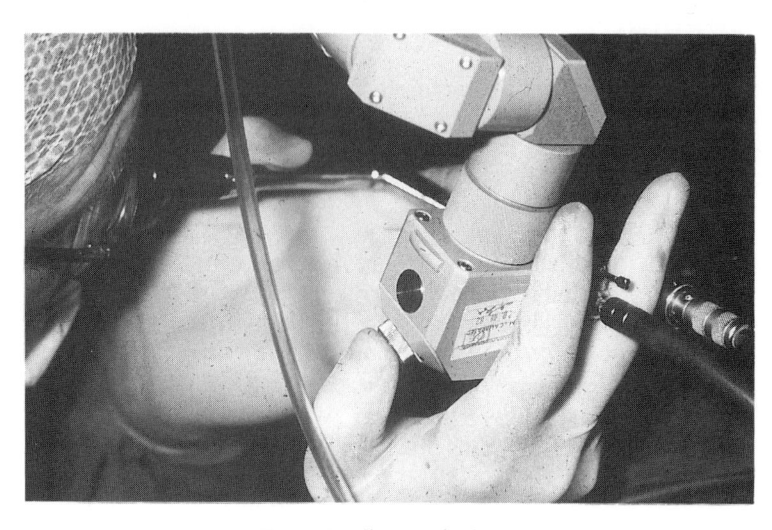

Figure 2. Micromanipulator.

second-puncture probes in the right or left iliac fossae due to the position of the patients legs when placed in semi-lithotomy.

Double-puncture technique

The main advantage of the double-puncture technique lies in the optimal visual conditions achieved using a standard 11 mm laparoscope. Once the extent and situation of the endometriosis has been assessed the second-puncture probes are inserted in the right or left iliac fossa in such a position that the laser beam can be directed as near as possible to a 90° angle of incidence to the implants that are to be vaporized (Figure 3). This is an

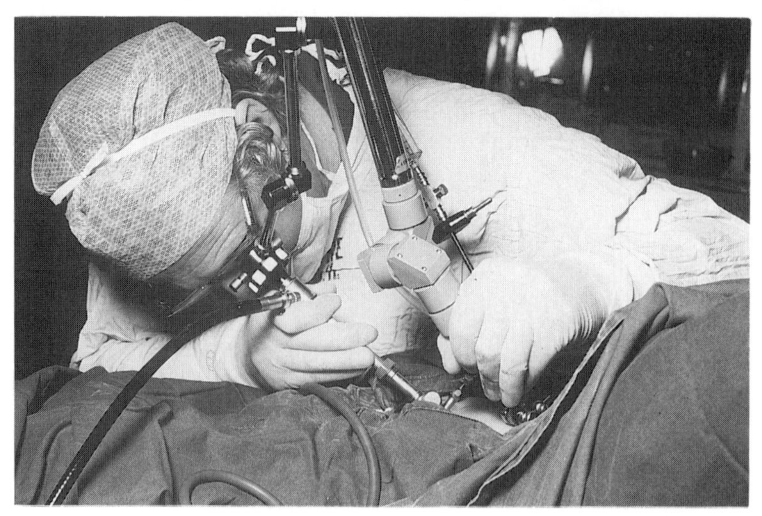

Figure 3. Double-puncture technique.

important practical point and failure to observe this simple rule may result in the laser beam being reflected off the shiny peritoneal surface, possibly resulting in injury to other structures such as bowel. Sometimes it is not possible to manoeuvre the probes into such a position and if the angle of incidence is too low it is necessary to use a different probe with a mirror set into the distal end at an angle of 45° so that laser light exits at 90° to the longitudinal axis of the probe.

In my opnion some of the commercially available second-puncture probes are far too long and this together with the constant need to adjust the focus with the joystick of the micromanipulator has inevitably attracted criticism that the technique is unwieldy and the equipment cumbersome when compared to the fibre lasers. We have therefore designed a much shorter probe only 160 mm in length with a fixed focus lens so that the focal point is 10 mm beyond the distal end of the probe (Rocket Ltd, London.) This obviates the need for a micromanipulator and the shortness of the instrument makes it less likely that the beam will bounce off the internal surface of the laser channel thus dissipating the power of the laser.

Carbon-dioxide laser fibre systems (infraguides)

Infraguide quartz fibres (LaserSonics, Santa Clara, California) have been introduced to avoid problems with beam alignment and coincidence by transmitting the CO_2 laser energy down a quartz fibre so that a spot size as low as 0.55 mm at a distance of 1 cm from the tip can be achieved. A true Gaussian distribution results in a smaller burn diameter, with less thermal damage and tissue necrosis which is relatively safer than using long focal lengths because there is a rapid fall off in power density beyond the focal point. This theoretically makes it a safer technique for beginners but although 90% of the CO_2 energy is transmitted, only 50% of the helium–neon (He–Ne) energy appears at the distal end, and this often makes the aiming beam difficult to visualize—especially with the accumulation of smoke that is an inevitable part of the procedure and the intense light sources that are necessary for television.

In practice I do not see any great advantage of these fibre guides over the short probes with fixed focal length lenses which we use. These rarely cause reflection of the beam off the inner side-walls of the probes and beam alignment is unaffected and I prefer to have a clear He–Ne aiming beam that is visible in strong light so that I can see the target area clearly before activating the laser.

Third-puncture probes for irrigation and retraction

In order to cool the tissues after laser vaporization and to remove any residual carbon debris it is essential to have a probe that will both flush the tissues with a jet of isotonic solution such as Ringer's lactate and also suck the excess of this solution out of the pelvis, together with any additional smoke that is not removed by the main smoke evacuation system. The Aquapurator designed by Semm (Karl Storz GmbH, Tuttlingen, West Germany) is suitable but is somewhat crude in construction whereas the Triton designed by Hubert Manhes (Micro-France, Bourbon L'Archambault, France) delivers a more powerful jet of fluid by a peristaltic pump or hydrostatic pressure and is also combined with an electrosurgical needle making it ideal for dealing with ectopic pregnancies. There are several other models available commercially; it is important to choose one without sharp edges since it also serves as an important retractor and the design must be such that it cannot harm delicate tissue, particularly bowel.

Smoke evacuation

One of the main disadvantages of CO_2 laser laparoscopy is the inevitable accumulation of smoke when tissue is vaporized. In order to retain visibility it is essential to have a system for evacuating smoke as fast as it is generated; for those using powerful lasers it is important to realize that the amount of smoke produced is directly proportional to the power density employed.

When we are performing laser laparoscopy the gas insufflator toggles are pulled down into the 'high-flow' position by the simple expedient of sealing them with adhesive tape for the duration of the procedure. Smoke is vented out by a smoke evacuator attached to the trochar sleeve of the second-portal probe and another smaller tube attached to the third-portal suction-irrigator which is controlled by the assistant. The main smoke evacuator is intermittently vented through a high-flow system into a charcoal filter and is controlled by the laser technician. The aim is to maintain sufficient pneumoperitoneum for the operation to continue without the 'roof coming down' on the endoscopist but at the same time to evacuate sufficient smoke to maintain visibility. Special insufflators and evacuators will soon be commercially available which will perform these various functions automatically but at the time of writing most of the available machines have been prototypes and all CO_2 laser laparoscopists eagerly await a machine that efficiently and inexpensively solves the vexed problem of smoke accumulation.

Ancillary equipment for arresting haemorrhage

The other main problem is the inability of the CO_2 laser to deal with anything more than small vessel haemorrhage—laser energy in this wavelength is absorbed by blood and the laser beam is thus rendered ineffective in the presence of significant bleeding.

Anyone seriously contemplating laser laparoscopy should already be a competent operative laparoscopist and should have haemostatic equipment available, in case of severe or ongoing haemorrhage. Depending on the amount of bleeding and the location this can be by unipolar or bipolar diathermy, endocoagulation or the use of various haemostatic clips or Roederer endoloops. For further details on these various techniques the reader is referred to the chapters on operative laparoscopy by Kurt Semm (Chapter 2) and Harry Reich (Chapter 13).

If bleeding persists but is not sufficiently severe to warrant laparotomy I tend to introduce a redi-vac drain into the pelvis through the suprapubic trochar to avoid the development of a pelvic haematoma postoperatively but also to enable the ward nurses to monitor the amount of ongoing intraperitoneal loss. In practice it tends to stop soon after the operation and most of these drains can be removed after 4 hours and the patient can still be discharged on the same day.

Video equipment

The ability to monitor and record the operation on television is not merely a luxury, but an essential component of laser laparoscopy. It allows the assistant to provide effective help for irrigation and retraction and also enables the nurses to anticipate instrument needs and the technician to help with smoke evacuation. If the procedure is unduly long it allows the surgeon to operate indirectly under television control thus preventing considerable back-strain due to the stooped and twisted position that has to be adopted when peering down a laparoscope. The definition and acuity of the human eye cannot yet be achieved by television and attempts to operate entirely by television are to be deprecated.

Television also offers the best method of documenting these procedures, particularly in patients who have a 'second-look' procedure since it is the only reliable method of assessing the progression of the disease and the effect of treatment. The advantage for teaching the technique to others and informing patients is self-evident and we also use it for patients who are attending other clinics for assisted conception since it often avoids the need for a further assessment laparoscopy.

GETTING STARTED IN LASER LAPAROSCOPY

The laser

Acquiring a laser purely for female fertility surgery may not appeal to the average District General Manager in these cost-conscious times, but most hospitals running a colposcopy service have been using lasers for the treatment of cervical intraepithelial neoplasia over the last decade. Nearly all lasers in current use can be adapted for laparoscopic work and the more modern lasers, particularly those with sealed tubes, can be transported from the colposcopy clinic to the operating theatre without any problem. (Some of the older ones do not take kindly to this treatment, however, and their mirrors go out of alignment.)

For laparoscopic use the laser should deliver between 5 and 55 W of power measured at the tissue, although for most practical purposes it is rarely necessary to go above 40 W. Some of the 20 W office lasers can be adapted for laparoscopic use but often need special extension tubes to give the necessary height for the articulated arm to attach to the laparoscopic delivery system. A superpulse facility is an advantage, particularly when dividing thick adhesions but is by no means essential; indeed, we have produced good results during our first 6 years of operation with a Sharplan 733 laser that was manufactured before the introduction of superpulse.

The theatre team

In order to convert from simple diagnostic or sterilization laparoscopy to operative laser laparoscopy it is essential to have co-operative nurses and technicians. We have been enormously helped by the enthusiastic support of our nurses and, in particular, our senior theatre nurse Annie Parker and the Operating Department Assistant, Dougie Bathie. The nurses need to be able to produce any conceivable combination of laparoscopic instruments at very short notice and by watching on the video screen the manoeuvres being performed should be able to anticipate the surgeon's needs. The laser technician needs to be able to operate and activate a variety of lasers at a moment's notice; in addition, should unforeseen complications arise during the procedure other treatment modalities such as unipolar or bipolar cautery or endocoagulation will be needed immediately. The technical aspects of laser laparoscopy have become so complicated that it really does require a separate laser technician to cope with all the equipment, although we have expected, somewhat unfairly, our ODA to look after the needs of the anaesthetist as well.

The surgeon

Before undertaking laser laparoscopy surgeons must make absolutely certain that they are familiar with the biological action of lasers on human tissues (Absten, 1989). In my opinion, they should also already have had considerable experience in using lasers on the lower genital tract. They should be aware of the different power densities required to achieve varying depths of destruction, the different actions made possible by varying the spot size and power, the use of defocused beams and reduction of power to stop unwanted bleeding. Only when they are fully confident of performing colposcopic laser surgery and dealing with the various complications encountered should they consider using the laser in the peritoneal cavity, first at open laparotomy and eventually via the laparoscope.

Surgeons should have: (i) a working knowledge of basic laser physics; (ii) attended the relevant courses in basic laser surgery and laser laparoscopy; (iii) become attached to a recognized laser laparoscopist for a number of sessions and preferably obtained some 'hands-on' experience. Acquiring experience in this type of surgery is vastly more difficult than in conventional surgery because teaching is indirect; the teacher is unable to perform rapid manoeuvres to rescue the student in time of difficulty, having to anticipate problems by way of the video monitor.

Initial experience should be acquired by means of a model simulating the female pelvis unless facilities are available for animal experimentation; for example, New Zealand White rabbits are used for teaching in the United States but such usage would be unlikely to be allowed in this country. I teach people to perform laser laparoscopy on my own mock-up of a pelvic trainer (Figure 4)—a plant propagator with three portals for the instruments and a human placenta lying in the seedling tray! The surface vessels are used to simulate endometriosis and the membranes are held up by a pair of watch-

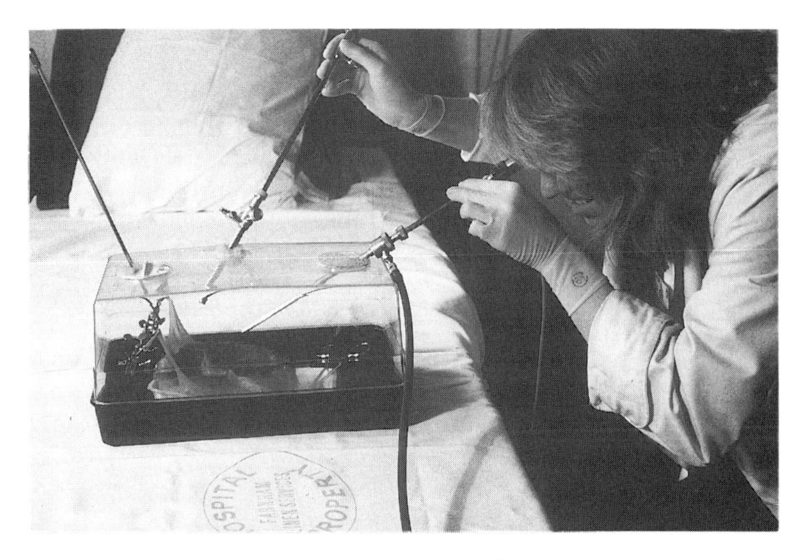

Figure 4. Pelvic trainer for laser laparoscopy.

makers' 'helping hands' to simulate adhesions which can then be divided by a laser probe with a backstop. Some operative laparoscopists would advise at least 3 months practice on such equipment before attempting to use the CO_2 laser on a live patient.

The hazards

Laser laparoscopy is essentially an exercise in the appreciation of pelvic anatomy whereby the operator recognizes the dangers and pitfalls and takes great care to avoid them. The most obvious hazard is damage to the bowel and until considerable experience has been gained the laser should not be activated in the vicinity of large or small bowel. It goes without saying that the laser foot switch should never be depressed unless a clear view is obtained down the laparoscope and any blood or debris obscuring the laparoscopic vision or any smoke accumulating in the peritoneal cavity must be cleared before the laser is fired. The golden rule is *never* to fire the laser unless you can see exactly the He–Ne aiming beam and you are certain that it is not overlying an anatomical structure which could be seriously injured if laser energy is allowed to penetrate it.

Another obvious hazard in the pelvis is the ureter, the course of which should constantly be borne in mind, with repeated attempts made to 'palpate' the ureter with one of the third-portal probes and visualize its course by the peristalsis that often betrays its presence. The other main hazards are the thin-walled veins which can bleed profusely if punctured; rather than having to use endocoagulators or diathermy equipment to stop the bleeding it is much more sensible to avoid these structures wherever possible. The chief danger areas as far as this is concerned are just lateral to the utero-sacral ligaments and also in the vascular area between the fallopian tube and the ovary and the large venous plexuses in the broad ligament just lateral to the uterus on either side.

If bowel is accidentally injured or if persistent bleeding occurs which cannot be stopped by laparoscopic methods the surgeon must be bold enough to proceed to laparotomy and repair the damage adequately using conventional surgical techniques. Ideally the patient should have consented

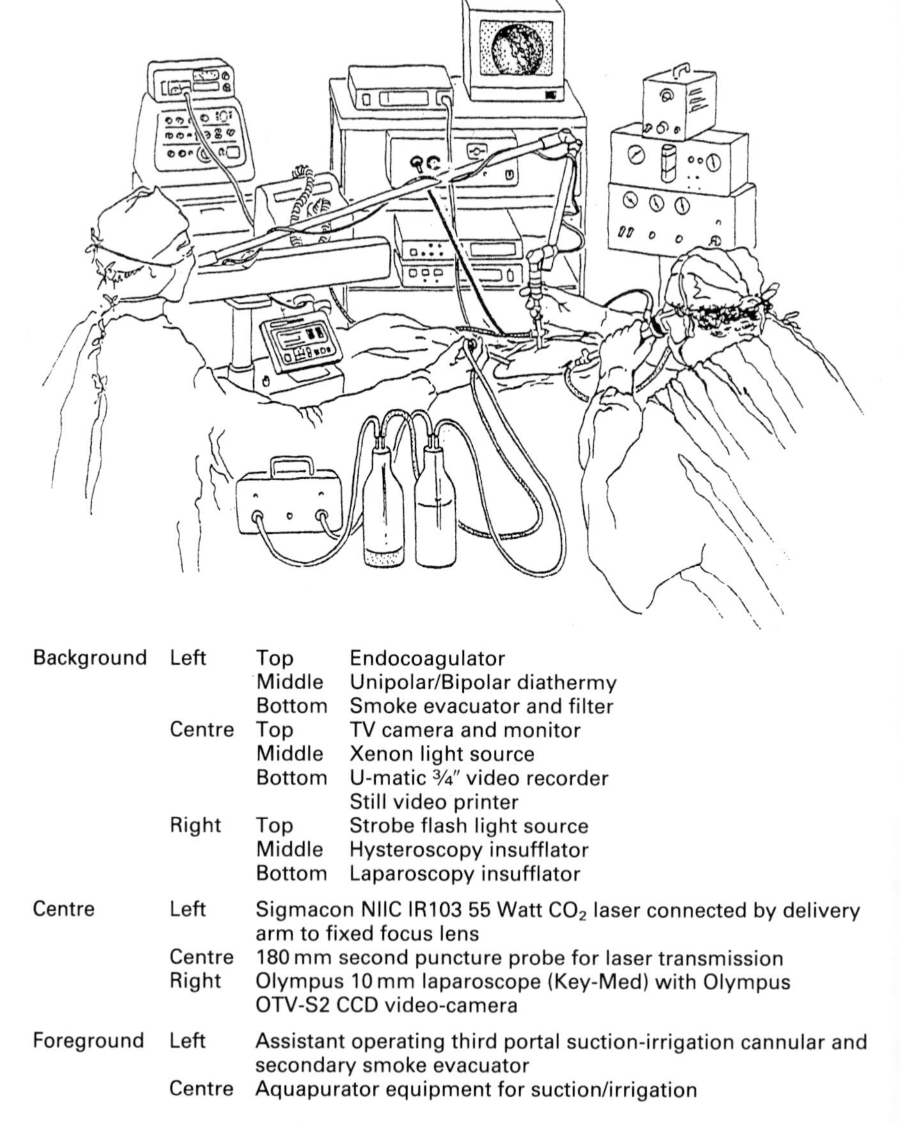

Background	Left	Top	Endocoagulator
		Middle	Unipolar/Bipolar diathermy
		Bottom	Smoke evacuator and filter
	Centre	Top	TV camera and monitor
		Middle	Xenon light source
		Bottom	U-matic ¾″ video recorder Still video printer
	Right	Top	Strobe flash light source
		Middle	Hysteroscopy insufflator
		Bottom	Laparoscopy insufflator
Centre	Left	Sigmacon NIIC IR103 55 Watt CO_2 laser connected by delivery arm to fixed focus lens	
	Centre	180 mm second puncture probe for laser transmission	
	Right	Olympus 10 mm laparoscope (Key-Med) with Olympus OTV-S2 CCD video-camera	
Foreground	Left	Assistant operating third portal suction-irrigation cannular and secondary smoke evacuator	
	Centre	Aquapurator equipment for suction/irrigation	

Figure 5. Instrumentation for CO_2 laser laparoscopy.

to this procedure beforehand. Most of the reported accidents from the use of lasers delivered laparoscopically have arisen from the failure of the surgeon to recognize the damage at the time that it was inflicted or, more likely, an ostrich-like hope that such damage would resolve spontaneously; performing an immediate laparotomy results in a certain loss of face for the surgeon but a far safer outcome for the patient.

Funding

The amount of equipment required for laser laparoscopy is illustrated in Figure 5. It may at first sight appear a little daunting but after the inevitable 'teething problems' and the co-operation of an enthusiastic theatre team it all works surprisingly well. The initial financial outlay is great and in a fast-developing field where new innovations and instruments are constantly being introduced, a support fund is required to make money available without any bureaucratic delay or harassment. We have been particularly fortunate in our hospital in having fundraisers who have worked hard and selflessly to raise the money for most of our laser equipment.

It should not, in fact, be necessary to rely on charitable funds to run a laser laparoscopy service since much of the surgery by this new technique has replaced major surgery and the prolonged hospital stay and recovery associated with it. The benefits in terms of health economics should sway any Hospital Manager worthy of their job.

THE GUILDFORD LASER LAPAROSCOPY UNIT

We were the first gynaecology department in the United Kingdom to start using laser laparoscopy, the equipment being installed in St Luke's Hospital, Guildford, in October 1982. Since then we have treated over 700 patients for a variety of conditions ranging from endometriosis and adhesions to neosalpingostomies, ovarian cysts, polycystic ovarian syndrome and unruptured ectopic pregnancies. Although some of these conditions could have been dealt with using operative laparoscopy or cautery many would have needed a formal laparotomy with the prolonged hospital stay and convalescence needed to recover from major abdomino-pelvic surgery.

By contrast, of the first 520 patients treated by laser laparoscopy, 124 were admitted on a day-case basis and 388 stayed for one night following the procedure, mainly for the convenience of nursing or ward administration. Four patients stayed for 48 hours for various reasons, usually associated with long or difficult procedures and a further two stayed for 3 days because of medical problems associated with diabetes and asthma.

There were only two serious complications. One patient required a laparotomy because of breakage of the metal backstop platform on the adhesiolysis probe which could not be retrieved via the laparoscope. The other problem involved a patient who developed surgical emphysema which took 10 days to resolve. In some of the early lasers, nitrogen was used to cool the lens and somehow this had managed to leak into the patient's subcutaneous tissues and was responsible for the slow resolution of a well-recognized complication of laparoscopy. In view of these complications the adhesiolysis probe was redesigned and we now use CO_2 to cool the lens so these two complications should not arise again. More importantly, we have not had any problems associated with the intraperitoneal use of laser energy.

RESULTS

Endometriosis treated by laser laparoscopy

We have recently reviewed 228 consecutive patients with endometriosis who were treated by laser laparoscopy between 1982 and 1987 and have been followed up for between 2 and 7 years (Sutton, 1989a). Patients were classified according to the presenting symptoms of pain, infertility or both and all had consented to laser treatment if endometriosis was found at the time of diagnostic laparoscopy. The results are summarized in Table 1.

Table 1. Results of Laser Laparoscopy in patients with endometriosis.

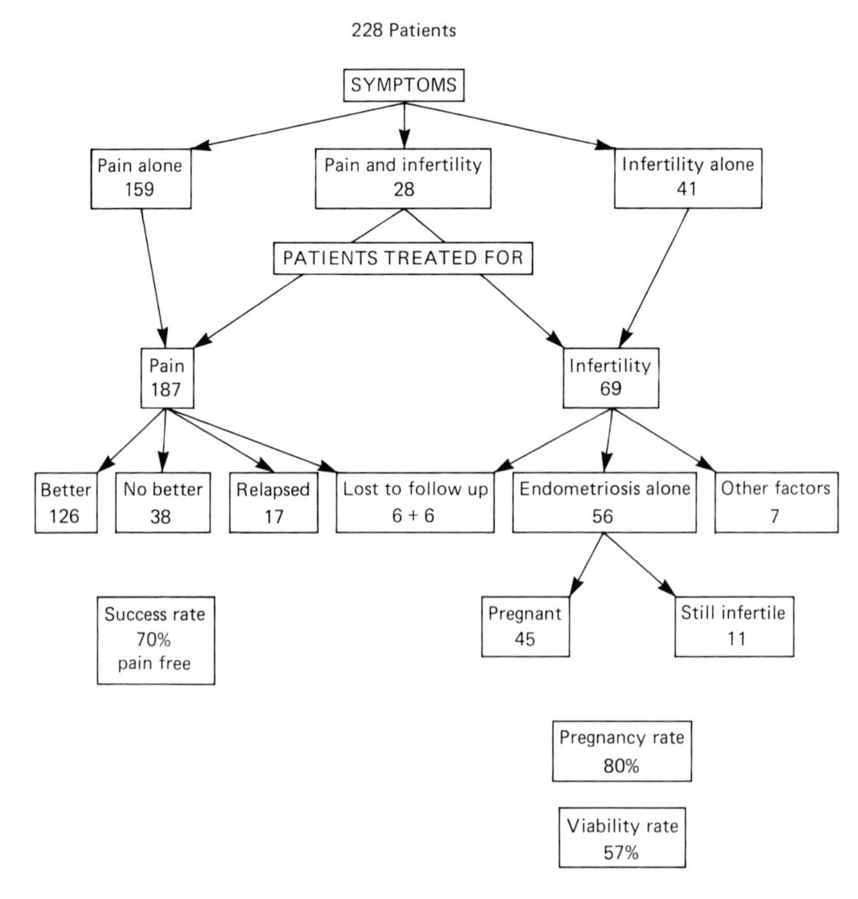

Endometriosis and pelvic pain

Symptomatic improvement was seen in 126 of 181 (70%) of patients complaining of pelvic pain and the benefit was sustained in all but 17 patients who relapsed, usually after 6–9 months. It is tempting to ascribe this success to the placebo effect of the laparoscopy but almost one third of these patients had undergone previous laparoscopies or medical therapy without relief of their pain. We managed to persuade 33 patients in this group to have a second-look procedure to evaluate the result of the original laser laparoscopy. In 15 patients there was no evidence of recurrent endometriosis although the charcoal deposits remaining from the laser vaporization could be seen clearly underneath the peritoneum. Careful inspection with the laparoscope lens held close to the peritoneal surface revealed a characteristic appearance with no inflammatory reaction and biopsy showed inactive carbon particles with no evidence of endometrial glands or stroma.

Eighteen patients had formed endometriosis at different sites but there was no evidence of endometriosis at the sites previously lasered. Obviously this group of patients required medical therapy, or definitive surgery if childbearing was no longer a consideration, to prevent further recurrence of the disease. The choice of medical therapy is, however, by no means easy. Danazol (Sterling-Winthrop), probably the most widely prescribed drug for endometriosis, has proven effective at reducing the majority of implants but nevertheless, a significant persistence or recurrence rate has been noted. Published data suggest a recurrence rate of 29–30% which is actually higher than that found following laser laparoscopy (Dmowski and Cohen, 1978; Greenblatt and Tzingounis, 1979; Puleo and Hammond, 1983). In addition it is neither wise nor practical to take danazol or luteinizing hormone releasing hormone (LHRH) analogues for longer than 6 months, not only because of the well-documented side-effects (Jelly, 1987) but also because of the adverse changes in serum lipids with danazol (Fahreus et al, 1984; Booker et al, 1986) and the loss of bone calcium and trabecular density with LHRH analogues (Matta et al, 1987).

In view of the above problems we tend to treat recurrent endometriosis following laser laparoscopy with continuous progestogen therapy, usually in the form of medroxyprogesterone acetate (Provera, Upjohn) at a relatively high dose of 25 mg t.d.s. We have been impressed by the lack of side-effects when this drug is used at an even higher dosage (200 mg b.d.) in patients with endometrial carcinoma whereas when prescribed at a low dose, side-effects including nausea, breast tenderness, fluid retention and depression are relatively common. These drugs act by causing initial decidualization of endometrial tissue with eventual atrophy and seem to be the drugs of choice when endometriosis occurs after laser vaporization and there is a need for long-term suppressive therapy.

Most of the published reports on laser laparoscopy deal exclusively with pregnancy, possibly because the end-point is easier to define than pelvic pain, which involves all sorts of subjective and even psychological factors. Daniell (1984) reported a 72% pain resolution rate after 12 months follow-up in 18 patients of all grades of severity treated with CO_2 laser laparoscopy and Keye and Dixon (1983) reported an impressive 92% reduction of pain in 50 patients with mild and moderate endometriosis treated with the argon laser. Nezhat et al (1988) divided a group of 120 women with all stages of endometriosis into three groups which were treated with the CO_2, argon and potassium titanyl phosphate (KTP)-532 lasers. Although the numbers in each group were small the best outcome in terms of pain relief and pregnancy was with the CO_2 laser.

Ovarian endometriomas are a pertinent cause of pelvic pain and are notoriously unresponsive to medical therapy. They are best treated by operative laparoscopy employing patient dissection to remove the cyst capsule to prevent recurrence (Reich and McGlynn, 1986) or by using the double-optic laparoscopic technique with an argon or KTP-532 laser to destroy the internal lining of the endometrioma. Details of this technique are described in Chapter 9 by Brosens and Puttemans.

Endometriosis and dysmenorrhoea

Dysmenorrhoea is common among sufferers of endometriosis and is usually of the congestive kind, preceding the period by a few days and often partially relieved or changing in character once the bleeding starts. These symptoms are particularly likely to be present when the endometriotic implants lie on or within the utero-sacral ligaments. This is not entirely surprising since the sensory parasympathetic fibres to the cervix and the sensory sympathetic fibres to the corpus traverse the cervical division of the Lee-Frankenhauser plexus which lies in, under and around the attachments of the utero-sacral ligaments to the cervix (Campbell, 1950).

For many years the operation of presacral neurectomy was employed for patients with intractable dysmenorrhoea but yielded disappointing results with failure rates around 11–15% in primary dysmenorrhoea and 25–40% in secondary dysmenorrhoea associated with endometriosis (Tucker, 1947; Ingersoll and Meigs, 1948; Polan and DeCherney, 1980). In 1952 White pointed out that the nerve supply to the cervix is not usually interrupted by the presacral neurectomy procedure (White, 1952) and then in 1963 Joseph Doyle described the procedure of paracervical uterine denervation that bears his name (Doyle and Des Rosiers, 1963). The operation was performed abdominally or vaginally and the results were extremely impressive with complete pain relief in 63 out of 73 cases (86%) and the results were equally good for primary or secondary dysmenorrhoea. With such a satisfactory outcome it is difficult to see why the operation sank into obscurity. Possibly the advent of powerful prostaglandin synthetase inhibitors and hormonal agents reduced the demand for relatively drastic forms of intervention. Interest in Doyle's work has recently revived with the development of surgical lasers which can be used endoscopically and will perform much the same tissue effect without the need for major surgery (Daniell and Feste, 1985; Sutton, 1989b).

During the past 5 years we have treated 126 patients with laser uterine nerve ablation (LUNA) laparoscopically (Sutton, 1989b). Twenty-six had primary dysmenorrhoea and 100 had secondary dysmenorrhoea associated with endometriosis. We did not include patients with secondary dysmenorrhoea due to other causes such as fibroids, adenomyosis or pelvic congestion.

In the endometriosis group six patients were lost to follow-up but 81 (86%) reported an improvement in symptoms even though 26 (32%) of them had a partial (unilateral) neurectomy. In three patients the symptoms returned at 6 months to 1 year following the procedure. No patients were made worse but 13 reported no improvement and, interestingly, nine of these had incomplete or partial neurectomies due to poor formation of the ligaments resulting in difficulty in localizing and vaporizing the nerve bundles. There were no serious complications in this group of patients and all were treated on a day-case or overnight stay basis. Troublesome bleeding was encountered in two patients requiring endocoagulation or haemostatic clips and the insertion of a redi-vac drain in the pelvis for several hours postoperatively.

Feste has recently reported on a larger series from Houston (Feste, personal communication). He performed laser neurectomy on 196 patients with intractable dysmenorrhoea who had failed to respond to traditional therapy. Of the 124 patients that he managed to follow-up the failure rate was only 12.9% which is almost exactly the same result as that obtained by us.

Both the above series suffer from the disadvantage that they are entirely retrospective and uncontrolled and sceptics can quite reasonably argue that there is a massive placebo effect with this kind of symptom, especially if it is treated with the sort of high-tech wizardry that is implicit in laser beam procedures. The study of Lichten and Bombard is therefore particularly interesting because it is one of the few (or indeed the only) randomized prospective double-blind study in the entire field of operative laparoscopy.

A relatively homogeneous group of women were selected who had severe or incapacitating dysmenorrhoea, who had no demonstrable pelvic pathology at laparoscopy and who were unresponsive to NSAIDS and oral contraceptives prescribed concurrently. Coexisting psychiatric illness was evaluated with the Minnesota Multiphasic Personality Inventory and those with an abnormal psychological profile were excluded from the study. The remaining 21 patients were randomized to uterine nerve ablation or control group at the time of the diagnostic laparoscopy. Neither the patient nor the clinical psychologist who conducted the interview at follow-up were aware of the group to which the patient had been randomized. No patient in the control group reported relief from dysmenorrhoea whereas nine of the eleven patients (81%) who had LUNA reported almost complete relief at 3 months and five of them had continued relief from dysmenorrhoea 1 year after surgery. Interestingly, those that reported surgical success also reported relief from the associated symptoms of nausea, vomiting, diarrhoea and headaches (Lichten and Bombard, 1987).

Endometriosis and dyspareunia

Patients with endometriosis complaining of deep dyspareunia are usually found to have active telangiectatic or vesicular implants in the cul-de-sac or deposits in the utero-sacral ligaments which are responsible for the nodular feeling when such patients are examined vaginally. When using the CO_2 laser to eradicate these nodules it is important to continue vaporization at a relatively high power density until no further haemosiderin is released and until the assistant confirms that no further nodules are palpable on vaginal and rectal examination (Figures 6 and 7).

Sometimes adhesions are present between the rectum and the posterior aspect of the cervix and this is often responsible for dyspareunia. In its

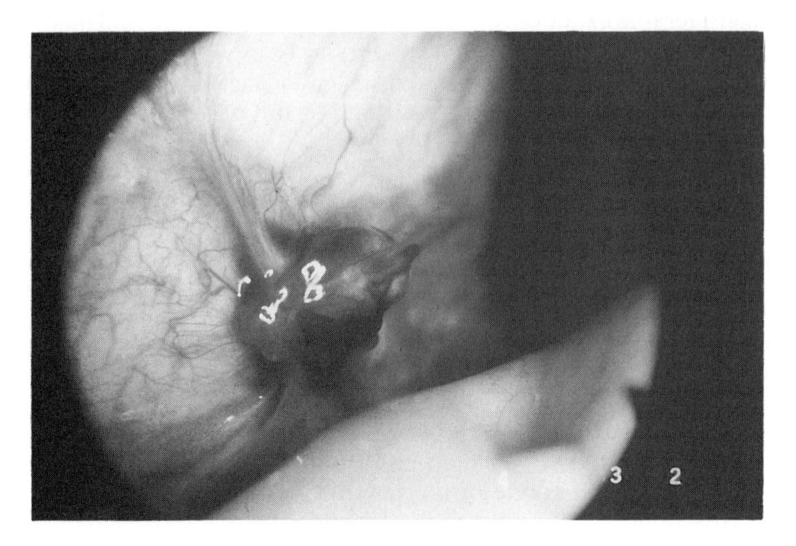

Figure 6. Deposit of endometriosis in cul-de-sac causing dyspareunia.

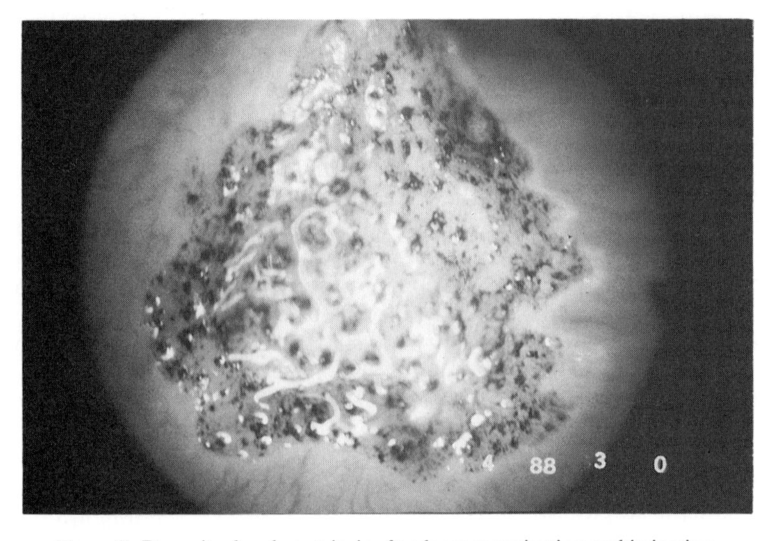

Figure 7. Deposit of endometriosis after laser vaporization and irrigation.

extreme form this eventually develops into partial or complete obliteration of the cul-de-sac giving rise to a high score on the AFS scale. Paradoxically, however, many patients with complete obliteration of the cul-de-sac do not mention dyspareunia among their symptoms whereas some patients with a few active deposits are acutely uncomfortable during deep penetration and the discomfort continues as a nagging ache well into the following day.

It is important to rid the cul-de-sac of all adhesions and implants in order to alleviate discomfort during intercourse. Care must be taken when using the laser over the rectum itself—the power density should be reduced and, until considerable experience has been amassed, the laser should be used on a pulsed mode with repeated irrigation to remove the charcoal and assess the depth of destruction in relation to the anatomy of the rectal wall. With experience the beam can be used on continuous mode with rapid hand movement to prevent penetration of the rectal mucosa. In patients with complete obliteration of the cul-de-sac it is necessary to use the laser to open up a plane of cleavage between the cervix and the rectum and to use aquadissection to extend this. These techniques of advanced operative laparoscopy are described in more detail by Harry Reich in Chapter 13.

In our retrospective study we did not specifically enquire about dyspareunia in our analysis of the results although our impression is that most patients with active disease in the posterior fornix have benefitted from laser treatment. Donnez reported on a series of 100 patients who have been followed for more than a year after LUNA. He found that most patients complaining of dyspareunia experienced relief from this symptom following the operation. We have noticed that even in the absence of visible endometriosis patients with very taut utero-sacral ligaments seem to complain of dyspareunia which is relieved by the simple act of dividing the ligaments with the laser. This may be a purely physical effect or it could be because 52% of patients with pelvic pain and no macroscopic evidence of endometriosis reveal endometrial glands and stroma on histological examination of biopsies from the utero-sacral ligaments (Nisolle, 1988). There is considerable controversy about the significance of random peritoneal biopsies but if it is eventually shown that endometriosis exists without its usual outward appearances it calls into question the whole philosophy of vaporizing the deposits with lasers or electrocautery and certainly explains some of our treatment failures.

Endometriosis and infertility

Most gynaecologists would agree that endometriosis is responsible for pelvic pain and dyspareunia but there is considerable controversy about the relationship between endometriosis and infertility. Although there is little doubt that the anatomical distortion caused by severe endometriosis is responsible for difficulties with ovum pick-up some authors have suggested that the relationship with early stage disease is casual rather than causal (Lilford and Dalton, 1987). Analysis of the data is further complicated by the fact that even a simple procedure such as laparoscopic chromopertubation involves several steps that may independently benefit the patient. For example, dilatation of the cervix may relieve cervical stenosis, at least temporarily, and this may be an important factor in the pathogenesis of endometriosis (Stillman and Miller, 1984); removal of peritoneal fluid from the cul-de-sac will decrease the macrophage content that has been implicated in infertility (Haney et al, 1983) and the simple act of insufflating the tubes has been claimed to enhance fertility (DeCherney et al, 1980; Olive et al, 1985). Since so-called 'expectant management' can be expected to give rise to a pregnancy rate of 25% (Olive and Haney, 1986), and treatment with danazol a pregnancy rate of 36.9% (range 0–60%) (Audebert et al, 1979; Chalmers and Shervington, 1979; Guzick and Rock, 1983; Buttram et al, 1985), laser laparoscopy must be shown to be an improvement on this. It must also be shown that it is safer than electrocautery, the use of which has been associated with damage to viscera (Chamberlain and Brown, 1978) and even the ureter (Cheng, 1976).

In the Guildford series there were 56 patients with endometriosis as the only abnormal factor implicated in their infertility which ranged from 6 months to 10 years. 45 (80%) of these patients have become pregnant following laser laparoscopy, without adjuvant drug treatment, the majority (73%) within 8 months of the procedure. The procedure–pregnancy interval and the relationship of the outcome to the severity of endometriosis are shown in Tables 2 and 3.

The Guildford data compare favourably with results from the United States (Daniell, 1984; Feste, 1985; Davis, 1986; Nezhat et al, 1986) and Europe (Donnez, 1987). Nezhat obtained 62 pregnancies in 102 patients which included one elective termination and nine spontaneous abortions. Unfortunately our abortion rate is even higher (24%). This probably reflects

Table 2. Guildford Laser Laparoscopy Project, October 1982–October 1987: procedure–pregnancy interval.

Number of months	Number of pregnancies
0–6	33 (73%)
8–12	7 (16%)
12–18	4 (9%)
>18	1 (2%)
TOTAL	45

Table 3. Guildford Laser Laparoscopy Project, October 1982–October 1987: Severity of endometriosis related to pregnancies.

Stage (AFS scale)		Number of patients	Other factors*	Number of pregnancies
Minimal	I	19	3	15 (94%)
Mild	II	25	1	17 (71%)
Moderate	III	16	3	11 (85%)
Severe	IV	2	0	2 (100%)
TOTAL		62	−7 = 55	45

* Other factors: Oligospermia, 6; cervical fibroid, 1.

the high abortion rate noted among endometriosis sufferers in general which has been reported in one series to be as high as 49% (Malinak and Wheeler, 1985). If the results are presented as pregnancies resulting in full-term infants our viability rate of 57% is exactly the same as that of Donnez in Belgium (Donnez, 1987). The results of several recent studies are given in Table 4. They can all be criticized on the basis that they are retrospective studies and there is a great need for a double-blind prospective study comparing laser treatment with placebo and accepted medical therapy.

Table 4. Results of laser laparoscopy for endometriosis.

Reference	Number of patients	Number of pregnancies	Viability
Feste (1985)	29	21 (72%)	n/s
Davis (1986)	65	37 (57%)	57%
Nezhat et al (1986)	102	62 (61%)	51%
Daniell (1984)	40	20 (20%)	n/s
Donnez (1987)	70	40 (n/s)	57%
Sutton (1989)	56	45 (80%)	57%
Nezhat et al (1989)	243	168 (69%)	n/s

n/s = not stated.

The only prospective study in the literature followed one group of 64 patients treated by CO_2 laser laparoscopy and compared them with another control group of 44 patients who were treated with drug therapy, laparoscopic electrocoagulation or expectant management. One criticism of this paper is that randomization appears to have depended on the availability or otherwise of a laser at the time of laparoscopy and the fact that there were too many variable treatment regimens in the control group. Nevertheless the laser group achieved pregnancy at a higher overall rate and also had shorter post-treatment intervals. Using life-table analysis the monthly fecundity rate for the laser group was 6.7% and the control group was 4.5% (Adamson et al, 1988).

When analysing the results of laser laparoscopy in infertility one of the most interesting observations is that the pregnancy rates seem to be excellent regardless of the severity of the disease. Olive and Haney (1986) have reported a series of 80 patients treated by laser alone with no pre- or postoperative medication with an overall fecundity rate of 3.25%. For mild and moderate disease the monthly fecundity rate was 3.33% and 2.51%, respectively, while for severe endometriosis the value was even higher at 5.79%. Nezhat has recently reported on 243 infertility patients treated by CO_2 laser laparoscopy of whom 168 (69.1%) became pregnant. The pregnancy rates were 71.8% in 39 patients with stage I disease, 69.8% in 86 patients with stage II disease, 67.2% in 67 patients with stage III disease and 68.6% in 51 patients with stage IV disease. The cumulative pregnancy rate computed by life-table analysis is shown in Figure 8 (Nezhat et al, 1989).

With results that are this good the rationale for conservative surgery must be seriously questioned. Although an overall pregnancy rate of 60.7% is claimed for conservative surgery (Olive and Haney, 1986), the only two studies providing monthly fecundity rates demonstrate a much lower rate of

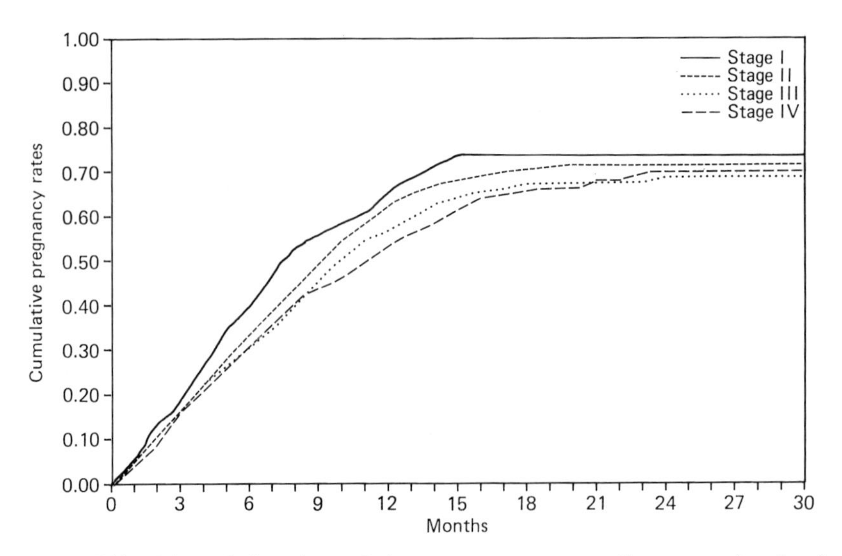

Figure 8. Life-table analysis and cumulative pregnancy rate according to severity of endometriosis.

conception in these patients than those treated by danazol or even expectant management (Rock et al, 1981; Olive and Lee, 1986). Even with the use of the CO_2 laser via an operating microscope at laparotomy, Chong and Baggish (1984) were only able to demonstrate a 61% pregnancy rate. Only 23 patients were included in this uncontrolled study and the results for stage III and IV disease at 35% and 0%, respectively, were far less impressive than the above series where the laser energy was delivered via the laparoscope.

There is now sufficient data in the literature to show clearly that CO_2 laser laparoscopy in the treatment of endometriosis-related infertility is both safe and effective. There is still, however, a complete lack of randomized prospective studies comparing this treatment modality with medical therapy or expectant management. Its real value probably lies in the ability to restore pelvic anatomical relationships without fibrosis, scarring or serious adhesion formation thus accounting for the excellent results in severe disease. Such procedures are very long and arduous and can only be performed by experienced and gifted surgeons with excellent hand and eye co-ordination.

The great advantage of laser laparoscopy in endometriosis is the ability to treat the disease at the same time as the diagnosis is made thus allowing the patient to try for conception without delay and avoiding major surgery or the use of expensive drugs many of which have extremely unpleasant side-effects.

Acknowledgements

The author thanks *Fertility and Sterility* for permission to reproduce Dr Camran Nezhat's data in Figure 8, and Margot Cooper for her illustration in Figure 5.

REFERENCES

Absten G (1989) Physics of light and lasers. In Sutton C (ed.) *Lasers in Gynaecology*. London: Chapman and Hall, in press.
Adamson GD, Lu J & Subak LL (1988) Laparoscopic carbon-dioxide laser vaporization of endometriosis compared with traditional treatments. *Fertility and Sterility* **50**(5): 704–710.
Allen JM, Stein DS & Shingleton HM (1983) Regeneration of cervical epithelium after laser vaporisation. *Obstetrics and Gynecology* **62:** 700–704.
American Fertility Society (1985) Classification of endometriosis. *Fertility and Sterility* **43:** 351–352.
Audebert AJ, Larne-Charlus S & Emperaire TC (1979) Danazol—endometriosis and infertility: A review of 62 patients treated with danazol. *Postgraduate Medical Journal* **55** (supplement): 10–15.
Bellina JH, Hemmings R, Voros IJ & Ross LF (1984) Carbon dioxide laser and electrosurgical wound study with an animal model. A comparison of tissue damage and healing patterns in peritoneal tissue. *American Journal of Obstetrics and Gynecology* **148:** 327.
Booker MW, Lewis B & Whitehead MI (1986) A comparison of the changes in plasma lipids and lipoproteins during therapy with danazol and gestrione for endometriosis. *Proceedings of the 42nd Annual Meeting of the American Fertility Society*, Birmingham, Alabama. p 66. Georgia: American Fertility Society.
Bruhat MA, Mage C & Manhes M (1979) Use of the carbon-dioxide laser via laparoscopy. In Kaplan I (ed.) *Laser Surgery III, Proceedings of the Third Congress of the International Society for Laser Surgery*, p 275. Tel Aviv: International Society for Laser Surgery.
Buttram VC, Reiter RC & Ward S (1985) Treatment of endometriosis with danazol: report of a six year prospective study. *Fertility and Sterility* **43:** 353–360.
Campbell RM (1950) Anatomy and histology of sacro-uterine ligaments. *American Journal of Obstetrics and Gynecology* **59:** 1–7.
Chalmers JA & Shervington PC (1979) Follow-up of patients with endometriosis treated with danazol. *Postgraduate Medical Journal* **55**(supplement): 44–49.
Chamberlain GVP & Brown JC (1978) *Gynaecological laparoscopy. The Report of the Working Party of the Confidential Enquiry into Gynaecological Laparoscopy*. London: Royal College of Obstetricians and Gynaecologists.
Cheng VS (1976) Ureteral injury resulting from laparoscopic fulguation of endometriosis implants. *American Journal of Obstetrics and Gynecology* **126:** 1045–1047.
Chong AP & Baggish MS (1984) Management of pelvic endometriosis by means of intra-abdominal CO_2 laser. *Fertility and Sterility* **41**(1): 14–19.
Daniell JF (1984) Laser laparoscopy for endometriosis. *Colposcopy Gynaecolic & Laser Surgery* **1:** 185–192.
Daniell JF & Brown DH (1982) Carbon dioxide laser laparoscopy: initial experience in experimental animals and humans. *Obstetrics and Gynecology* **59:** 761.
Daniell JF & Feste JR (1985) Laser laparoscopy. In Keye WR (ed.) *Laser Surgery in Gynaecology and Obstetrics*, pp 147–163. Boston: G K Hall.
Davis GD (1986) Management of endometriosis and its associated adhesions with the carbon dioxide laser laparoscope. *Obstetrics and Gynecology* **68:** 422–425.
DeCherney AH, Kort H, Barner JB et al (1980) Increased pregnancy rate with oil soluble hysterosalpingography dye. *Fertility and Sterility* **33:** 407–409.
Dmowski WP & Cohen MR (1978) Antigonadotrophin (danazol) in the treatment of endometriosis. Evaluation of post-treatment fertility and three-year follow-up data. *American Journal of Obstetrics and Gynecology* **130:** 41.
Donnez J (1987) Carbon dioxide laser laparoscopy in infertile women with endometriosis and women with adnexal adhesions. *Fertility and Sterility* **48:** 390–394.
Doyle JB & Des Rosiers JJ (1963) Paracervical uterine denervation for relief of pelvic pain. *Clinical Obstetrics and Gynecology* **6:** 742–753.
Fahraeus L, Larsson-Cohn U, Ljungberg S & Wallentin L (1984) Profound alterations of the lipo-protein metabolism during danazol treatment in premenopausal women. *Fertility and Sterility* **42:** 52–57.
Feste JR (1985) Laser laparoscopy. *Journal of Reproductive Medicine* **30:** 414.

Greenblatt RB & Tzingounis V (1979) Danazol treatment of endometriosis: Long-term follow-up. *Fertility and Sterility* **32:** 518.
Guzick DS & Rock JA (1983) A comparison of Danazol and conservative surgery for the treatment of infertility due to mild to moderate endometriosis. *Fertility and Sterility* **40:** 580–584.
Haney AF, Misukonis MA & Weinberg JB (1983) Macrophages and infertility: Oviductal macrophages as potential mediators of infertility. *Fertility and Sterility* **39:** 310.
Ingersoll F & Meigs JV (1948) Presacral neurectomy for dysmenorrhoea. *New England Journal of Medicine* **238:** 357.
Jansen R & Russell P (1986) Nonpigmented endometriosis: Clinical, laparoscopic and pathologic definition. *American Journal of Obstetrics and Gynecology* **155:** 1154–1159.
Jelly RJ (1987) Multicentre open comparative study of buserilin and danazol in the treatment of endometriosis. *British Journal of Clinical Practice* **41** (supplement 48): 64–68.
Keye WR & Dixon J (1983) Photocoagulation of endometriosis by the argon laser through the laparoscope. *Obstetrics and Gynecology* **62**(3): 383–386.
Lichten EM & Bombard J (1987) Surgical treatment of primary dysmenorrhoea with laparoscopic uterine nerve ablation. *Journal of Reproductive Medicine* **32**(1): 37–41.
Lilford RJ & Dalton ME (1987) Effectiveness of treatment for infertility. *British Medical Journal* **295:** 6591.
Malinak LR & Wheeler JM (1985) Association of endometriosis with spontaneous abortion; prognosis for pregnancy and risk of recurrence. *Seminars in Reproductive Endocrinology* **3:** 361–369.
Martin DC (1985) Carbon dioxide laser laparoscopy for the treatment of endometriosis associated with infertility. *Journal of Reproductive Medicine* **30:** 409–412.
Matta WH et al (1987) Hypogonadism induced by luteinising hormone releasing hormone agonist analogues: effects of bone density in premenopausal women. *British Medical Journal* **294:** 1523–1524.
Meigs JV (1938) Endometriosis, a possible aetiological factor. *Surgery, Gynaecology and Obstetrics* **67:** 253 (editorial).
Meyer R (1919) Uber den Staude der Frage der adenomyosites Adenoma in allgemeinen und Adenomyometitis Sarcomastosa. *Zentralblatt fur Gynakologie* **36:** 745–759.
Nezhat C, Crowgey SR & Garrison CP (1986) Surgical treatment of endometriosis via laser laparoscopy. *Fertility and Sterility* **45:** 778–783.
Nezhat C, Winer W & Nezhat F (1988) A comparison of the carbon-dioxide, Argon and KTP/532 lasers in the videolaseroscopic treatment of endometriosis. *Colposcopy Gynaecologic & Laser Surgery* **4:** 41–47.
Nezhat C, Winer W, Crowgey S & Nezhat F (1989) Videolaseroscopy for endometriosis. *Fertility and Sterility* **51:** 237–240.
Nisolle M (1988) Utero-sacral biopsy in women with pelvic pain. In Donnez J (ed.) *Operative laser laparoscopy and hysteroscopy*. Belgium: Nauvelaerts Publishers.
O'Connor DT (1987) Endometriosis. In Singer A & Jordan JA (eds) *Current Reviews in Obstetrics and Gynaecology*. Edinburgh: Churchill Livingstone.
Olive DL & Haney AF (1986) Endometriosis-associated infertility: a critical review of therapeutic approaches. *Obstetrical and Gynaecological Survey* **41:** 538–555.
Olive DL & Lee KL (1986) Analysis of sequential treatment protocols for endometriosis associated infertility. *American Journal of Obstetrics and Gynecology* **154:** 613–619.
Olive DL, Stohs GF, Metzger DA et al (1985) Expectant management and hydrotubations in the treatment of endometriosis associated with infertility. *Fertility and Sterility* **44:** 35.
Polan ML & DeCherney A (1980) Presacral neurectomy for pelvic pain in infertility. *Fertility and Sterility* **34:** 557.
Puleo JG & Hammond CB (1983) Conservative treatment of endometriosis externa: The effects of danazol therapy. *Fertility and Sterility* **40:** 164.
Redwine DB (1987) Age-related evolution in colour appearance of endometriosis. *Fertility and Sterility* **48:** 1062.
Reich H & McGlynn F (1986) Treatment of ovarian endometriomas using laparoscopic surgical techniques. *Journal of Reproductive Medicine* **31:** 577–584.
Rock JA, Guzick DS, Sengos C et al (1981) The conservative surgical treatment of endometriosis: Evaluation of pregnancy success with respect to the extent of disease as categorized using contemporary classification systems. *Fertility and Sterility* **35:** 131.

Sampson JA (1927a) Peritoneal endometriosis due to menstrual dissemination of endometrial tissue into peritoneal cavity. *American Journal of Obstetrics and Gynaecology* **14:** 422.
Sampson JA (1927b) Metastatic or embolic endometriosis due to menstrual dissemination of endometrial tissue into the venous circulation. *American Journal of Pathology* **18:** 571–592.
Schneider GT (1983) Endometriosis: an update. In Studd JWW (ed.) *Progress in Obstetrics and Gynaecology*, vol. 3, pp 246–256. Edinburgh: Churchill Livingstone.
Semm K & Mettler L (1980) Technical progress in pelvic surgery via operative laparoscopy. *American Journal of Obstetrics and Gynecology* **138:** 121–127.
Shaw RW (1988) LHRH analogues in the treatment of endometriosis—comparative results with other treatments. *Bailliere's Clinical Obstetrics and Gynaecology* **2**(3): 659–676.
Stillman RJ & Miller LC (1984) DES exposure in utero and endometriosis in infertile females. *Fertility and Sterility* **41**(3): 369–372.
Sutton CJG (1985) Initial experience with carbon dioxide laser laparoscopy. *Lasers in Medical Science.* **1:** 25–31.
Sutton CJG (1989a) The treatment of endometriosis. In Studd JWW (ed.) *Progress in Obstetrics and Gynaecology*. London: Churchill Livingstone, in press.
Sutton CJG (1989b) Laser laparoscopic uterine nerve ablation. In Donnez J (ed.) *Operative laser laparoscopy and hysteroscopy*. Louvain, Belgium: Nauwelaerts Publishers.
Sulewski JM, Curcio FD, Bronitsky C et al (1980) The treatment of endometriosis at laparoscopy for infertility. *American Journal of Obstetrics and Gynecology* **138:** 128.
Tadir Y, Kaplan I & Zuckerman K (1981) A second puncture probe for laser laparoscopy. In Atsumi K & Nimsakul N (eds) *Laser Surgery IV, Proceedings of the Fourth Congress of the International Society for Laser Surgery*, pp 25–26. Tokyo: Japanese Society for Laser Medicine.
Thomas EJ & Cooke ID (1987a) Impact of gestrinone on the course of asymptomatic endometriosis. *British Medical Journal* **294:** 272–274.
Thomas EJ & Cooke ID (1987b) Successful treatment of endometriosis: does it benefit infertile women? *British Medical Journal* **294:** 1117–1119.
Tucker AW (1947) Evaluation of pre-sacral neurectomy in the treatment of dysmenorrhoea. *American Journal of Obstetrics and Gynecology* **53:** 226.
Vernon MW, Beard JS, Graves K & Wilson EA (1986) Classification of endometriotic implants by morphologic appearance and capacity to synthesise prostaglandin F. *Fertility and Sterility* **46:** 801–806.
White JC (1952) Conduction of visceral pain. *New England Journal of Medicine* **246:** 686.

5

CO_2 laser laparoscopic surgery

Adhesiolysis, salpingostomy, laser uterine nerve ablation and tubal pregnancy

J. DONNEZ
M. NISOLLE

Laser endoscopy has been in established use in otolaryngology and gastroenterology for some years and is currently being investigated for clinical use in orthopaedics, urology, and gynaecology. Prototype instruments for CO_2 laser laparoscopy were developed independently on three continents (by Bruhat et al, 1979; Tadir et al, 1981; Daniell and Brown, 1982; Kelly and Roberts, 1983). The initial prototypes proved to be inadequate because of loss of carbon dioxide, accumulation of intraperitoneal smoke, and inability to keep the beam focused in the centre of the channel. With the development of new laparoscopic instrumentation for CO_2 laser use, the majority of these technical problems have now been overcome.

INSTRUMENTATION AND OPERATIONAL INSTRUCTIONS

Single puncture laser laparoscopy

The operating laparoscope for laser laparoscopy is 12 mm in diameter with a 7.3 mm operating channel (Eder, USA; Wolff, Storz, West Germany). To use the CO_2 laser through the laparoscope, the operator simply attaches the articulated arm of the laser to the black coupler containing the alignment mirror and focusing lens which transmits the laser beam through the operating channel of the laparoscope (Figure 1).

The laser coupling assembly (Figure 2) consists of the following:

1. Coupler housing:
   (a) joystick control for manual adjustment of the laser beam within the lumen of the laparoscope tube;
   (b) screw thread for quick and easy attachment and release of the laparoscope tube.

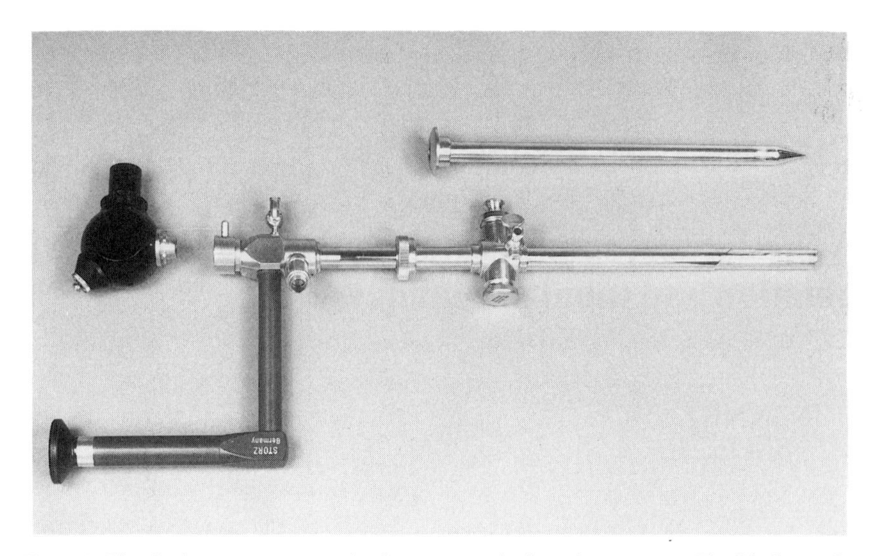

Figure 1. The single-puncture operating laparoscope for laser laparoscopy. The black coupler containing the alignment mirror and focusing lens is attached to the operative channel of the laparoscope.

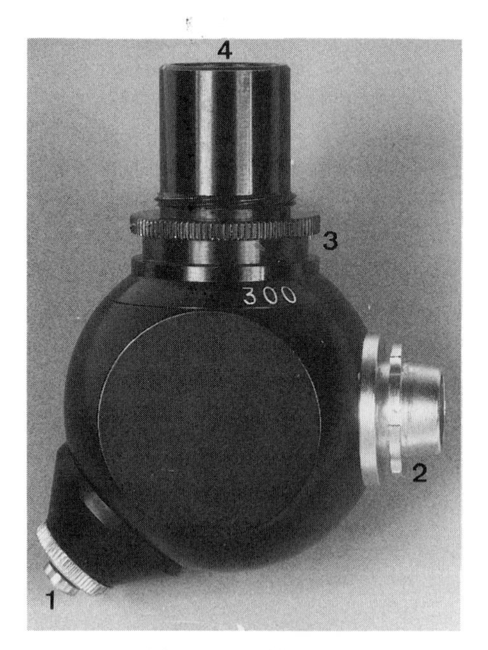

Figure 2. Laser coupler assembly: (1) joystick, (2) tube attachment, (3) lens, (4) laser arm attachment.

2. Interchangeable lens housing:
   (a) 200 mm working distance lens housing to match beam focal length to nominal length of standard second-puncture tube, giving spot size of diameter of 0.64 mm;
   (b) 300 mm working distance lens housing to match beam length to nominal length of single-puncture tube (and optional 300 mm second-puncture tube), giving spot size diameter of 0.70 mm;
   (c) each lens housing has a groove around it for convenient attachment of a sterile drape.

Laser coupler adjustments and beam focus/defocus

1. Turn on the laser system. Aim the Helium–Neon (He–Ne) beam at an appropriate thermal barrier such as a moistened tongue depressor positioned approximately 1 cm distal to the tube.
2. With the external illumination turned off, adjust the coupler joystick to obtain a full, round He–Ne spot without wall reflection effects. The halo around the He–Ne spot should be symmetrical as well. Turn the external illumination back on.
3. Viewing through the eyepiece, position the laparoscope away from the target site so that the He–Ne beam spot appears on the horizontal diameter of the viewing field, two thirds of the way to the right of the viewing field centre point, as shown in Figure 3. In this position the CO_2 beam is in focus 10 mm distal to the laparoscope tube.
4. To obtain a defocused CO_2 beam on the target site, move the laparoscope tube away from the tissue. The He–Ne beam will move towards the centre of the viewing field. At a distance of 80 mm from tissue site, the He–Ne beam spot will appear at the centre of the field of vision.

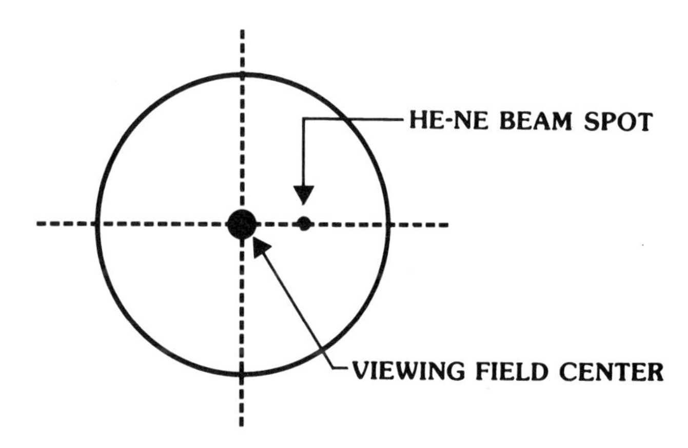

Figure 3. He–Ne beam spot two thirds of the way to the right from viewing field centre, indicating beam focus at 10 mm distal to laparoscope tube.

Smoke evacuation

To allow for the flow of fresh carbon dioxide down the beam channel, the CO_2 insufflation tubing is attached to this operating channel thus displacing smoke which can reduce the power of the beam from the laser channel and also avoids fogging the mirror and lens in the black coupler.

To evacuate smoke, a Veress needle can be inserted suprapubically under direct vision and transillumination, directing it towards the target site and connected to the smoke evacuation system. Auxiliary kits (Sharplen Industries, Tel-Aviv) are available for synchronizing smoke evacuation to laser emission, providing automatic smoke evacuation from the target site. With the automatic smoke evacuation kit installed, smoke evacuation begins with actual laser emission and remains active 3 seconds after laser emission ceases.

If smoke disturbs the field of vision, the smoke evacuation flow can be increased, taking care not to cause collapse of the pneumoperitoneum. The equilibrium state will be reached when the insufflation system is able to provide the amount of gas that the smoke evacuation port is releasing. If the smoke evacuation kit is installed, the expulsion of gas (smoke) can be regulated using a sterile infusion drip kit.

Second-puncture probes

The second-puncture probe currently used for combining the CO_2 laser with the laparoscope is a double-ring probe, 8 mm in external diameter with a 5.6 mm operating channel. The second-puncture laparoscope is based on two concentric tubes. The inner tube contains the operating channel and the insufflation port as well as the locking device for securing it to the outer tube. Two distinct outer tubes are provided: open-ended and with a backstop (adhesiolysis probe) (Figure 4). The outer tube includes a smoke evacuation port with stopcock. This assembly provides the user with a double-lumen, second-puncture laparoscope that is easily disassembled for cleaning. The adhesiolysis outer tube is recommended for use in clinical situations that require a backstop to protect healthy tissue beyond the treatment site. The probe attaches to the same laser coupler assembly that is used with the operative laparoscope using a 200 mm focal length lens.

Wave guides (Figure 5)

Rigid stainless steel CO_2 laser probes (outer diameter 4.9 mm) have been developed recently (Baggish and Elbakry, 1986; Tadir et al, 1988). The probe is attached to the articulated arm of a CO_2 laser system. Optical transmission through these probes is not affected by manipulating the articulated arm. A conventionally used He–Ne aiming beam is coaxially transmitted through the probe. The short focal length (focal length >0.4 mm <2 cm from the probe top) yields a beam that defocuses within a small distance beyond the focal plane. This is expressed by a sharp drop of power density and may serve as an optical backstop.

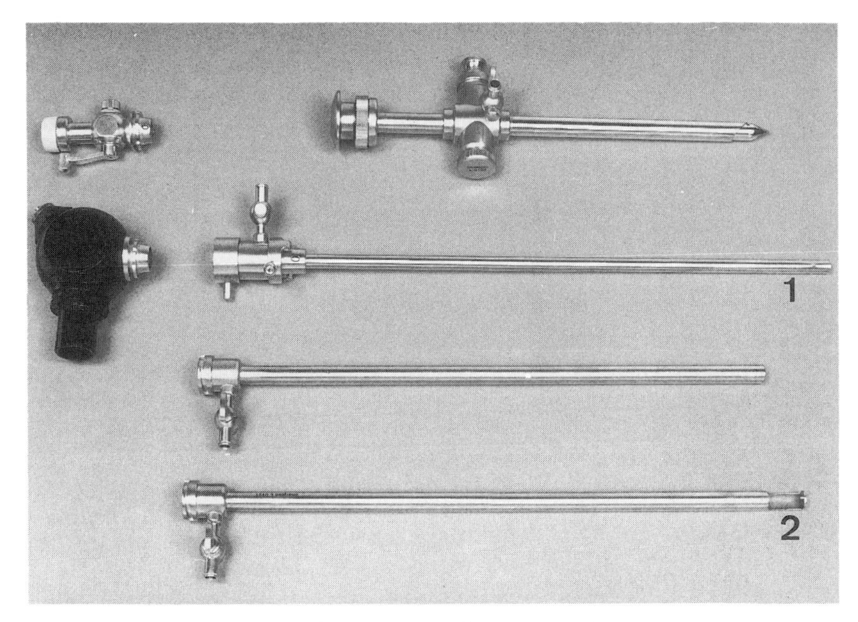

Figure 4. Second-puncture probes. (1) Open-end. (2) Hook-tipped.

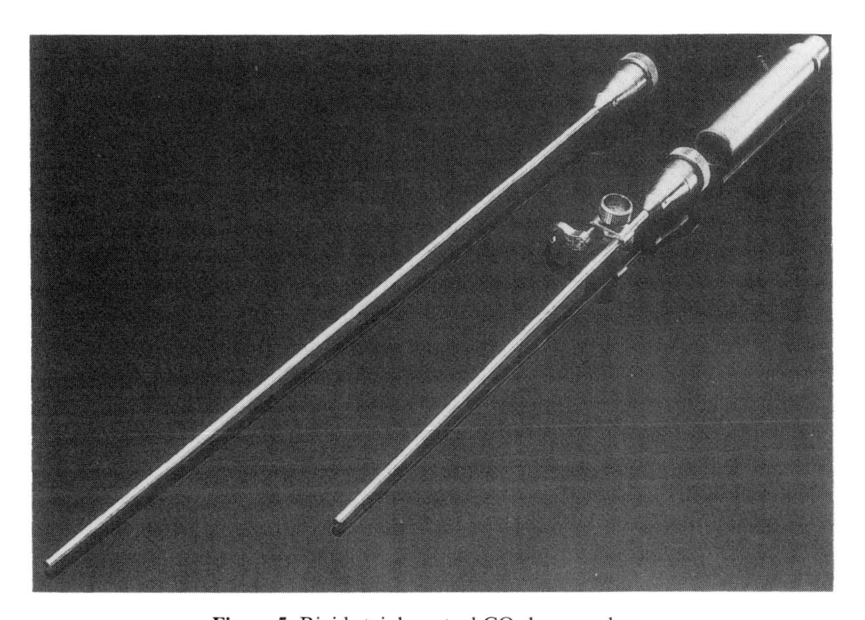

Figure 5. Rigid stainless steel CO_2 laser probes.

Accessories (second- and third-puncture probes) (Figure 6)

The following operating instruments were developed in our department.

1. Atraumatic probe.
2. Hook for fimbrioplasty.

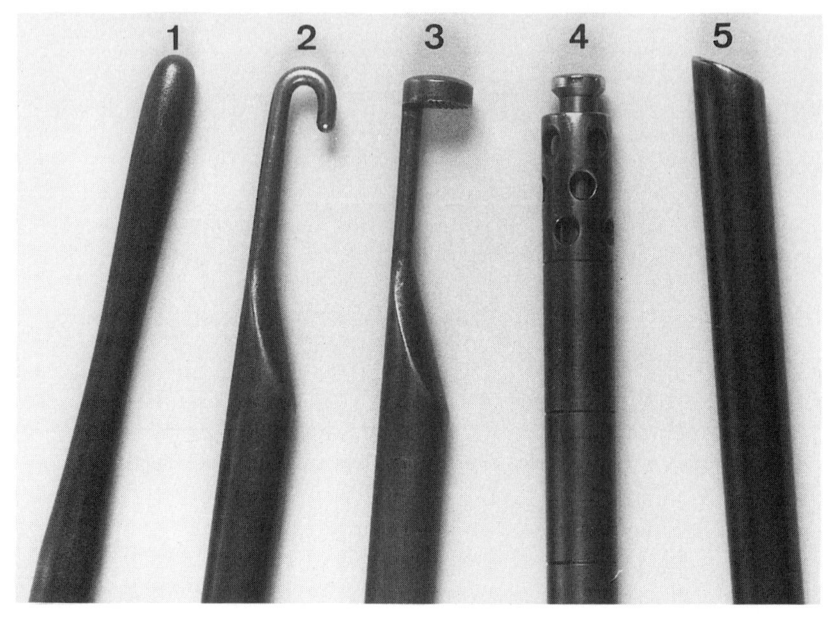

Figure 6. Third-puncture probes. (1) Atraumatic probe. (2) Hook for fimbrioplasty. (3) Probe with backstop. (4) Smoke suction and rinsing tube. (5) Double-channel probe for rinsing and suction.

3. Probe with backstop for use in vaporizing adhesions near the blood vessels.
4. Smoke suction and irrigation tube.
5. Double-channel probe for suction and irrigation of the pelvis.

CLINICAL APPLICATIONS FOR CARBON DIOXIDE LASER LAPAROSCOPY

The most frequent procedures carried out with CO_2 laser laparoscope include:

1. Vaporization of peritoneal and ovarian endometriosis.
2. Pelvic adhesiolysis, salpingolysis and ovariolysis.
3. Utero-sacral ligament ablation.
4. Fimbrioplasty and salpingostomy.
5. Salpingotomy in cases of tubal pregnancy.
6. Vaporization of small uterine fibroids.

1450 CO_2 laser laparoscopies were carried out in our department between July 1983 and December 1988. The most frequent indication is endometriosis (Table 1); mild, moderate and severe endometriosis can be treated. Endometriosis is discussed in detail in Chapter 4.

Table 1. Indications for CO_2 laser laparoscopy. From Université Catholique de Louvain, Brussels.

Indications	Number of patients
Laser neurectomy	151
Tuboplasty	212
Fimbrioplasty	169
Neosalpingostomy	43
Endometriosis	735
Mild (peritoneal only)	354
Moderate (ovarian endometrioma) } Severe (ovarian endometrioma)	381
Pelvic adhesions	382
Salpingolysis	172
Salpingo-ovariolysis	210
Tubal pregnancy	20
	1450

Adhesiolysis

In many patients, postoperative or postinfectious adhesions are amenable to vaporization by laser laparoscopy. When compared to the standard technique with cautery and the use of laparoscopic scissors or blunt dissection, there is probably no difference in the outcome when the adhesions are small and avascular. With more vascular adhesions or particularly thick tubo-ovarian adhesions, however, the CO_2 laser allows more precise destruction of the adhesions with minimal injury to the adjacent normal tissue. Filmy peritubular and periovarian adhesions are easily vaporized with the operative laser laparoscope. The adhesiolysis probe with its backstop should be used to make the procedure safer.

The adhesion is positioned across the 'firing' platform when the laser is activated to prevent damage to any tissues distal to the adhesion (Figure 7). Using a power output of 25 W (power density of 7500 W/cm^2), adhesions can be both coagulated and incised. For beginners, single or repeat-pulse modes should be used for laser vaporization of adhesions until confidence in the technique is gained. Short exposure times of 0.05 or 0.10 s are usually adequate to vaporize the adhesions around the fallopian tubes and ovaries and will prevent the laser beam from penetrating to a depth of more than 100–200 μm. Great care should be taken when dividing adhesions between the tube and the ovary because this area is very vascular and accidental venepuncture with the laser beam can cause troublesome bleeding which can be difficult to stop in this location due to the proximity of the fallopian tube.

Salpingolysis is usually performed by applying traction to adhesions with atraumatic grasping forceps placed suprapubically and by another probe

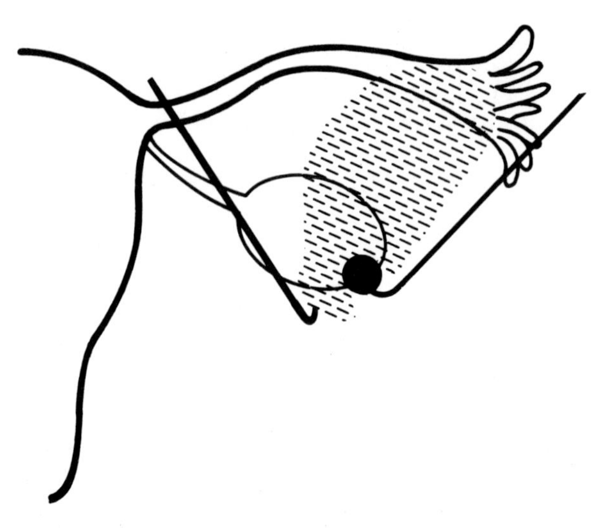

Figure 7. Filmy peritubal and periovarian adhesions. When the probe with its backstop is used, the adhesion is placed across the 'firing' platform and the laser is fired to vaporize the band.

(smooth manipulating probe, hook, probe with its backstop) (Figure 8). Frequently, adhesions are incised without the need of a separate backstop but the surgeon must be constantly aware of the anatomy of the situation for laser energy will continue to vaporize tissue until the energy is absorbed. Manipulating the fallopian tube should be avoided as much as possible.

Ovariolysis is performed by applying torsion to the utero-ovarian ligaments with atraumatic tubal forceps. Elevation and rotation of the ovary is made while continuing traction and torsion (Figure 9). Adhesions can be easily dissected from the ovarian surface by superficial vaporization. Care must also be taken not to apply too much traction, for fear of tearing the ovarian ligament from its attachment which can result in copious bleeding that can only be stopped by haemostatic clips or endocoagulation.

Precautions

1. During adhesiolysis, the use of the probe with a backstop eliminates the risk of inadvertent injury to other intraperitoneal structures, particularly bowel.
2. Irrigation fluid can be introduced into the pelvis as an aquatic backstop to protect the bowel from inadvertent damage by scatter of the laser beam.
3. At the end of the procedure, the peritoneal cavity is irrigated with heparinized Ringer's solution to remove carbonized particles. Thereafter, following the removal of fluid from the cul-de-sac, 100–200 cm^3 of 32% dextran 70 is instilled into the peritoneal cavity, as previously reported by Donnez and Casanas-Roux (1986) describing microsurgical techniques by laparoscopy.

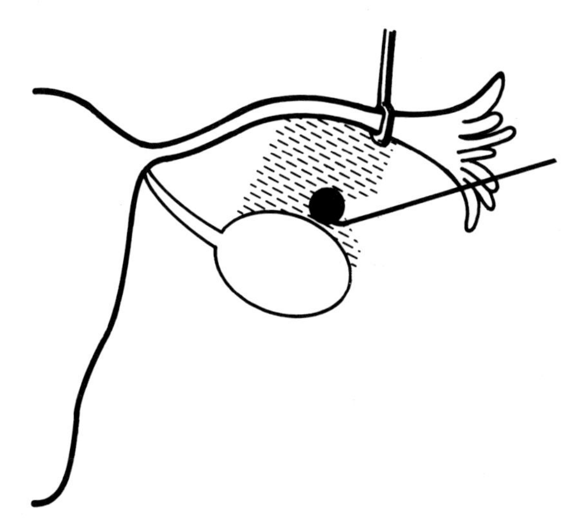

Figure 8. Salpingolysis: traction to adhesions is applied by atraumatic grasping forceps and another probe.

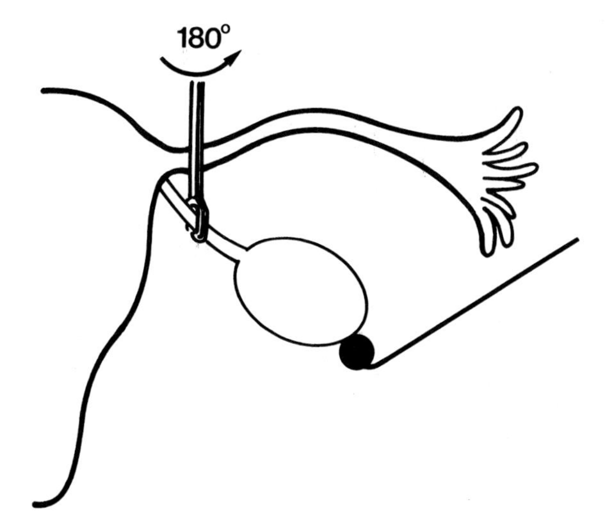

Figure 9. Ovariolysis: elevation and rotation of the ovary by applying torsion to the utero-ovarian ligament with the atraumatic forceps.

Results

In our series of 186 infertile patients followed over 18 months after adhesiolysis for degree I (filmy and avascular) and degree II (dense and vascular) adhesions, pregnancy rates were 64 and 50% respectively (Table 2).

Table 2. Results of CO_2 laser laparoscopy in infertility. Viable pregnancy rate in 311 patients for a follow-up period of 18 months. From Université Catholique de Louvain, Brussels.

	Number of patients	Number of pregnancies
Adhesiolysis		
Degree I	102	65 (64%)
Degree II	84	43 (50%)
Total	186	108 (58%)
Fimbrioplasty	100	61 (61%)
Neosalpingostomy	25	5 (20%)

Second-look

The finding of carbon black pigments at the site of laser vaporization probably results from insufficient irrigation of the pelvic cavity. Nevertheless, no adhesions were found around the deposits re-epithelialized by the peritoneal surface. The absence of lymphocyte infiltration suggested complete healing without any inflammatory reaction. In an experimental study (Donnez et al, 1987a, b) mouse ovaries were vaporized to evaluate both the formation of adhesions and luteal function. When microsurgical techniques such as glass rods and irrigation were used, complete ovarian healing without sequelae occurred a few weeks after laser vaporization and ovarian function was unaltered.

Other advantages found in the study were: (i) The precision achieved by the CO_2 laser allows the experienced operator to vaporize adhesions close to the ureter or even on the bowel. (ii) The magnification obtained with the laparoscope and the precision of the CO_2 laser allow precise removal of diseased tissue in many sites often unapproachable by electrocautery.

In cases of laser adhesiolysis, the pregnancy rate is similar to that obtained after microsurgical salpingolysis by laparotomy. However, laser procedures cannot replace microsurgical procedures where the indications remain true. Laser procedure permits incision of numerous adhesions by laparoscopy, but adhesiolysis of very dense and fibrous adhesions (degree III) between the fimbria and the ovary must be carried out by microsurgical procedures.

In our series of 1500 infertile women operated on with the CO_2 laser laparoscope, no case required laparotomy for bleeding and no bladder or bowel injury was reported. During the operation, some technical difficulties arose due to smoke obscuring the He–Ne beam or due to back-strain associated with operating directly through the laparoscope. One problem is associated with the high intensity of the light source necessary for photographic purposes which obscures the visibility of the He–Ne beam. To avoid back-strain it is often helpful to operate directly from the video monitoring system.

We believe that in selected patients, CO_2 laser laparoscopy will become the preferred procedure for resection of postoperative or postinfectious adhesions. Very dense adhesions are still best treated by conventional microsurgical techniques.

Neosalpingostomy and fimbrioplasty

The results of microsurgical salpingostomy for hydrosalpinx are poor (Donnez and Casanas-Roux, 1986). At best a 20–30% term pregnancy rate is generally reported. CO_2 laser laparoscopic salpingostomy therefore seemed a reasonable alternative in selected patients who desired pregnancy but did not wish to undergo a major surgical procedure for hydrosalpinx.

Laparoscopic salpingostomy is more complicated than the microsurgical procedure, and its use is still controversial. It can be performed with the CO_2 laser and is indicated in cases of thin wall hydrosalpinx where proximal tubal patency has been confirmed by hysterosalpingogram (Figure 10A). Routine steps preceding laparoscopic salpingostomy must include cervical cannulation to provide a route for the intraoperative injection of dye to distend the tubes. Two grasping forceps are introduced for traction and manipulation at

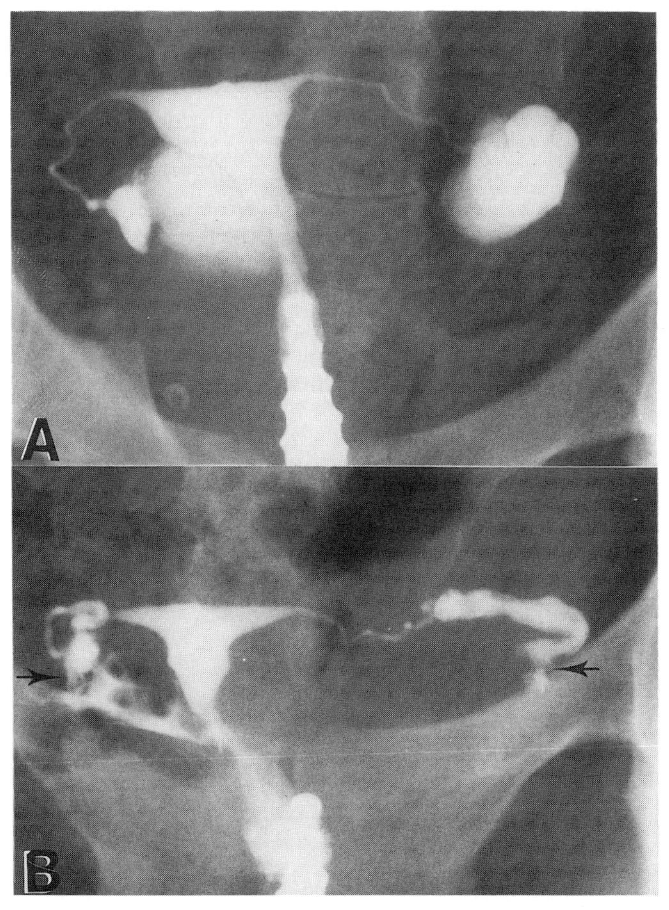

Figure 10. Hysterosalpingography: (A) hydrosalpinx; (B) three months after CO_2 laser laparoscopic salpingostomy.

the ampullary–fimbrial segment. The blocked tube is held so that the focused laser beam can be aligned at 90° to the dimple (Figure 11). The laser is set on continuous mode at 25 W (power density 7000 W/cm^{-2}) and two linear incisions are made, cutting from anterior to posterior along the blood vessels. As soon as the lumen is entered, the tube collapses, and continuous dye injection keeps it distended. Only then is the incision enlarged. At this point, the grasping forceps gently hold the incision edges and a reduced power, defocused beam is used to contract and evert the serosal aspect of the incised edge. In an initial series of 20 patients (Daniell and Feste, 1985) a 6-week postoperative patency rate of 80% was achieved. Three intrauterine pregnancies, one ectopic pregnancy, and one spontaneous abortion were obtained.

In our department, hysterosalpingography was systematically performed 3 months after the procedure. Recovery of a normal tubal pattern was found (Figure 10B) when postoperative patency was achieved. The same postoperative patency rate was achieved with an intrauterine pregnancy rate of 20% in a first series of 25 patients. This rate is similar to that obtained by laparotomy and microsurgery (Donnez and Casanas-Roux, 1986). Additional follow-up of these patients is necessary before any conclusions concerning the efficacy of this new operative procedure are possible, but CO_2 laser salpingostomy is likely to be the ideal procedure for management of patients with large, thin-walled hydrosalpinx.

We also carry out fimbrioplasty during laparoscopy. If fimbrial adhesions are found when the blue dye begins to spill through the open tube, these adhesions between fimbrial folds are carefully grasped with the probe with a hook passed through a third-puncture trocar and cut in a bloodless fashion with the finely focused CO_2 beam set at about 20 W (6500 W/cm^{-2}) (Figure 12). By pulling the probe back from the tissue 4–5 cm, the beam is defocused and then aimed at the peritoneum of the fimbrial folds, a few millimeters

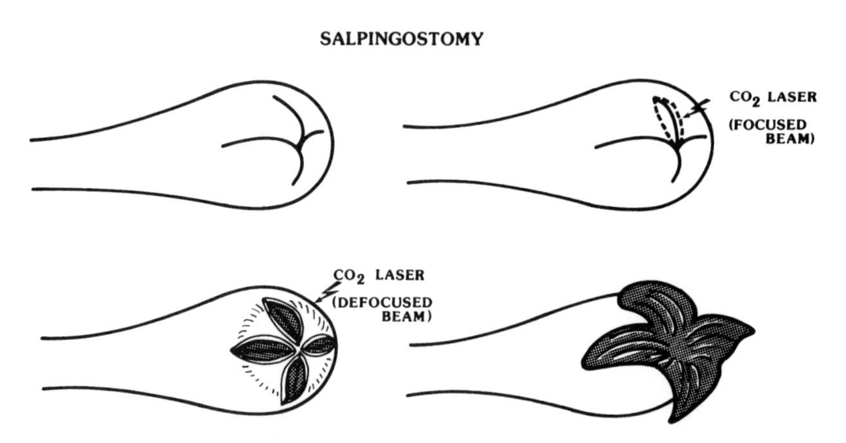

Figure 11. Salpingostomy for hydrosalpinx. The finely focused CO_2 beam is fired to open the fallopian tube. The beam is then defocused and aimed at the peritoneum of the fimbrial folds, a few millimeters proximal to the incised edges, to cause contraction of the serosa.

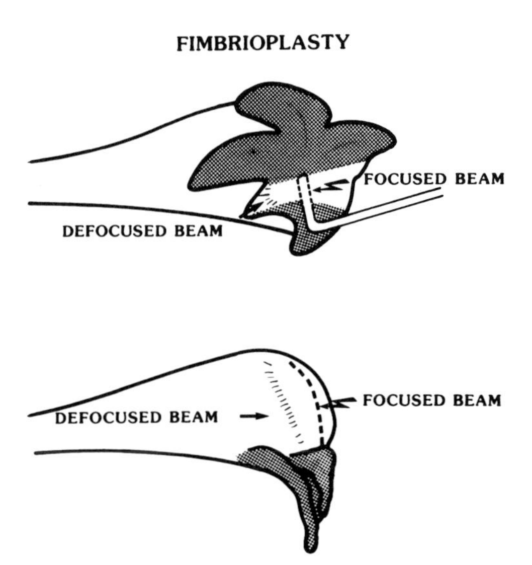

Figure 12. Fimbrioplasty: (a) fimbrial adhesions; (b) phymotic ostium.

proximal to the incised edges, to cause contraction of the serosa. It is usually sufficient just to cause blanching of the serosa to obtain the desired effect, this allows adequate eversion of the mucosa and avoids recurrence of adhesions. The postoperative pregnancy rate is 61% in a first series of 100 patients. This rate is similar to that obtained in a series of 142 fimbrioplasties carried out by microsurgery (Donnez and Casanas-Roux, 1986).

Utero-sacral neurectomy

The excision of utero-sacral ligaments adjacent to the cervix has been used as a treatment for dysmenorrhoea and dyspareunia (Daniell and Feste, 1985; Sutton, 1985). The vaporization of the utero-sacral ligaments at their attachment to the posterior portion of the cervix is a simple and rapid procedure with the operative laser laparoscope or laser probe. A segment 2–3 cm long and 1 cm in depth is vaporized over the vascular portion of the ligament (Figure 13). It is important to vaporize more medially than laterally, however, because of vessels located just lateral to the attachment of utero-sacral ligament. This technique essentially destroys the sensory nerve fibres and the secondary ganglia within the ligaments. The procedure takes less than 10 minutes to perform.

Results in a series of 100 patients who had been followed for more than 1 year are as follows: complete relief or symptoms was found in 50% of cases; mild or moderate relief of dysmenorrhoea or dyspareunia occurred in 41% of cases; in 9% of patients, no relief was found.

In a series of 136 patients with laparoscopically diagnosed endometriosis, biopsies were taken from peritoneal endometriotic implants (positive sites,

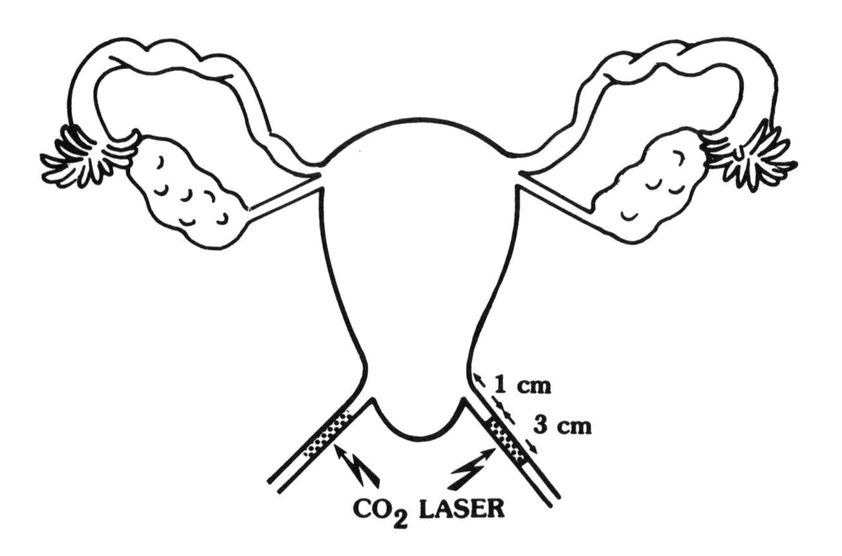

Figure 13. Vaporization of the utero-sacral ligaments. A segment 2–3 cm long and 1 cm in depth is vaporized over the vascular portion of the ligament.

$n = 99$) and/or from the visually normal peritoneum of the utero-sacral ligaments (negative sites, $n = 71$). Histology revealed the presence of both endometrial epithelium and stroma in 93% of positive sites and in 13% of negative sites (Nisolle, 1988).

In another group of 43 women with pelvic pain, endometriosis was diagnosed by laparoscopy in 26 of them. In the 17 remaining patients, no endometriosis was suspected macroscopically elsewhere in the pelvis. Nevertheless, biopsies taken from completely normal uterosacral ligaments revealed the presence of microscopic endometriosis in two cases (11%) (Nisolle, 1988). This study could be the rationale for vaporizing uterosacral ligaments (LUNA) in all women suffering from pelvic pain with or without endometriosis.

It seems that in the absence of any demonstrable pathology, relief of symptoms can be accomplished in many patients by this simple technique. On several occasions, patients who have had laparoscopic laser neurectomy have had subsequent laparoscopy and examination of the neurectomy site has shown reperitonealization without any substantial adhesion formation. Further investigation of this rapid procedure is continuing to prove the long-term efficacy. Controlled and randomized prospective trials carried out carefully over the next few years will clearly define the place of laser neurectomy in the treatment of dysmenorrhoea.

Linear salpingotomy for tubal pregnancy

In addition to the indications for the laser laparoscope previously discussed, there are other occasional situations in which the controlled destruction of tissue is possible with the proper focused CO_2 laser beam.

Linear salpingotomy for tubal pregnancy and ablation of small uterine fibroids and ovarian fibromas can be easily performed with the CO_2 laser. Unruptured tubal pregnancy can be treated laparoscopically with the CO_2 laser, especially if it is located on the ampullary segment. A longitudinal incision is made on the side opposite to the mesosalpinx, using a focused beam (Figure 14). After irrigation, removal of products of conception is performed with a suction cannula. If bleeding is observed after aspiration, haemostasis is achieved by compression with atraumatic forceps or by application of a bipolar coagulator or by injection of vasopressin solution (5 IU diluted in 20 ml of sterile saline solution) into the mesosalpinx. The salpingotomy is left open. An intraperitoneal drain is left in the pouch of Douglas for 24 h.

In our department, most tubal pregnancies are treated using laparoscopic techniques as described by Bruhat et al (1980). With the use of 7 mm Triton (Microfrance) a 10–15 mm incision is made in the antimesenteric portion of the haematosalpinx with the retractable monopolar needle electrode. Vasopressin is injected into the broad ligament only in case of persistent bleeding. This procedure is necessary in less than 5% of cases, reducing the risk of side-effects induced by this drug. In a first series of 300 tubal pregnancies, bleeding at the site of the salpingotomy occurred in two cases (± 300 ml) in the immediate (<2 h) postoperative period. No laparotomy was necessary. The bleeding stopped spontaneously. The presence of a suction catheter in the pouch of Douglas allowed drainage and evaluation of the amount of blood loss. Failures of treatment occurred in two cases (0.66%) secondary to incomplete removal of the trophoblast and required a laparotomy with conservative treatment. These two failures occurred in the first 50 patients. Concentrations of human chorionic gonadotrophin (HCG) were not controlled in the postoperative period in this group of patients.

The postoperative follow-up evaluation period now includes HCG assay, 48 h and 72 h after the laparoscopic procedure. If the HCG concentration remains higher than 60% of the prelaparoscopy value after 2 or 3 days, methotrexate (40 mg/IM) is administered. If the HCG concentration is greater than 20% of the initial value 4 days later, methotrexate is given again intramuscularly. In our series, injection of methotrexate was necessary in 15 cases (5%) (Figure 15). The control of HCG is continued until it is undetectable (<5 mUI/ml), and this systematic control meant that neither a second laparoscopic procedure nor a laparotomy was necessary for removing residual trophoblast.

Hysterosalpingography (HSG) was performed 3 months after the procedure. Among 120 patients who wished to become pregnant, an intrauterine pegnancy rate of 63% was achieved. Recurrent tubal pregnancy occurred in 8% of cases (Table 3). In a group of 18 women with a history of microsurgical tuboplasty, the postoperative intrauterine pregnancy rate was lower and the recurrent tubal pregnancy rate was higher than those observed in the group of women without a history of infertility.

Among patients with a 'solitary' tube, the intrauterine pregnancy rate is

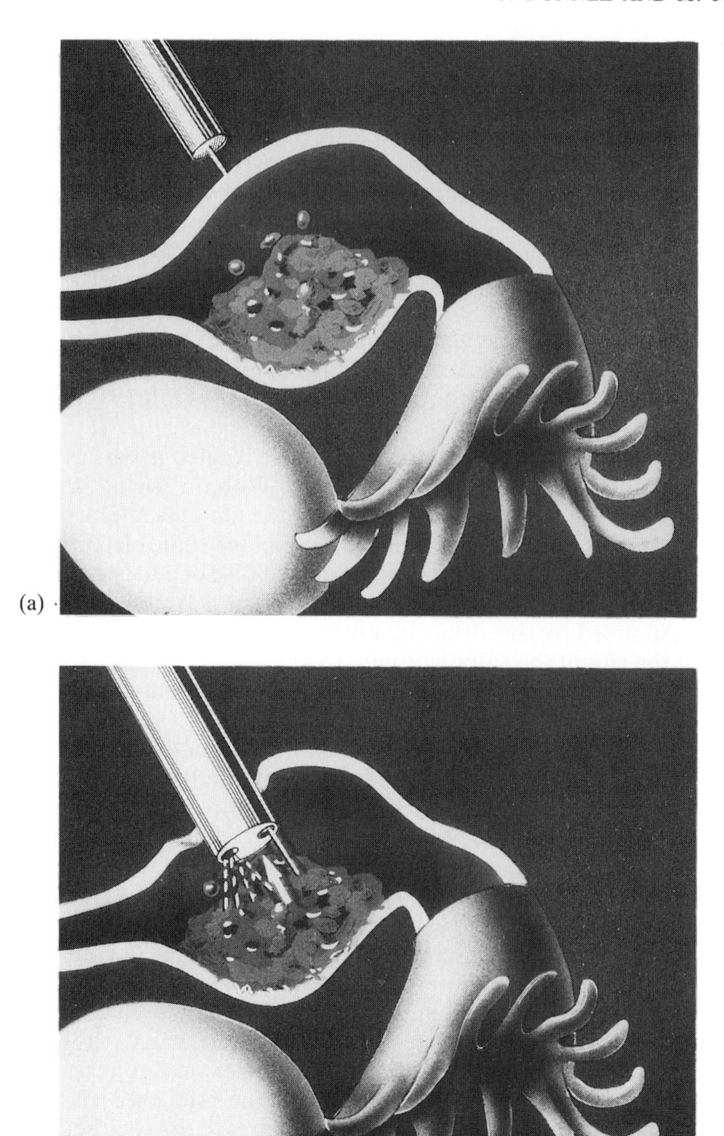

Figure 14. Salpingotomy in a case of unruptured tubal pregnancy. (a) Incision in the antimesenteric area of the dilated ampullary portion (proximal site). (b) Irrigation with saline solution for rinsing the tubal lumen and removal of trophoblast by suction.

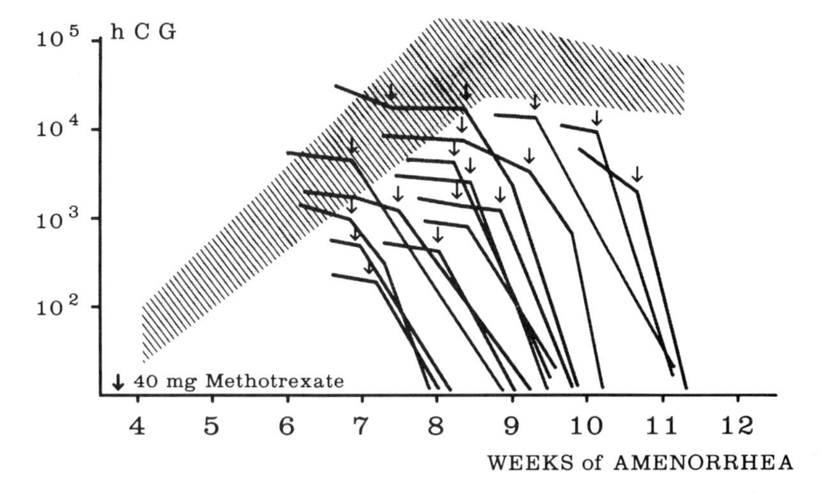

Figure 15. Concentrations of HCG in 15 patients after administration (↓) of methotrexate (40 mg/iM) for persistently high HCG concentrations after trophoblast removal.

Table 3. Postoperative fertility after conservative management of unruptured ampullary tubal pregnancy by laparoscopy.

	Number of patients	Intrauterine pregnancy	Ectopic pregnancy
No history of infertility	120	65 (63%)	10 (8%)
After microsurgical tuboplasty	18	5 (27%)	4 (22%)*

* ($p < 0.005$)

52% (11/21) with a recurrent tubal pregnancy rate of 22% (5/21). In our department (see Table 1) the incision was carried out most frequently with the needle electrode and not with the CO_2 laser beam. Indeed preliminary results from experimental data show no significant difference in the subsequent healing process. For the sake of safety, salpingotomy for tubal pregnancy, a procedure often occurring during the night, is carried out preferentially with the needle electrode.

SUMMARY

Used endoscopically, the CO_2 laser offers some advantages over other operative techniques for endometriosis and adhesions but, in spite of the continuing development of new instrumentation there are still problems with the system. The technique needs specialized equipment requiring ongoing biomedical maintenance and specialized technical care in the operating room. Some problems such as the intraperitoneal accumulation of smoke, gas leakage, and difficulty with maintenance of proper beam alignment still occur.

In spite of these problems the advantages are numerous: the system allows precise bloodless destruction of diseased tissue and eliminates the risks of cautery. In the hands of an experienced laparoscopist, it appears safe and effective in vaporization of endometriotic lesions, utero-sacral neurectomy, adhesiolysis and salpingostomy. The judicious use of these techniques, combined with carefully planned further investigations by well-trained and experienced laparoscopists and continuing improvements in the delivery systems, will soon reveal the true efficacy of the CO_2 laser laparoscope. If studies continue to show pregnancy rates and pain relief to be equivalent to those patients treated by laparotomy, CO_2 laser laparoscopy will become the preferred procedure for the management of pelvic endometriosis and its associated adhesions, distal tubal occlusion, pelvic pain and tubal pregnancy.

With the exception of using the argon laser to treat endometriosis, the selective absorption characteristic of lasers has not been greatly utilized. While the CO_2 laser is heavily absorbed by water and hence vaporizes most cells in a rather indiscriminate fashion, this is not true for other wavelengths, such as argon, Nd-YAG, KTP, krypton, xenon, copper and gold vapour lasers. The energy form of each of these lasers has different properties of penetration, absorption, reflection and heat dissipation. Many of these lasers have not yet been evaluated in human subjects. An exciting, although not new, area of possible laser application involves the use of photo-sensitizers and fluorescing agents (Dougherty et al, 1978). Some recent experimental studies (Schellhas and Schneider, 1986; Schneider et al, 1988) may lead to new therapeutic possibilities.

The surgical laser is not, however, a panacea. Only controlled trials carried out carefully over the next few years will clearly define its potential. In the meantime it is incumbent upon all of us to investigate the clinical, gynaecological and surgical applications in a careful, methodical and scientific manner.

REFERENCES

Acosta AA, Buttram CJ Jr, Besch PK et al (1973) A proposed classification of pelvic endometriosis. *Obstetrics and Gynecology* **42:** 19–24.

Baggish MS & Elbakry MM (1986) A flexible CO_2 laser fiber for operative laparoscopy. *Fertility and Sterility* **46:** 16–20.

Bruhat M, Mage G & Manhes M (1979) Use of the CO_2 laser in laparoscopy. In Kaplan I (ed.) *Proceedings of the Third International Society for Laser Surgery, September 24–28, 1979*, pp 235–238. Tel-Aviv: International Society for Laser Surgery.

Bruhat M, Manhes H, Mage G & Pouly JL (1980) Treatment of ectopic pregnancy by means of laparoscopy. *Fertility and Sterility* **33:** 411–414.

Daniell JF & Brown DH (1982) Carbon dioxide laser laparoscopy: Initial experience in experimental animals and humans. *Obstetrics and Gynecology* **59:** 761–763.

Daniell JF & Feste JR (1985) Laser laparoscopy. In Keye WR (ed.) *Laser Surgery in Gynecology and Obstetrics*, pp 147–163. Boston.
Donnez J (1984) In Donnez J (ed.) *La Trompe de Fallope: Histophysiologie normale et Pathologique*, p 105. Leuven: Nauwelaerts Printing.
Donnez J (1985) Microchirurgie et fécondation in vitro: méthodes concurrentes ou complémentaires? *Revue Medicale de Bruxelles* **6:** 627–633.
Donnez J (1987) CO_2 laser laparoscopy in infertile women with endometriosis and women with adnexal adhesions. *Fertility and Sterility* **48:** 390–394.
Donnez J (ed.) (1987) *CO_2 Laser in Intraepithelial Neoplasia and in Infertility*. Leuven: Nauwelaerts Printing.
Donnez J (1989) CO_2 laser laparoscopy in endometriosis. In Sutton C (ed.) *Lasers in Gynaecology*. London: Chapman & Hall, in press.
Donnez J & Casanas-Roux F (1986) Prognostic factors of fimbrial microsurgery. *Fertility and Sterility* **46:** 200–205.
Donnez J, Lemaire-Rubbers M, Karaman Y, Nisolle-Pochet M & Casanas-Roux F (1987a) Combined (hormonal and microsurgical) therapy in infertile women with endometriosis. *Fertilily and Sterility* **48:** 239–242.
Donnez J, Fernandez C, Willems T & Casanas-Roux F (1987b) Experimental ovarian CO_2 laser surgery. In Donnez J (ed.) *CO_2 Laser in Intraepithelial Neoplasia and in Infertility*, pp 25–31. Leuven: Nauwelaerts Printing.
Donnez J, Nisolle M & Casanas F (1989) CO_2 laser laparoscopy in infertile women with adnexel adhesions and women with tubal occlusion. *Journal of Gynecologic Surgery* **5:** 47–53.
Donnez J, Nisolle-Pochet M & Casanas-Roux F (1989) Endometriosis-associated infertility: evaluation of preoperative use of Danazol, Gestrinone and Buserelin. *International Journal of Fertility*, in press.
Dougherty TJ et al (1978) Photoradiation for the treatment of malignant tumors. *Cancer Research* **38:** 2628–2631.
Johnston M, Huether S & Dixon JA (1983) Spectrophotometric and laser doppler evaluation of normal skin and post wine stains treated with argon laser. *Lasers in Medicine and Surgery* **3:** 149–155.
Kelly RW & Roberts DK (1983) Experience with the CO_2 laser in gynecologic microsurgery. *American Journal of Obstetrics and Gynecology* **146:** 585–589.
Nezhat C, Crowgey SR & Garrison CP (1987) Surgical treatment of endometriosis via laser laparoscopy. *Fertility and Sterility* **45:** 778–783.
Nisolle M (1988) Utero-sacral biopsy in women with pelvic pain. Presented at the IIIth International Symposium on Laser Surgery, Brussels, 1988.
Nisolle M, Casanas-Roux F & Donnez J (1988) Histologic study of ovarian endometriosis after hormonal therapy. *Fertility and Sterility* **49:** 423–427.
Nisolle M, Paindaveine B, Bourdon A et al, Peritoneal endometriosis in infertile women and in women with pelvic pain. *Fertility and Sterility*, submitted.
Pouly JL, Manhes H, Mage G & Bruhat MA (1986) Conservative laparoscopic treatment of 321 ectopic pregnancies. *Fertility and Sterility* **46:** 1093–1097.
Schellhas HF & Schneider DF (1986) Hematoporphyrin derivative photoradiation therapy applied in gynecology. *Colposcopy Gynecologic & Laser Surgery* **2:** 53–58.
Schneider DF, Schellhas HF, Wesseler TA, Chen IW & Moulton BC (1988) Hematoporphyrin derivative uptake in uteri of estrogen-treated ovariectomized rats. *Colposcopy Gynecologic & Laser Surgery* **4:** 67–71.
Sutton CJG (1985) Initial experience with carbon dioxide laser laparoscopy. *Lasers in Medical Science* **1:** 25–31.
Sutton CJG (1989) Laser laparoscopic uterine nerve ablation. In Donnez J (ed.) *Operative Laser Laparoscopy and Hysteroscopy*. Belgium: Nauwelaerts Publishers.
Tadir Y, Kaplan J, Zuckerman Z et al (1981) Laparoscopic CO_2 laser sterilization. In Semm K & Mettler L (eds) *Human Reproduction*. Amsterdam.
Tadir Y, Karni Z, Fisch B & Ovadia J (1988) Carbon dioxide laser probe for operative laparoscopy. *Colposcopy Gynecologic & Laser Surgery* **4:** 87–94.

6

Fibreoptic laser laparoscopy

JAMES F. DANIELL

THE DEVELOPMENT OF FIBREOPTIC LASERS FOR LAPAROSCOPY

The first person to evaluate clinically the argon laser at laparoscopy was Keye at the University of Utah. Working with a local manufacturer (HGM, Salt Lake City, Utah), he investigated an argon laser that could be transmitted through flexible fibres. He reported his initial experience with animals and the clinical use of this fibreoptic laser for vaporization of endometriosis (Keye et al, 1983). Since then, others have reported different uses for the argon laser at laparoscopy (Diamond et al, 1986). The neodymium-yttrium aluminium garnet (Nd-YAG) laser introduced into gynaecology for hysteroscopic endometrial ablation has also been used via flexible fibres at laparoscopy (Lomano, 1983). In 1985, the potassium titanyl phosphate (KTP) laser (Laserscope, Santa Clara, California) became available in North America for clinical investigation in gynaecology. Initial evaluations were carried out in rabbits (Daniell, 1986) and later used for laparoscopic treatment of endometriosis as well as other pelvic conditions (Daniell et al, 1986). These two visible light lasers, the argon and the KTP, now are available commercially and used widely by operative laparoscopists.

PHYSICS AND TISSUE INTERACTION OF THE ARGON AND KTP LASERS

Both the KTP and argon lasers generate visible light. The wavelength of KTP is 532 nm and that of the argon is 488 (argon blue) and 515 nm (argon blue). Argon laser light is bluish-green while the KTP is a lime-green colour. These lasers can pass through flexible fibreoptic fibres which allow easier delivery to the tissues. They can pass through clear fluids and their primary tissue effect is coagulation. The depth of tissue penetration is less than with the Nd–YAG but more than with the CO_2 laser.

The argon laser beam is generated from a resonator chamber filled with argon gas, whereas the KTP laser beam is produced by pumping a Nd-YAG laser at 50 watts through a crystal of KTP. From this crystal is generated a green beam which at 532 nm is double the wavelength of the Nd-YAG. Thus the KTP laser is sometimes referred to as a frequency-doubled YAG laser.

For laparoscopic surgery, the energy of these two types of laser can be delivered through flexible fibres without focusing tips. Argon laser energy is delivered through either a 600 or a 300 μm fibre, and the KTP energy is delivered through a 400 or 600 μm fibre. These fibres can be used repeatedly since a worn tip can be cleaved with a knife or special cleaving instrument. Since these lasers generate bright visible light with significant backscatter from tissue impact, it is necessary to work with safety filters in order to protect the operator's eyes and allow observation of the effects of the laser when fired. Tissue penetration does not exceed 2 mm and vaporization and incisions are possible with high power densities accomplished by using smaller fibres and close tissue approximation.

Although the Nd-YAG laser has been tested for laparoscopy with use of bare fibres since 1983, it has never been approved by the Federal Drug Administration (FDA) because of the risk of damage to vital structures by the raw Nd-YAG unfocused beam which can penetrate to depths of 4–5 mm. The development of synthetic focusing tips made of sapphire that allow contact use of Nd-YAG energy now has led to wider use of the Nd-YAG in laparoscopy. Different types of tips are available commercially for cutting or coagulating. The tips are expensive but can be reused if treated carefully.

ADVANTAGES AND DISADVANTAGES OF FIBREOPTIC LASERS FOR LAPAROSCOPY

In our experience the fibreoptic lasers have distinct advantages over CO_2 lasers for laparoscopy (Table 1). The main advantage of fibreoptic lasers is

Table 1. Advantages of fibres for laparoscopy.

Simplified delivery to tissue
Backstop only necessary occasionally
Effective in a wet field
Reduced smoke formation
Excellent haemostasis
Both vaporization and coagulation possible
Shortened operating time

the ease with which their energy can be delivered to tissue compared with the cumbersome coupling devices needed for the CO_2 laser. The fibre is delivered simply either through the operating channel of the laparoscope or through an alternate port into the pelvis, and using a guidance probe, placed on or close to the impact site. There are no cumbersome alignment steps needed for the application of laser energy. Since fibreoptically delivered laser energy passes through clear fluids, the amount of smoke generated is considerably reduced. This simpler delivery system combined with less smoke generation shortens operative procedures. Another advantage of fibreoptic lasers is the ability to either incise, vaporize or photocoagulate very rapidly by merely altering the distance of the fibre from the tissue. Since these lasers have greater haemostatic effects than the CO_2 laser, there is less potential for intraoperative bleeding. Finally, they can be also used for certain hysteroscopic procedures if desired.

As with all developments in technology, there are also disadvantages of these three lasers for laparoscopy. These include the necessity for running water to cool the laser generators and the need for a special three-phase electricity supply for argon and KTP lasers. In addition, an eye safety filter must be placed over the laparoscope before firing, and this reduces the field of view and adds an extra encumbrance to the eyepiece of the laparoscope. Early filters developed by the manufacturers somewhat obscured the view, but newer filters which do not impede the view of the operator or video monitors are now available. Another disadvantage of these three lasers for laparoscopic surgery is that they are more expensive than CO_2 lasers.

In spite of these disadvantages, the ease and simplicity of their use in certain procedures combined with the reduced operative time far outweigh the disadvantages. In addition, the better haemostatic properties and the reduced need for a backstop to protect underlying structures seem to increase the safety of laparoscopic surgery in our hands. This has led us to discard use of the CO_2 laser for laparoscopic surgery except for certain specific procedures or when training physicians in use of the CO_2 laser.

DELIVERY TECHNIQUES

Since the energy from Nd-YAG, KTP and argon lasers can be delivered through flexible fibres or probes with sapphire tips, it becomes very simple to deliver the energy into the peritoneal cavity for laparoscopic surgery. When only a minimum amount of laser firing is planned, the easiest method is to pass the fibre down the coaxial channel of a standard operating laparoscope. The advantage of this is that it does not require an extra puncture in the abdomen, and it allows the operator to have a good angle of attack in the pelvis. The disadvantage is that an operating laparoscope has a reduced light output due to a small optical channel and the depth perception of the operator is altered because the fibre is passed down the line of sight.

Alternatively a standard diagnostic laparoscope can be used and the fibre passed through another port. The KTP or argon fibres can be passed through the central channel of a 5 mm probe usually used for suction and irrigation at CO_2 laser laparoscopy. These are available from most manufacturers of endoscopic instruments. Recently, a 5 mm steerable probe (Gynescope, Willoughby, Ohio) has been designed which allows suction and irrigation of smoke as well as passage of the fibre (Figure 1). The tip of the probe can be moved between 90° and 180° so that the fibre can be directed at different angles. This probe is particularly helpful for treating the posterior surfaces of the ovary. Alternatively, this probe can be used as a backstop for the fibre or to accomplish traction on tissues in the pelvis. It is particularly helpful in advanced laparoscopic procedures such as salpingostomy, extensive adhesiolysis, or treatment of advanced stages of endometriosis. The Nd-YAG fibre with appropriate sapphire tip can only be passed through a 3 mm probe.

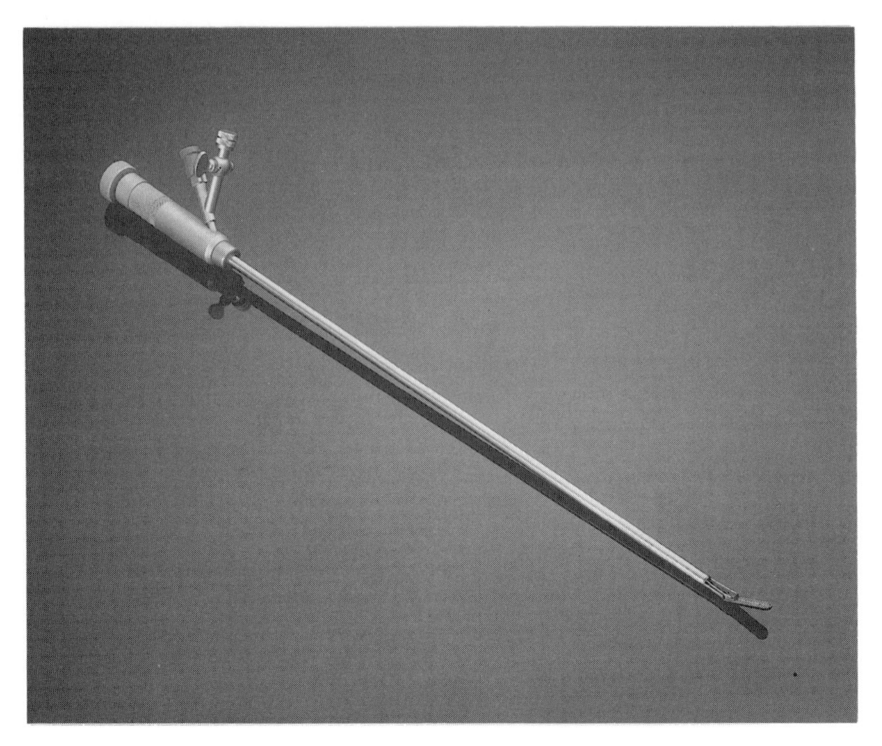

Figure 1. A steerable probe that allows simultaneous suction of smoke and irrigation. This multiple purpose probe also can be used for traction, manipulations in the pelvis, as a backstop, or to allow bending of the fibre to target hard-to-reach areas in the pelvis.

Advanced operative laparoscopic techniques demand the placement of extra probes and the location of the ports of entry should be chosen carefully. Normally we introduce our first handling probe in the midline suprapubically and use this with 5 mm instruments for retraction, irrigation, suction, and dissection as necessary (see Figure 4). If indicated, we usually place a third probe 2–3 inches lateral to the umbilicus on the side opposite the major portion of pelvic disease. If a fourth probe is needed, it is placed on the opposite side. Occasionally, three probes can be placed in the midline, but this often leads to problems with clashing of the instruments during pelvic manipulations. Care should be taken to avoid the inferior epigastric vessels when placing the lateral probes by transluminating the abdominal wall with the laparoscope and identifying the vessels in a briefly darkened operating room. Multiple ancillary instruments have been developed for laparoscopy, and many have specific uses. We feel that the minimum necessary is at least three 5 mm trochars with scissors, atraumatic grasping forceps, and cautery forceps for both unipolar and bipolar use. Any gynaecologist who plans to undertake extensive operating using laser laparoscopy should first be experienced with multiple punctures and trained in the use of both unipolar and bipolar cautery at laparoscopy.

Table 2. Advantages of video use for gynaecological endoscopy.

Better assistance is possible
Assistants can be allowed to do more
Greater involvement by operating room team
Teaching potential improved
Educational tapes can be produced
Patient enlightenment and information
Medicolegal record

The use of video can be very helpful during operative laparoscopy with lasers (Table 2). Since multiple punctures for extensive operative procedures require more than two hands, it is mandatory to have a coordinated, knowledgeable assistant. The only way that an assistant can reasonably be expected to help is by being able to visualize what is actually occurring endoscopically, to anticipate the actions necessary to optimize the results. The use of video may be with a direct coupler which requires the operator to work while looking directly at the TV monitor, or with a beam splitter which gives the option of either looking directly through the laparoscope or at the monitor. We prefer using a beam splitter, since it gives the operator the chance to look into the pelvis with the human eye directly when necessary. A 90–10 beam splitter which directs 90% of light to the video monitor and 10% through to the eye of the operator has been adequate for us, giving good diameter of vision on the monitor as well as enough light for good visibility on the monitor and for recording purposes (Wolf Instrument Company, Chicago, IL). If the operator prefers to work directly off the video monitor, it is best to place the monitor between the patient's legs so that the orientation is the same as the operator would have if looking directly into the pelvis. Although the term 'videolaseroscopy' has been coined in North America, we feel that this is a silly term which has no real bearing on what is being performed. A better and more accurate term would be 'laparoscopic surgery performed under video control'. The notion that a flat video monitor being viewed by two eyes would give one better depth of perception and finer colour discrimination than that of the human eye looking through the laparoscope seems impossible to accept. In my opinion, no monitor or camera system will ever approach the optics of the human eye. Because of this, we like to always retain the ability to look directly into the pelvis when we feel we are in a tight spot or doing a particularly difficult dissection. A video beam splitter makes this very simple and saves the need to remove and replace the camera intermittently.

SPECIFIC LAPAROSCOPIC PROCEDURES

Almost every procedure that has been done laparoscopically with scissors, cautery and CO_2 lasers has now been carried out using the three fibreoptic lasers. This list includes treatment of polycystic ovaries, correction of hydrosalpinx, conservative treatment of ectopic pregnancy, extensive adhesiolysis, treatment of stage IV endometriosis, and myomectomy.

Treatment of polycystic ovaries

Following reports of the successful use of laparoscopic ovarian cautery (Gjønnæss, 1984), and ovarian biopsy to treat polycystic ovaries (Campo et al, 1983), we began investigating the use of laser energy to treat polycystic ovaries in 1984. Initially, we used the carbon dioxide laser for this technique but the large volume of tissue vaporized produced a tremendous amount of smoke. Thus this procedure required a fairly long operating time. With the availability of KTP, argon and Nd-YAG lasers, we began to use these lasers for laparoscopic treatment of polycystic ovaries. We have been able to reduce operating time while still selectively destroying portions of the ovarian stroma satisfactorily. In a recent report of 85 patients, we have been able to produce spontaneous ovulation postoperatively in 71% and successful pregnancy in 56% of these patients (Daniell, 1989).

Our present technique for treating patients with polycystic ovarian disease (PCOD) involves laparoscopy with a three-puncture technique. A 5 mm grasping forceps is used to fix the ovary and the fibre from either the argon, KTP or Nd-YAG laser is introduced and used to vaporize multiple sites symmetrically over each ovary. Some of the subcapsular cysts are opened and the follicular fluid removed and aspirated. In addition, part of the ovarian stroma is also vaporized. Small craters in the range of 3–5 mm are thus developed on the ovarian surface with laser energy. The procedure can usually be accomplished in less than an hour and the majority of the patients are discharged from hospital within 8 hours. We feel that this is an excellent procedure in those patients desiring immediate pregnancy who have failed to respond to clomiphene in the correct dosage, or who have responded to clomiphene but need a laparoscopy to complete their infertility evaluation. It gives these patients a ‘window of opportunity’ during which they might conceive without the need for expensive ovulation induction therapy or wedge resection. The effect is transient, as almost all patients not conceiving have reverted back to anovulatory status within one year after the laparoscopic treatment. We have had no complications from this procedure in over 120 cases and now recommend it for all of our PCOD patients who meet the criteria of failure to respond to clomiphene or otherwise need a laparoscopy while desiring immediate postoperative pregnancy.

Switching from the use of CO_2 lasers to fibreoptic lasers has made this an easier, safer, quicker procedure at laparoscopy, particularly for obese patients. The advantages to these patients are considerable compared to the risks and discomfort that they would experience from a laparotomy for wedge resection. The expense involved with ovulation induction is minimized as well as the complications of ovarian hyperstimulation and the risks and inconvenience of multiple pregnancies.

Laparoscopic neosalpingostomy

The treatment of hydrosalpinx has had uniformly poor results with even the best surgeons reporting no more than 30% pregnancy rates with long-term follow-up in controlled series (Bateman et al, 1987). Laparoscopic treatment of hydrosalpinges has been attempted since the late 1970s with the first reports by Gomel (1977), Mettler et al (1979) and Fayez (1983). Following the reports of Mage and Bruhat (1983) using the CO_2 laser for repair of hydrosalpinx at laparotomy, we began investigating the use of laser energy through the laparoscope for treatment of hydrosalpinges (Daniell and Herbert, 1984). More recently we have switched to visible-light laser fibres for this technique and have obtained better results by being more selective in our attempts at salpingostomy and by refining our techniques using the fibreoptic laser delivery systems. The problems that we encountered with the CO_2 laser were bleeding that often required cautery to the opened edges of the tubes and the inability in some tubes to evert the edges successfully. Using the small diameter visible-light laser fibres with four puncture techniques, we find salpingostomy easier to perform, with less bleeding. A small linear incision is made on the distal end of the tube and either one or two radial cuts performed using the smallest laser fibre. After the tube is opened, the 5 mm steerable probe is placed into the tube and used as a backstop and for traction so that the thinner portions of the tube can be identified and the proper site for the next incisions selected. After the tube is opened, the laser fibre is then held 2 cm from the lateral edges of the peritoneum of the open fimbria and defocused laser energy used to constrict the peritoneum. This causes the tubes to evert like the petals of a flower. This 'Bruhat technique' is much easier, in our opinion, to accomplish laparoscopically using a fibre than with the CO_2 laser. It is not possible to do this specific procedure with sapphire tips on a Nd-YAG laser since only contact firing is possible at laparoscopy with Nd-YAG fibres.

Our recent results in patients in which the primary treatment of their tubal blockage was carried out laparoscopically using the KTP laser with minimum 18 month follow-up are given in Table 3. As can be seen, a reasonable pregnancy rate has been obtained with an acceptable level of ectopic pregnancies in these patients. It is our opinion that in this age of availability of office-based ultrasound in vitro fertilization (IVF) with increasing pregnancy rates, laparotomy for hydrosalpinges should only be offered to those patients who cannot afford or do not desire IVF and in whom the fallopian tubes cannot be repaired by a laparoscopic approach. Certainly the advantages to the patients in reduced discomfort, minimum recuperation time, and reduction of cost and time off from work are tremendous. Although further confirmation by other investigators is needed, it appears that laparoscopic treatment of hydrosalpinges using laser

Table 3. Results of laparoscopic neosalpingostomy with KTP lasers, West Side Hospital, Nashville, Tennessee (18-month minimum follow-up).

Laser type	Years	Total patients	Patent tubes at 6 weeks HSG	Attempting pregnancy	Pregnancy results		
					IUP	Abortion	Ectopic
KTP	1985–86	36*	24/28 (86%)	32	10 (31%)	3 (9%)	5 (16%)

* Only three procedures were recurrent hydrosalpinges.
IUP, intrauterine pregnancy; HSG, hysterosalpingography.

energy is a reasonable alternative to laparotomy in the hands of experienced operative laparoscopists.

Laparoscopic treatment of tubal pregnancy using laser energy

Although laparoscopic cautery appears effective for the treatment of tubal pregnancy, we do feel that the techniques that we have used with fibreoptic laser energy have some advantages in the treatment of ectopic pregnancies. Certainly there have been reports of successful treatment of ectopic pregnancies using laparoscopic techniques by Pouly et al (1986), Reich et al (1987) and Loffer (1987). The risk of bleeding from the tube is reduced when using fibreoptic laser energy compared with that of the CO_2 laser. In addition, the trauma to the tube appears to be less with the laser fibres than when using needle electrodes or scissors. Table 4 lists our results at West Side Hospital in Nashville, Tennessee using laser energy for the treatment of unruptured ectopic pregnancies by laparoscopy. All cases after 1985 were performed with fibreoptic laser energy. We agree with Brumsted et al (1988) that laparoscopic treatment of ectopic pregnancy is well tolerated by patients and very cost-effective when compared to the older techniques.

Table 4. Laparoscopic treatment of ectopic pregnancies, HCA West Side Hospital, Nashville, Tennessee, January 1984–January 1988.

Total patients	36
Ruptured tubes	2
Salpingectomy	6
Salpingostomy	30
Laparotomies done	0
Tubal patency on HSG	18 of 20 tested (90% postoperatively)
Repeat ectopics	2 of 20 attempting pregnancy (10%)
Intrauterine pregnancies	8 of 20 (40%)

HSG, hysterosalpingography.

Operative laparoscopy at the time of egg recovery in assisted conception

Many patients who are infertile also have other symptoms related to either endometriosis and/or adhesions. These patients often come to laparoscopy either because of persistence of their infertility or recurrence or persistence of pain or a combination of both. The ability to offer patients an attempt at conception by gamete intrafallopian transfer (GIFT) and simultaneous treatment for their primary disease (operative laparoscopy with adhesiolysis, vaporization of endometriosis, etc.), seems very appealing. The main hazard during a laparoscopy done with GIFT is that the ovaries have been stimulated and therefore are enlarged and tend to bleed if excess manipulation is attempted. In addition, uterine manipulators should not be used and chromotubation cannot be carried out. Because of this, the laparoscopist is limited somewhat as to what can be accomplished at the time of a GIFT procedure. The use of visible light laser energy is particularly helpful for adhesiolysis around ovaries in these patients because of the increased vascularity related to the multiple follicles that have been stimulated before the laparoscopy. After aspirating the follicles the surgeon has an opportunity to perform indicated laparoscopic procedures while the laboratory personnel are identifying and preparing the gametes for transfer into the tube. The laser fibres can be easily brought in through one of the accessory probes and used for adhesiolysis and/or vaporization of endometriosis. This often does not prolong the anaesthesia time and if the surgeon is careful, will not increase risks of bleeding from manipulation in the pelvis. It is even possible to transect the uterosacral ligaments in these patients if one is careful to reflect the ovaries laterally and lift the uterus up with accessory probes. We feel that this ability to give the chance of conception to the patient via GIFT as well as accomplish treatment of her pelvic pathology is logical and intelligent and an option that many patients will choose if given the opportunity.

Treatment of endometriosis and adhesions

The techniques for treating endometriosis depend on the location and amount of disease present. Surface implants can usually be photocoagulated using the larger fibres held close to the tissue. If vaporization is desired, the tip can actually touch the endometriotic tissue. An alternative method is to use accessory forceps to grasp the implants of endometriosis, put them on traction and dissect them from the area of implantation using the tip of the laser fibre. Davis and Brooks (1989) have reported excellent relief of pain associated with endometriosis with this technique in a series of 66 patients. With endometriosis it is important to remember that some active disease that is not visible to the naked eye may be located in the margins of visible implants. Because of this, we treat each implant in a similar fashion to viral lesions on the perineum using an 'airbrush' technique to photovaporize the periphery of the lesions. Care must be taken when working over the bladder and bowel or close to the ureter. In other areas, laser energy can be used with little risk to underlying tissues.

Although others have reported the treatment of bowel endometriosis using laser energy through the laparoscope, we have no experience with this condition. Since most bowel implants are somewhat oedematous and ill-defined, we feel that the risk of bowel perforation is greater than the potential for successful destruction of the entire lesion. For this reason, we limit laparoscopic treatment of bowel endometriosis to those lesions that are exophytic or on epiploic fat or on the tip of the appendix. We will perform an appendectomy through the laparoscope if the tip of the appendix is affected with endometriosis and if we feel we can safely get an endoloop around the proximal appendix and mobilize it enough for removal in one piece through the laparoscopic 10 mm trocar. We do not remove infected appendices or perform elective appendectomy through the laparoscope, as we feel this is better left to general surgeons at laparotomy.

Ovarian endometriomas

Endometriomas must be carefully dissected from their usual attachments to the lateral pelvic sidewalls. In our experience, it has been the sidewall that usually bleeds and not the ovary itself, so putting gentle traction on the ovary and using laser energy to vaporize the ovary free of the sidewall is usually more effective than bluntly mobilizing the ovary. Care must be taken to identify and avoid the ureter and to protect the major vessels lateral to the ovary. Once the ovary is freed from the sidewall, the endometrioma can be opened and the chocolate contents aspirated or irrigated. The method of handling the endometrioma depends on whether or not the capsule can be stripped from the ovarian stroma. By using grasping forceps, if it is possible to tease the capsule free, it can usually be removed from the ovary with gentle traction. This is basically a non-laser technique. If the capsule is too adherent to the ovarian stroma, we then use the fibreoptic laser fibres to vaporize the capsule by holding the fibre very close to the surface of the inside of the endometrioma and gently passing it over the entire surface. The endometrioma bed, if under 5–6 cm, will usually constrict with the ovarian surfaces touching. Laparoscopic sutures can be placed if necessary. Endometriomas larger than 8 or 9 cm are probably still best handled by laparotomy because of the large open ovarian surface areas that result from opening the cyst.

Adhesions associated with endometriosis

Adhesions associated with endometriosis are handled in a similar fashion to other adhesions. The advantage of the visible light laser fibres is that the energy dissipates from the tip very rapidly so that any structures more than 2 cm beyond the tip will not be affected by impact of the laser beam. This means that it is not necessary to maintain a backstop behind adhesions that are not closely overlying vital structures. However, when working close to the bowel, bladder, or the tube, it is necessary to use a backstop because of the potential for damage beneath the beam. The best instrument for providing this extra safety is a 5 mm steerable probe with a titanium tip (Gynescope, Willoughby, Ohio) which can be placed through a second puncture site (5 mm) and manipulated as needed to provide both a backstop and traction behind the adhesion while firing the laser. Gentle traction is usually necessary on the adhesion so that the bands can be easily vaporized. The KTP and argon lasers are particularly advantageous for this technique because of the speed with which the adhesions can be incised, with minimal risk of bleeding and with minimal smoke production. A scalpel tip on the Nd-YAG laser can also be used but must be kept in contact with the tissue to be effective.

There has not been an organized prospective study using second-look laparoscopy to evaluate early healing after laparoscopic surgery of any type. A multicentre study is now underway evaluating the early second-look laparoscopic appearance in patients undergoing extensive operative laser laparoscopy. Hopefully this study will shed some light on the actual type, amount, and location of adhesions that occur following laparoscopic adhesiolysis with various techniques, both laser and non-laser.

Perihepatic lesions

Perihepatic adhesions are often seen in patients who have had infectious pelvic pathology. Some of these may be symptomatic (Fitzhugh–Curtis syndrome); however in most cases they are an incidental finding. We routinely vaporize these adhesions using the visible light laser fibres. In this case, since the pathology is high in the upper abdomen, we introduce the fibre through the operating channel of the laparoscope which is swung around into the upper abdomen. Since the energy dissipates from the tip of the fibre very rapidly, there is no need for a backstop and one does not need to be concerned about damaging the diaphragm. Additionally, the haemostatic properties of the beam reduces the potential for bleeding from the liver.

Postsurgical adhesions

Laparoscopic bowel adhesiolysis following postsurgical or infectious processes can also be accomplished successfully in many cases using fibreoptic laser energy. A significant number of patients over the last decade have been referred to us for attempts at laparoscopic adhesiolysis after multiple abdominal operations. Many of these patients have had previous bowel obstructions and are at extremely high risk for potential complications at attempted laparoscopy. We routinely counsel these patients concerning the risks of bowel injury and the possible need for immediate laparotomy and/or diverting colostomy. We do a standard bowel preparation and restrict them to clear fluids for 48 hours before surgery. We will not perform surgery on these patients without having a consenting adult present in the waiting area to give us immediate consent for laparotomy if indicated and without having a general surgeon standing by to repair any bowel injuries that might occur during attempted enterolysis through the laparoscope. We do not routinely do an open laparoscopy, but initially will try to accomplish pneumoperitoneum in a standard fashion, and then introduce a 5 mm laparoscope for initial visibility. After confirming that we are in the proper peritoneal space and noting the proper site for placement of the 10 mm laparoscopic trocar, the larger laparoscope is inserted. The accessory probes for the laser fibres are introduced under direct vision and placement is based on the location of any abdominal wall adhesions. Many of these patients can be helped, but some have such extensive adhesions with bowel so adherent to the intra-abdominal wall that it is impossible to accomplish a complete adhesiolysis via the laparoscope. However, those patients with pain from postsurgical adhesions who undergo successful laparoscopic lysis do have improvement in the majority of cases. We have not yet had any late complications and have had only one bowel perforation that required immediate laparotomy in a series of 40 patients treated with extensive laparoscopic bowel adhesiolysis since 1984.

Removal of adnexal structures with laparoscopic laser energy

We have had good experience with the use of endoloop sutures for oophorectomy, salpingectomy, or removal of periadnexal structures. In these cases, the technique is mainly non-laser. However, we will occasionally use the KTP or argon laser to excise the ovary away from its pedicle, or to vaporize the pedicle after the bulk of the tissue has been removed. These lasers can be very helpful for cutting dense pedunculated fibroids into smaller pieces after the fibroid has been constricted with endoloop sutures for subsequent removal with forceps.

Uterosacral ligament transection

One of the more common operations that we perform is transection of the uterosacral ligaments using laparoscopic laser energy (LUNA). We offer this procedure to all patients who have dysmenorrhoea and who are undergoing laparoscopy. Doyle (1955) was the first to report successful relief from dysmenorrhoea by dividing the uterosacral ligaments. Data from Feste (1984) and Lichten and Bombard (1987) suggest that laser transection via laparoscopy can be successful therapy for dysmenorrhoea, either with or without endometriosis. We initially used the CO_2 laser for LUNA, but encountered several cases of bleeding that required cautery. At the time of writing, there have been at least two deaths in North America resulting from bleeding from uterosacral ligaments that occurred when these were transected with CO_2 laser energy. To date neither of these case reports have been published.

We feel that the haemostatic properties of visible light laser energy add some degree of safety when the uterosacral ligaments are transected. Our technique is to identify the uterosacral ligaments, trace them out to the pelvic brim, locate the ureters and note the proximity of the uterine artery to the lateral cervix. We then take a 5 mm probe and push against the posterior cervix to tent up the uterosacral ligaments. The laser fibre is then used to transect the ligaments at right angles just as the ligaments insert into the posterior cervix. Sometimes the ligaments will be attenuated and difficult to identify. In these cases we may refrain from cutting if we feel it is unsafe or the landmarks cannot be identified. Occasionally, rectosigmoid obliteration of the cul-de-sac in cases of endometriosis will preclude the ability to cut the uterosacrals in this area. Our results have been satisfactory in the majority of

Table 5. LUNA results with KTP laser—6-month follow-up.

	Worse	Same	Improved
Endometriosis (80 patients)	3 (4%)	17 (21%)	60 (75%)
Primary dysmenorrhoea (20 patients)	2 (10%)	6 (30%)	12 (60%)
Totals (100 patients)	5 (5%)	23 (23%)	72 (72%)

LUNA, laparoscopic uterosacral nerve ablation.

patients with at least 70% having reduction in their menstrual pain (Table 5). Most patients will have a somewhat painful initial period postoperatively, which probably reflects early tissue swelling. We have not noted any effect on bowel or bladder function in these patients, and no patients have reported any reduction in ability to enjoy intercourse or obtain orgasm. It is important to counsel these patients carefully preoperatively and make certain that they are aware that success is not guaranteed in all cases.

FUTURE DEVELOPMENTS

Since the KTP laser contains a 50 watt Nd-YAG laser, the option now exists for accessing either the ND-YAG or the KTP energy sources independently from this one laser (Figure 2; Figure 3). This opens up the possibility of using the Nd-YAG component for ablation of the endometrium at hysteroscopy as well as using the Nd-YAG with the same fibre with sapphire tips laparoscopically in selected indications. The combined Nd-YAG and KTP laser has just been approved for use by the FDA, and has only now become

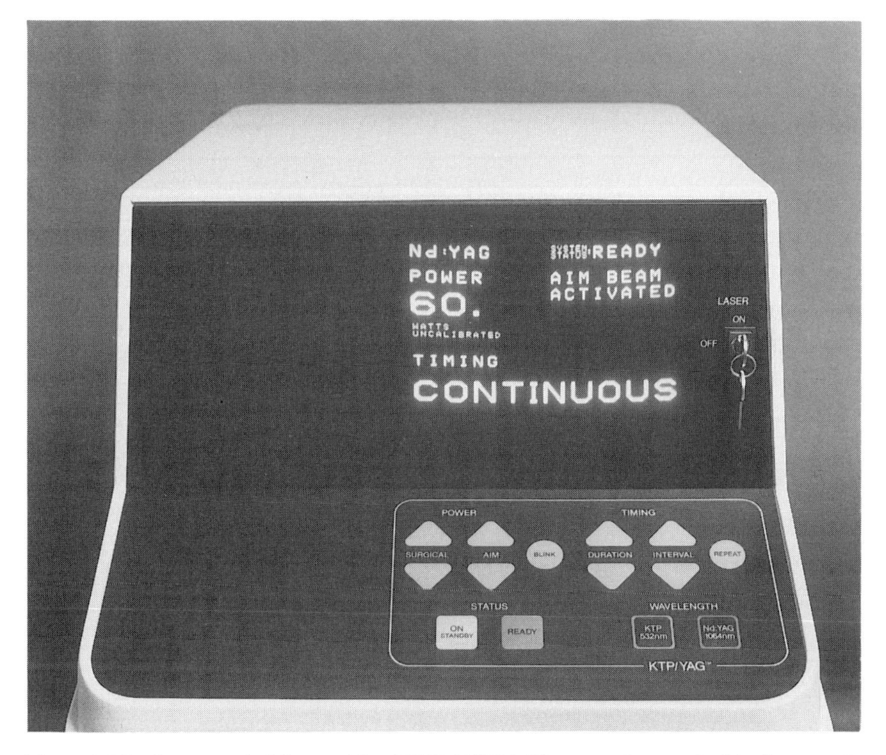

Figure 2. The front panel of the combined KTP–Nd-YAG laser can be seen in this photograph. The machine can be changed from one mode to another in 30 s and is delivered from the same port and through the same fibre. This allows very simple intraoperative switching from one form of laser energy to the other as clinically indicated.

available to us for clinical evaluation. The mechanics of the dual delivery system have been engineered to alleviate concerns of the FDA concerning safety precautions for failsafe use of either the Nd-YAG or the KTP laser separately from the one unit.

Other lasers may become available for laparoscopic use in the future. Some of these include the carbon monoxide laser which has tissue effects similar to those of the CO_2 laser, but which can be delivered through a fibre. A new flexible fibre has also been recently developed to transmit CO_2 laser

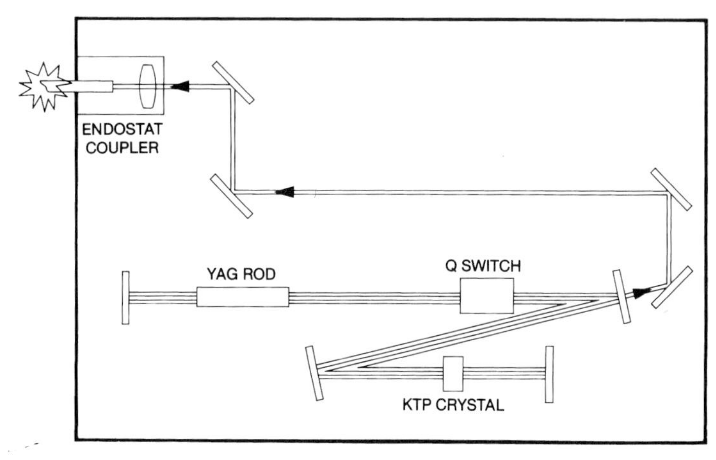

KTP/532 Laser

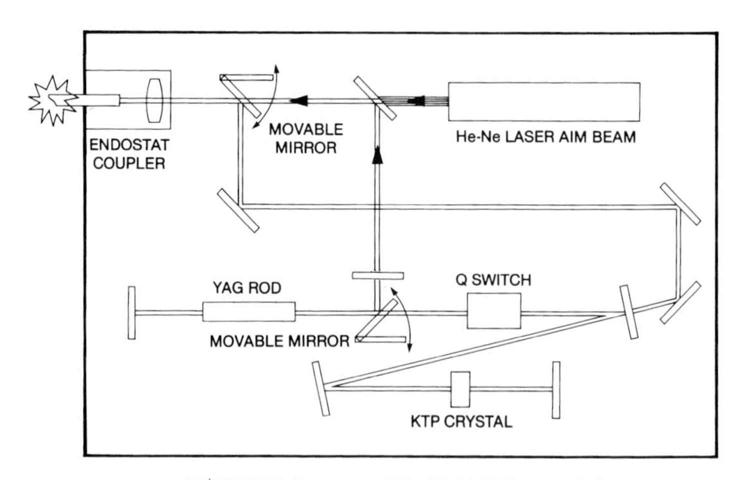

KTP/532 Laser with Nd:YAG module

Figure 3. These two schematic drawings demonstrate how the KTP energy can be diverted to allow direct use of the primary 50 watt Nd-YAG laser present in each KTP machine. The lower drawing shows the beam pathway with Nd-YAG and associated helium–neon aiming laser use, while the upper sketch demonstrates the original KTP beam pathway.

energy and is presently undergoing clinical evaluation in the UK. In addition, the gold vapour laser, tuneable dye laser, the free electron laser and excimer laser all have future potential uses through the laparoscope. At the time of writing, none of these have been evaluated either experimentally or in humans for laparoscopic surgery.

SAFETY IN FIBREOPTIC LASER LAPAROSCOPY

Hazards to the eyes

Proper use of these fibreoptic lasers at laparoscopy includes the use of eye filters and protection for the patient, the surgeon, and assistants in the operating room. Since the laser energy from the argon and KTP is a visible beam, it is less likely that damage will be done to the operator's eyes. Any inadvertent firing of the laser without eye filters will be immediately recognized because of the bright green colour that is seen. This improves the safety of use of these lasers compared to the Nd-YAG which is infrared and therefore not visible when fired. When working in a closed abdominal cavity, we do not require people in the operating room to wear safety glasses. The fibre has a special coating which protects leakage of the energy except from its tip. The operator is the only person at risk when the beam is being fired intraperitoneally through the laparoscope, and his eyes are protected by the eye filter that is placed over the eyepiece of the laparoscope. With both the argon and the KTP laser, the laser cannot be fired if the eye filter is not working properly. The Nd-YAG manufacturers, however have not yet produced built-in eye safety filters, so special care is necessary to use proper filters or goggles. If an attempt is made to override the eye filter (this can be done for instance by placing the eye filter on another laparoscope that might be on the table), the operator will immediately be aware of intense brightness when he attempts to fire the laser into the pelvis.

Hazards from the smoke

There must be evacuation of smoke from the operating room because of possible harmful effects from its inhalation. We vent off the smoke through a specially designed disposable suction-irrigation system that is used to aspirate fluid and pass it through a filter into standard disposable floor canisters (PumpVac, Gynescope, Willoughby, Ohio; Figure 4). By using in-line filters, we protect the hospital filter system from being blocked by particulate matter in the plume.

Other problems

Fibre breakage or loss of sapphire tips from the Nd-YAG laser is another potential problem. This risk can be reduced by checking YAG tips for fit and never advancing more of the fibre into the peritoneal cavity than is necessary to visualize the tip during firing.

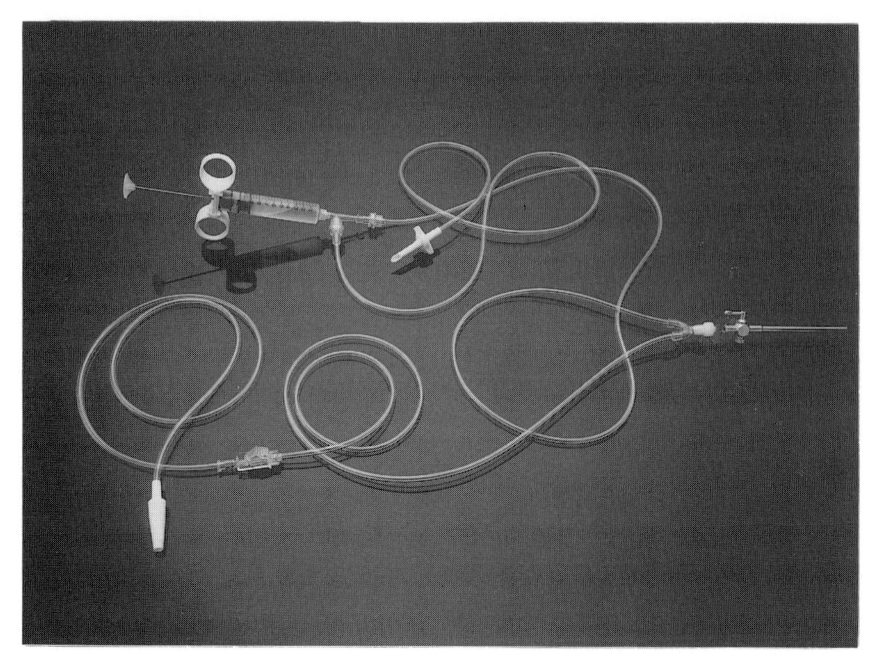

Figure 4. The disposable PumpVac system for rapid smoke or fluid suction and irrigation at operative laparoscopy. It attaches to floor suction tubing and an intravenous bag containing irrigation solution allows aquadissection as well as simple control of smoke production. It can be operated with ease either by the surgeon or an assistant.

Other safety precautions are those that one would undertake with any sort of operative laparoscopy, such as gentle tissue handling, use of instruments specially designed for certain situations, and correct use of both bipolar and unipolar cautery when necessary. With proper attention to safety the careful endoscopist can perform extensive operative laparoscopic procedures with good results in the majority of cases with minimal complications and few postoperative problems.

CREDENTIALING AND CERTIFICATION FOR ADVANCED OPERATIVE LAPAROSCOPIC LASER SURGERY

The American Fertility Society has recently published guidelines for credentialing surgeons for intra-abdominal and endoscopic laser surgery in gynaecology. Basically, these guidelines consist of three stages. First, the surgeon must be trained and certified to perform the procedure for which he wants to utilize lasers (i.e. the surgeon must be a skilled operative laparoscopist before undertaking laser laparoscopy). Secondly, the applicant must have completed a formal course with exposure to didactics, safety, and tissue effects of the specific laser which he wants to use for laparoscopic surgery. Finally, the physician must complete a preceptorship and have 'hands' on use of the laser under the tutelage of a person already experienced in that specific laser used for laparoscopic surgery. We feel that this three-step credentialing process is probably the most reasonable way of trying to maintain quality control and promote safe use of various laser energies at laparoscopy. It is important to remember that just because one is competent and skilled in use of the CO_2 laser does not imply expertise or familiarity with use of the argon, KTP, or Nd-YAG laser. The same learning curve must be followed with each specific wavelength of laser energy that one wishes to use for specific procedures. It is mandatory that any gynaecologist who wants to use the laser laparoscopically first becomes very comfortable and skilled at using multiple puncture techniques with both unipolar and bipolar cautery at laparoscopy.

To undertake any sort of extensive operative laparoscopy without the proper safety precautions, training, equipment, and assistance, can result in unnecessary complications and its tragic sequelae. It behoves all of us who are interested in operative laser laparoscopy to be careful and selective in the techniques that we undertake to perform. This will protect us, our hospitals and our patients.

SUMMARY

Many gynaecologists are now doing more aggressive operative laparoscopic surgery. We feel that procedures which in the past required open laparotomy to be successfully performed, can now be done with fibreoptic laser energy. This chapter reviews our experiences with argon, KTP and Nd-YAG lasers for advanced laparoscopic surgery. We feel that these fibreoptic lasers allow us to obtain good results with less risk, shortened operating room time and with reduced difficulty during surgery.

In this time of concern for cost containment in medicine, it seems reasonable for interested physicians to reduce costs without cutting corners or compromising patient care. Careful, intelligent, selective use of fibreoptic lasers as well as non-laser laparoscopic techniques in gynaecology may help in cost containment by allowing compatible results while avoiding major surgery with its concomitant expense, increased risks, morbidity and discomfort for patients. All forward-thinking gynaecologists should investigate the potential for fibreoptic laparoscopic laser surgery in their practices.

REFERENCES

Bateman BG, Nunley WC & Kitchin JD (1987) Surgical management of distal tubal obstruction—are we making progress? *Fertility and Sterility* **48:** 523–542.

Brumsted J, Gibson C, Gibson M et al (1988) A comparison of laparoscopy and laparotomy for the treatment of ectopic pregnancy. *Obstetrics and Gynecology* **71:** 889–892.

Campo S, Garcea N, Caruso A et al (1983) Effect of coelioscopic ovarian resection in patients with polycystic ovaries. *Gynecologic and Obstetric Investigation* **15:** 213–222.

Daniell JF (1986) Laparoscopic evaluation of the KTP/532 laser for treating endometriosis—Initial report. *Fertility and Sterility* **46:** 373–377.

Daniell JF (1989) Polycystic ovaries treated by laparoscopic laser vaporization. *Fertility and Sterility* **51:** 232–236.
Daniell JF & Herbert CM (1984) Laparoscopic salpingostomy utilizing the CO_2 laser. *Fertility and Sterility* **4:** 558–563.
Daniell JF, Meisels S, Miller W et al (1986) Laparoscopic use of the KTP/532 laser in nonendometriotic pelvic surgery. *Colposcopy Gynecologic & Laser Surgery* **2:** 107–111.
Davis GD & Brooks RA (1989) Excision of pelvic endometriosis with the CO_2 laser laparoscope. *Obstetrics and Gynecology* **72:** 816–819.
Diamond MP, DeCherney AH & Polan ML (1986) Laparoscopic use of the argon laser in nonendometriotic reproductive pelvic surgery. *Journal of Reproductive Medicine* **31:** 101–104.
Doyle JB (1955) Paracervical uterine denervation by transection of the cervical plexus for the relief of dysmenorrhea. *American Journal of Obstetrics and Gynecology* **70:** 1–16.
Fayez JA (1983) An assessment of the role of operative laparoscopy in tuboplasty. *Fertility and Sterility* **39:** 476–479.
Feste JR (1984) CO_2 laser neurectomy for dysmenorrhoea. *Lasers in Surgery and Medicine* **3:** 327–331.
Gjønnæss H (1984) Polycystic ovarian syndrome treated by ovarian electrocautery through the laparoscope. *Fertility and Sterility* **41:** 20–25.
Gomel V (1977) Salpingostomy by laparoscopy. *Journal of Reproductive Medicine* **18:** 265–268.
Keye WR, Matson GA & Dixon J (1983) The use of the argon laser in the treatment of experimental endometriosis. *Fertility and Sterility* **39:** 26–29.
Lichten EM & Bombard J (1987) Surgical treatment of primary dysmenorrhoea with laparoscopic uterine nerve ablation. *Journal of Reproductive Medicine* **32:** 37–41.
Loffer FD (1987) Outpatient management of ectopic pregnancies. *American Journal of Obstetrics and Gynecology* **156:** 1467–1472.
Lomano JM (1983) Laparoscopic ablation of endometriosis with the YAG Laser. *Lasers in Surgery and Medicine* **3:** 179–183.
Mage G & Bruhat MA (1983) Pregnancy following salpingostomy: comparison between CO_2 laser and electrosurgery procedures. *Fertility and Sterility* **40:** 472–475.
Mettler L, Giesel H & Semm K (1979) Treatment of female infertility due to tubal obstruction by operative laparoscopy. *Fertility and Sterility* **32:** 384–389.
Pouly JL, Mahnes H, Mage G et al (1986) Conservative laparoscopic treatment of 321 ectopic pregnancies. *Fertility and Sterility* **46:** 1093–1097.
Reich H, Freifeld ML, McGlynn F et al (1987) Laparoscopic treatment of tubal pregnancy. *Obstetrics and Gynecology* **69:** 275–279.

7

Laparoscopic treatment of polycystic ovarian syndrome

JÖRG KECKSTEIN

Polycystic ovarian disease (PCOD) is a syndrome of unknown aetiology. In 1935 Stein and Leventhal described a clinical syndrome with the characteristics of anovulation, infertility, hirsutism, obesity and bilateral polycystic ovaries (Stein and Leventhal, 1935) (Figure 1). The pathogenesis of the PCOD has been variously ascribed to primary abnormalities of the ovaries, of gonadotrophin secretion and of the adrenal glands (Kirschner et al, 1976; Yen, 1980).

Treatment considerations must be tailored according to the patient's fertility requirements. For those patients who want to conceive, induction of ovulation is usually performed with drug therapy. An alteration of the luteinizing hormone: follicle stimulating hormone (LH:FSH) ratio and

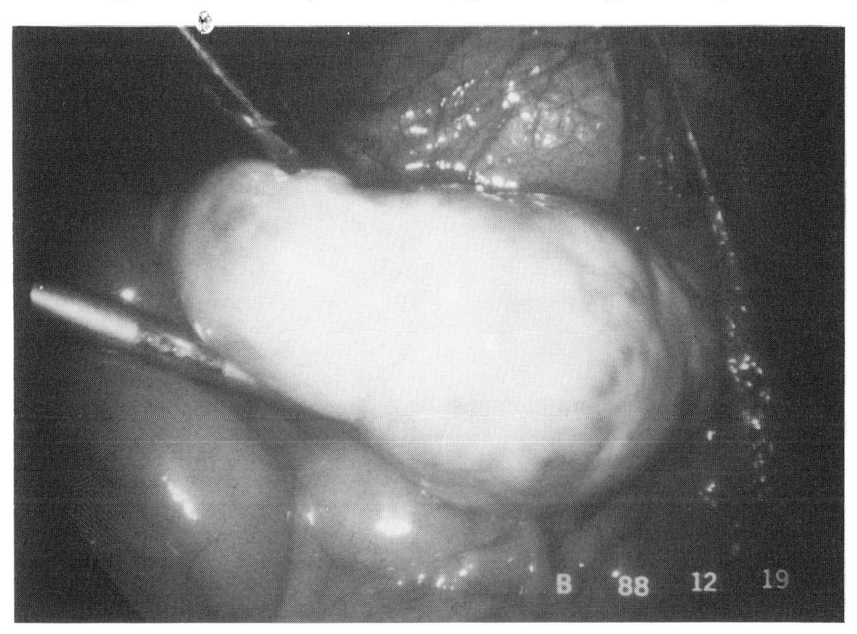

Figure 1. Typical appearance of an ovary in PCOD.

androgen level has to be achieved. Clomiphene citrate is the primary drug of choice. If this fails, two other methods—low-dose FSH or exogenous gonadotrophins after pituitary desensitization with luteinizing hormone releasing hormone (LHRH) analogues—may be successful (Fleming et al, 1985; Franks et al, 1987).

Some patients, however, do not respond to hormone stimulation. For these women, ovarian wedge resection represented a viable alternative for many years. The effectiveness of this procedure was first thought to result from removal of the collagenous ovarian capsule. Others have suggested that coring out the androgen-producing hilus or the oestrogen-producing atretic follicles alters the endocrine milieu. Various investigators have shown that in PCOD patients profound hormonal alterations occur after ovarian wedge resection (Judd et al, 1976; Katz et al, 1978).

The pitfall of this therapeutic procedure is the development of post-operative adhesions. In a series of 173 wedge resections reported by Buttram and Vaquero (1975), 34 patients underwent a second-look endoscopy or laparotomy. All these patients had developed periovarian adhesions. For this reason, less extensive surgical techniques performed by operative laparoscopy have been suggested for the treatment of anovulation in patients with PCOD.

LAPAROSCOPIC SURGICAL TECHNIQUES

1. Ovarian biopsy (Yuzpe and Rioux, 1975; Campo et al, 1983; Portuondo et al, 1984)
2. Electrocautery (Gjønnæss, 1984; Greenblatt and Casper, 1987; Van der Weiden and Alberda, 1987; Sumioki, 1988)
3. Laser: vaporization or photo-coagulation
   (a) CO_2 laser vaporization (Daniell and Miller, 1989)
   (b) Neodymium-yttrium aluminium garnet (Nd-YAG) laser coagulation (Keckstein et al, 1988a)
   (c) Nd-YAG laser incision (Huber et al, 1989)
   (d) Nd-YAG laser vaporization (Grochmal, 1988)
   (e) Argon laser (Daniell and Miller, 1989)
   (f) Potassium titanyl phosphate KTP-532 laser (Daniell and Miller, 1989)

Ovarian biopsy

In this technique the multiple puncture method is applied. All biopsies are obtained using the Palmer biopsy forceps. The resection of the ovarian tissue is performed along the longitudinal axis of the ovaries on the opposite surface to the hilum. The size of the fragments removed is 0.5–1.5 mm in diameter. Any bleeding from the puncture sites is coagulated by electrocautery or thermocoagulation.

Electrocautery

In this technique, first described by Gjønnæss (1984), no ovarian tissue is

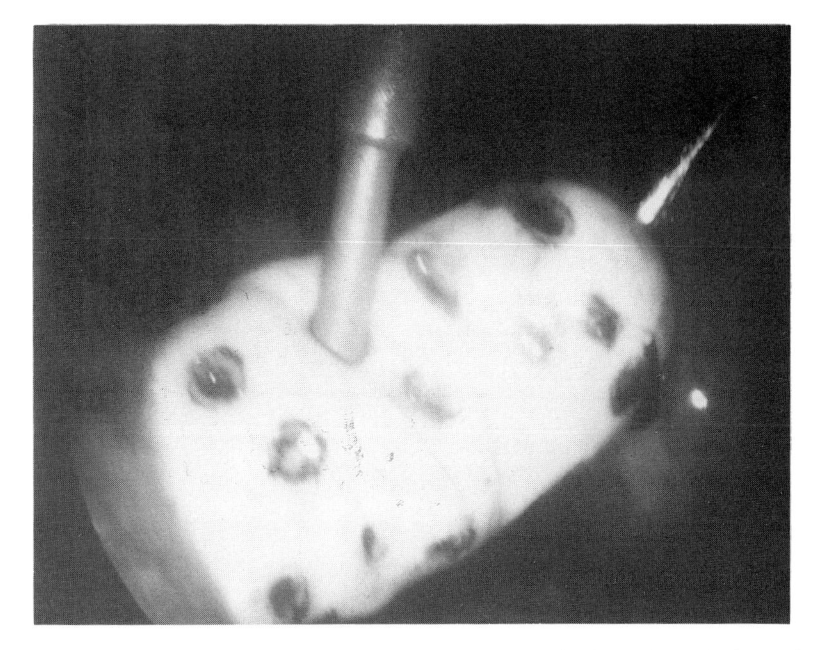

Figure 2. Coagulation and penetration of the ovarian surface by the thermal coagulation probe.

removed; the aim is to destroy part of the atretic follicles.

Unipolar biopsy forceps are held against the ovarian surface. To prevent injury to the neighbouring organs it is very important to fix the ovary in position. With a power between 200 and 300 W the electrode is pressed against the ovary to penetrate the ovarian capsule. The dimensions of the perforations depend on the thickness of the ovarian capsule and the size of the underlying atretic follicles. The number of the perforations range between 10 and 15, on each side. The same procedure may also be performed with the thermocoagulation probe described by Semm (1980) (Figure 2).

The well-known risk of using laparoscopic unipolar cautery (see Chapter 2) was one of the reasons to introduce various laser techniques in the treatment of the PCOD. The ability to transmit laser beams through rigid endoscopes or small flexible optical fibres makes them well-suited to endoscopic procedures. Under appropriate conditions laser instruments can not only cut but will also coagulate or vaporize. So far the CO_2, Nd-YAG, KTP and argon lasers have all been used in the therapy of PCOD.

Lasers

CO_2 laser

The user of the CO_2 laser aims to minimize the number of the atretic follicular cysts in the ovary and to destroy androgen-producing tissue. It may

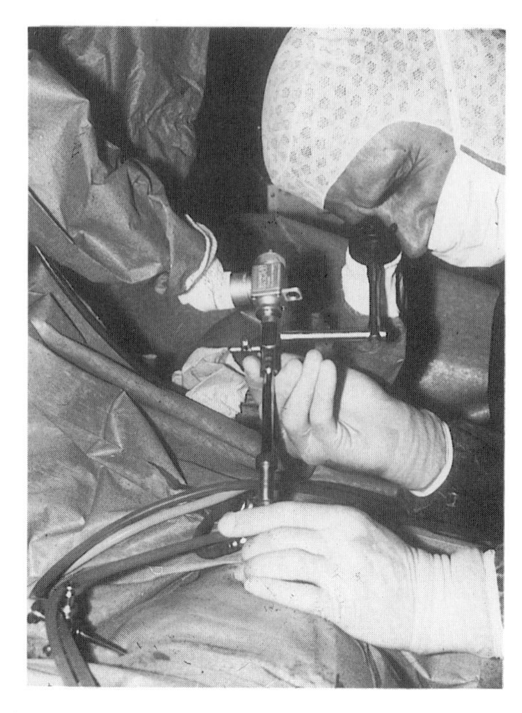

Figure 3. Laser laparoscopy. The rigid laser arm is attached to the operative laparoscope.

be used through the operative channel of the laparoscope (Figure 3) or through a special CO_2 laparoscopic laser probe which is introduced through a 5 mm trocar sheath. The ovaries are manipulated with atraumatic 5 mm grasping forceps. By holding the ovarian ligament, good fixation and control of the laser beam is achieved.

The laser power is set at 10–20 W in continuous mode. The laser beam is focused with a spot size of 0.2 mm (power density 32 000–60 000 W/cm^2). The surface of the ovary is vaporized in a dotted fashion (Figure 4). After opening the cysts the follicular fluid spills out and is partially vaporized by the CO_2 laser (Figure 5). Each ovary is treated by vaporizing 10–30 atretic follicles. The interior walls of the opened follicles have to be destroyed completely. The drilling should not be performed too deep otherwise bleeding may occur. Due to the vaporized follicular fluid an excessive amount of laser plume may be generated which unfortunately hampers visualization. This may be eliminated to some extent by a special laser-plume filtering system (Fa. Wolf, Knittlingen, West Germany) without any loss of intraperitoneal gas pressure. Physiological saline solution or ringer lactate is used to irrigate the ovarian surface. Significant bleeding has to be controlled by the defocused laser beam or with additional instruments such as a thermocoagulation probe.

The disadvantages of this technique lie in its unwieldiness due to the rigid arms of the delivery system, the high amount of laser plume produced during the operation, and poor haemostatic effect of the CO_2 laser. For these reasons, other laser systems have been introduced for the treatment of the PCOD.

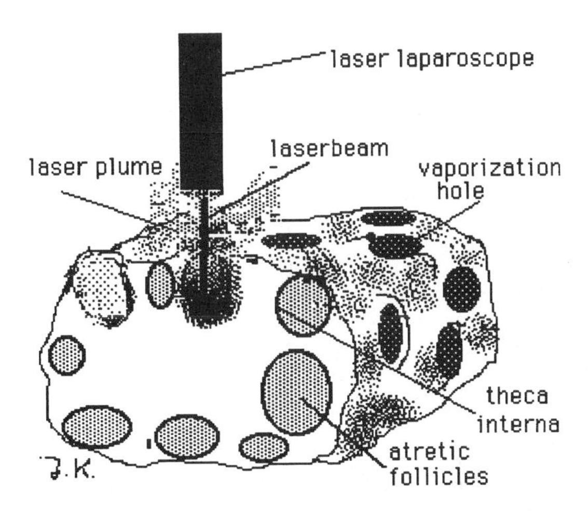

Figure 4. The effect of CO_2 laser vaporization of the polycystic ovary. The atretic follicles are opened by the laser beam. After drainage of the follicular fluid, the interior walls are vaporized. The lateral tissue damage is minimal.

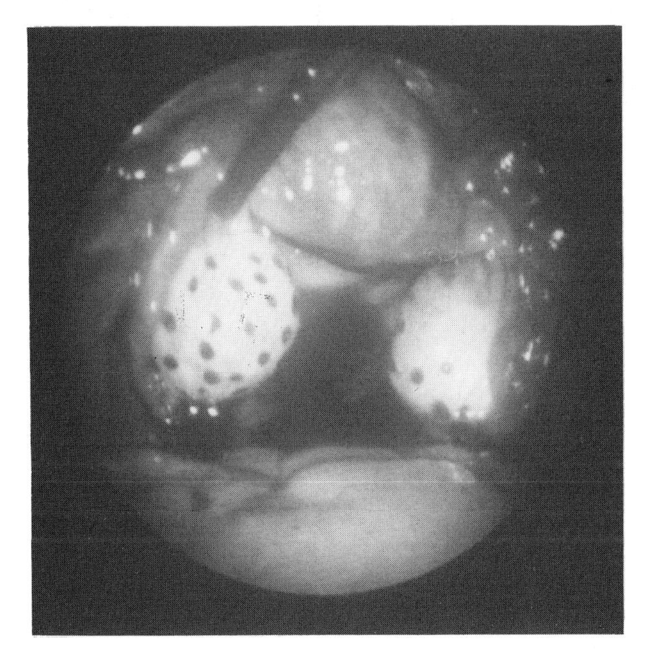

Figure 5. View of the ovaries after drilling by CO_2 laser vaporization. Each ovary is treated by 10–30 surface penetrations. Visualization is hampered by laser plume.

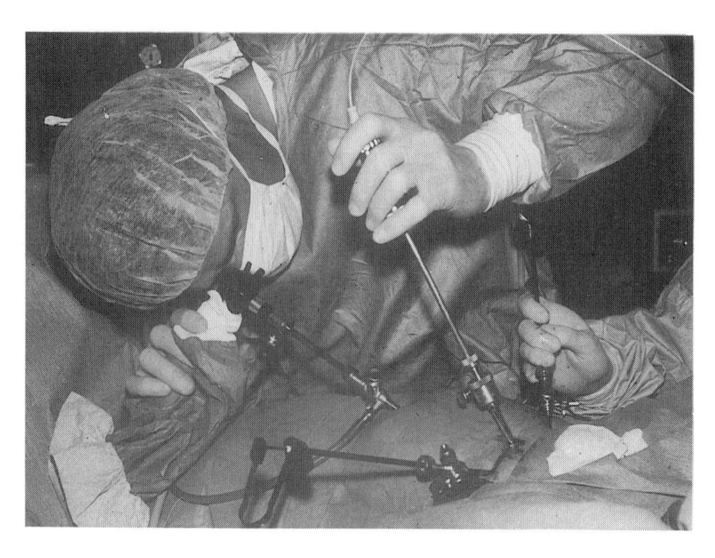

Figure 6. Laser laparoscopy using the Nd-YAG laser. The laser beam passes through a flexible quartz fibre. A special laser-fibre steering device allows the deflection of the fibre tip.

Nd-YAG laser

The advantage of this technique derives from its ability to deliver high power output of laser energy via fine quartz fibres (Figure 6). The wavelength of the Nd-YAG laser light coagulates tissue without vaporization at low powers when used in the non-contact mode. It is diffusely absorbed by body tissue, thus permitting deep penetration of laser energy. The depth of penetration of the laser light depends on the power being used and the application time. With the use of special laser probes the Nd-YAG laser may also be used in the contact mode.

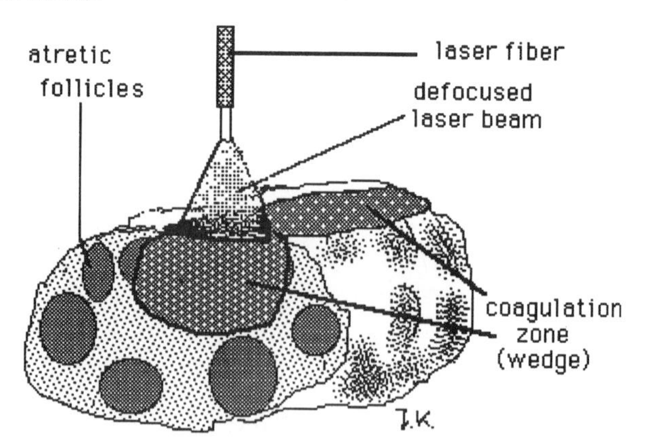

Figure 7. Effect of the Nd-YAG laser used in the non-contact mode. The laser light causes coagulation of the ovarian tissue in a wedge shape. If necessary adjacent atretic follicles may be opened with raised power levels.

Non-contact technique with the Nd-YAG laser. The aim of the non-contact Nd-YAG treatment of polycystic ovaries is to achieve deep coagulation in a wedge-like shape. A large amount of atretic, androgen-producing (-containing) follicles should be denaturated by this technique.

The sterile laser fibre is passed through the operating channel of the laparoscope or via a second puncture probe. A special laser fibre steering device (Fa.Wolf, Knittlingen, West Germany) with a deflectable tip gives maximum mobility to the fibre during the operation. The defocused laser beam is moved slowly across the anti-mesenteric surface of the ovary (Figures 7 and 8) at a distance of 5–10 mm. The power ranges between 45 and 70 W. The laser effect is controlled by a colour change of the ovarian surface. The ovarian tissue is coagulated to a depth of 4–10 mm. During laser application, the tissue is heated up slowly, allowing the surgeon to choose between coagulation and vaporization. When carbonization of ovarian tissue occurs, the absorption of the beam in the blackened tissue allows the Nd-YAG laser to cut. By application of this technique, part of the atretic follicles can also be opened and drained.

Contact technique with the Nd-YAG laser. Specially designed artificial sapphire tips have been developed and used successfully for coagulation and vaporization in the same procedure. The contact laser probes screw onto a metal connector that fastens to the 2.2 mm optical quartz fibres (Figure 9).

For the treatment of PCOD, a 2-mm round or flat contact tip is used. The

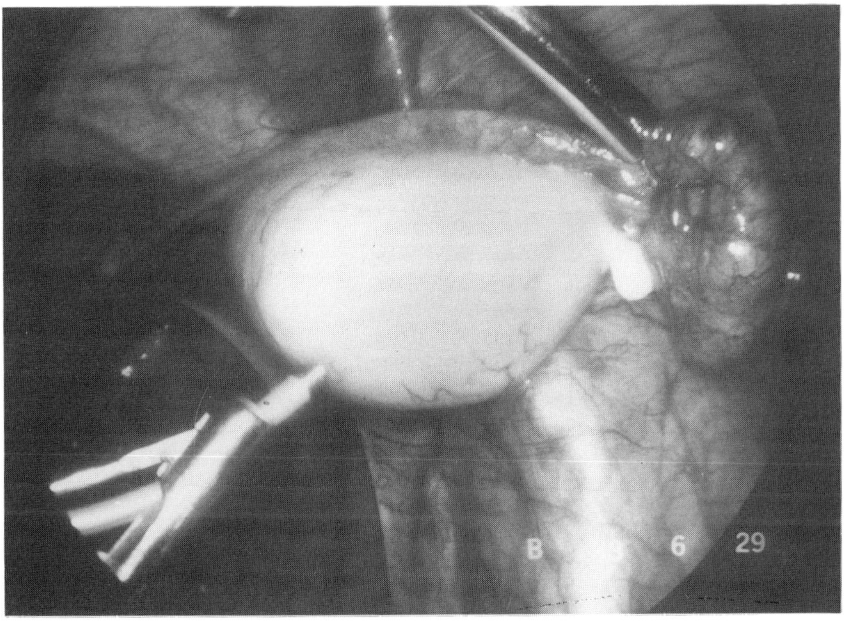

Figure 8. Non-contact Nd-YAG laser coagulation of the ovary. The flexible fibre is deflected by a special steering device and directed on the ovarian surface.

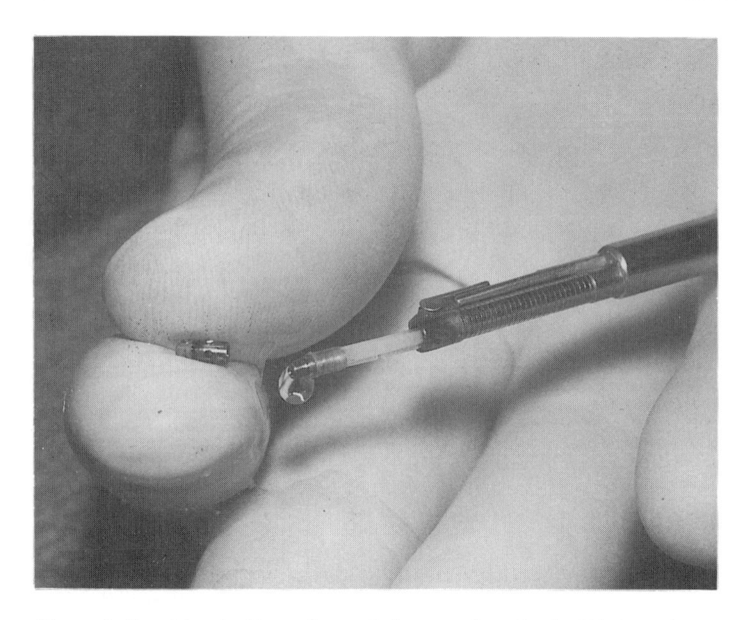

Figure 9. Sapphire tip (2 mm flat probe) screwed on the flexible laser fibre.

probe is pressed against the ovarian surface (as in electrocautery) until vaporizaton starts. As the ovarian cysts are opened the probe is advanced into the stroma (Figures 10 and 11). The laser light will then be absorbed by the debris which sticks to the sapphire tip. This results in heating of the contact tip up to 200–400C, which leads to thermal necrosis of the cysts. Because of the combination of laser and thermal effect bleeding rarely occurs.

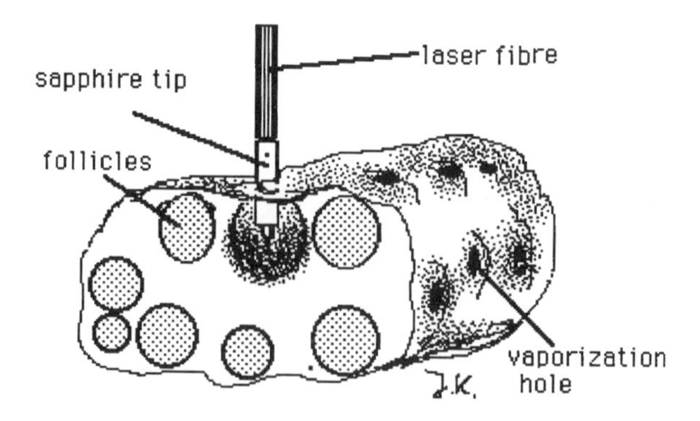

Figure 10. Contact Nd-YAG laser application. After penetration of the ovarian surface the probe is advanced into the stroma or atretic follicle. Laser light and heating up of the probe lead to destruction of surrounding tissue.

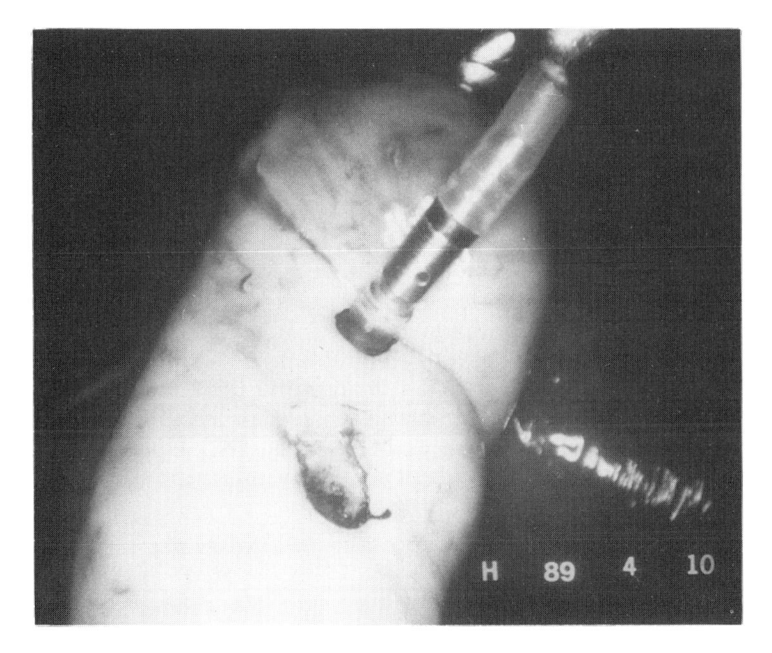

Figure 11. Sapphire tip pressed on the ovarian surface. Notice the opened atretic follicle at the bottom.

Argon and KTP-532 lasers

Recently the argon and KTP-532 laser have been introduced for the laparoscopic treatment of PCOD (Daniell and Miller, 1989). Although these lasers produce deeper tissue effects than the CO_2 laser, the coagulation property is less than that achieved by the Nd-YAG laser (Keckstein et al, 1988a). Using the argon laser with the bare fibre technique, good vaporization and coagulation effects have been achieved (Keckstein et al, 1988b). The fibre is advanced close to the ovarian surface. With power levels between 6 and 12 W the atretic follicles are opened and vaporized completely. Since the argon beam is not absorbed by clear fluids there is reduced smoke production during the procedure.

EFFICACY OF THE TECHNIQUES

Laparoscopic techniques have already proved efficacious in the treatment of PCOD: endocrine responses and ovulation rate after these procedures resemble those seen after wedge resection.

Pattern of menstrual cycle

The effectiveness of the laparoscopic approach can be demonstrated by the resumption of the normal pattern of the menstrual cycle. Excluding three women who became pregnant within 7 weeks, 51 (86.4%) of 59 patients established regular menstrual cycles after electrocautery (Gjønnæss, 1984). In our study of 19 patients treated with the CO_2 laser, all patients ($n=6$) with secondary amenorrhoea had vaginal bleeding within the first postoperative month. Seventy-two percent of the patients with severe oligomenorrhoea had regular periods for longer than 6 months.

Ovulation

The results of inducing ovulation after laparoscopy are encouraging (Table 1). Within the first 6 months we found an ovulation rate of between 71.4 and 87.5% after CO_2 laser vaporization and 73% after Nd-YAG laser coagulation. All these patients had failed to respond to clomiphene preoperatively. These results are similar to those achieved by electrocautery or using Nd-YAG laser incision (Aakvaag and Gjønnæss, 1985; Huber et al, 1989). Gjønnæss and Norman (1987) did not notice any influence of ovarian size on

Table 1. Ovulation rate after operative laparoscopy. (a) Patients ovulating on clomiphene before treatment. (b) Patients not ovulating preoperatively.

Operative technique	Investigator	Patients n (a/b)	Patients ovulating after treatment (spontaneously)
Electrocautery	Gjønnæss	62 (?/19)	57 (?/6)
Nd-YAG incision	Huber	8 (0/8)	5 (0/5)
Nd-YAG coagulation	Keckstein	11 (0/11)	8 (0/8)
CO_2 laser vaporization, argon or KTP	Daniell	85 (47/38)	60 (40/20)
CO_2 laser vaporization	Keckstein	14 (0/14)	10 (0/10)

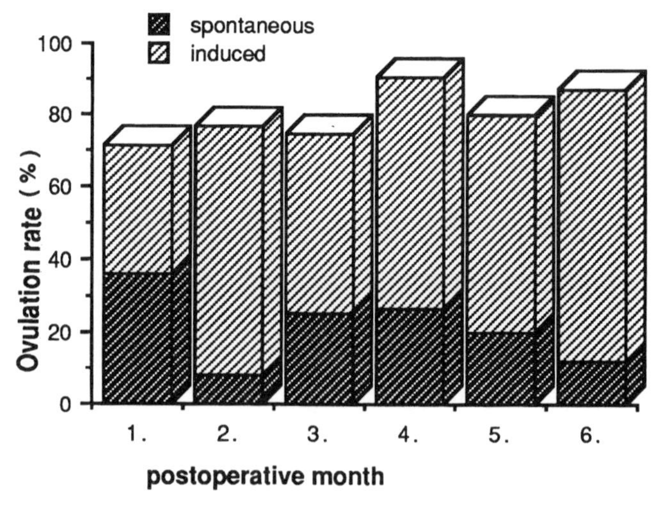

Figure 12. Ovulation rate after CO_2 laser vaporization (follow-up in 14 patients). All patients did not respond on clomiphene or HMG preoperatively.

the effect of electrocautery. However, the number of points cauterized is almost certainly related to the ovulation rate.

Observation of the patients who did not become pregnant shows that the effects of laser therapy or electrocautery are probably of limited duration. In our series of 19 patients treated with the CO_2 laser 14 patients were serially monitored for ovulation. The rate of spontaneous ovulations decreased over a period of 6 months (Figure 12). Gjønnæss (1984) followed 12 of 32 patients who did not become pregnant after electrocoagulation for more than 2 years; in only three women did the treatment effect last more than this time.

Fertility

The pregnancy rates reported after laparoscopic treatment of PCOD range from between 0 and 75% (Table 2). A direct comparison of these results is only partially valid because of variable follow-up periods and the lack of homogeneity of the treated patient population.

Table 2. Fertility rate after laparoscopic treatment of PCOD.

Operative technique	Investigator	Number of patients	Number of pregnancies
Laparoscopic biopsy	Portuondo	16	9
Laparoscopic biopsy	Campo	12	7
Electrocautery	Gjønnæss	35	24
Nd-YAG incision	Huber	8	–
Nd-YAG coagulation	Keckstein	11	3
CO_2 laser vaporization, argon or KTP	Daniell	85	49
CO_2 laser vaporization	Keckstein	16	8

Hormonal response

Androstendione and testosterone

The hormonal change observed after ovarian wedge resection has been studied by various authors (Judd et al, 1976; Katz et al, 1978). It is suggested that the mechanism responsible for ovulation following surgery is a reduction of intraovarian androgens, caused by a removal of androgen-producing tissue, which is mainly found in the atretic follicles (Mori et al, 1982). Although the tissue destruction achieved by multiple punch biopsies, or electrocautery is much smaller than by wedge resection, the hormonal effect is similar.

Aakvaag and Gjønnæss (1985) studied 59 patients with PCOD before and after electrocautery of the ovaries. Serum levels of testosterone and androstendione were reduced significantly within the first 3 days. Greenblatt and Casper (1987) also demonstrated a dramatic fall of androstendione, testosterone and dihydrotestosterone levels in the early postoperative period. Gjønnæss (1984) was able to demonstrate that the postoperative effect depends on the number of sites being cauterized. With the multiple punch biopsy described by Sumioki (1988) parts of thickened capsule overlying the follicles were removed. Although he found a decrease of the serum level of androgens, he could not demonstrate a relationship between the hormonal changes and the amount of ovarian tissue resected, or the number of the ovarian follicles destroyed.

In methods delineated thus far, two different effects are achieved. On one hand, the cauterization of the ovarian surface leads to a drainage of the follicular fluid which contains a high level of androgen. On the other hand the electrocautery causes a destruction of the interior wall of the atretic follicles and the adjacent hormone producing tissue. Both effects in combination achieve a reduction of postoperative androgen levels in the serum. That each of these effects solely can lead to an altered ovarian function was demonstrated in two of our studies with different laser systems:

1. When applying the non-contact Nd-YAG laser a large portion of the ovary is destroyed, without opening of the atretic follicles. Experimental studies demonstrated that a significant portion of the ovarian tissue is reduced by Nd-YAG laser (Keckstein et al, 1988a). Eleven patients in our clinical study showed a dramatic fall of the androgen levels within the first 2 days after Nd-YAG laser coagulation without draining of atretic follicles. Before operation the mean serum androstendione level was 3.4 ± 0.4 ng/ml and that of testosterone was 1.1 ± 0.1 ng/ml. The postoperative decrease was significant ($p < 0.01$) with values of 2.2 ± 0.2 ng/ml and 0.5 ± 0.3 ng/ml, respectively (Figure 13).
2. In contrast to the aforementioned Nd-YAG laser effects, the CO_2 laser has only little coagulation property and vaporization is limited by the presence of follicular fluid or blood. The dot-like vaporization of the ovaries leads to a drainage of the atretic follicles and thus to a decrease of the intraovarian androgen level. The preoperative androstendione level (mean $\pm$ SD) of 2.8 ± 1.0 ng/ml decreased to a level of 2.17 ± 0.7 ng/ml.

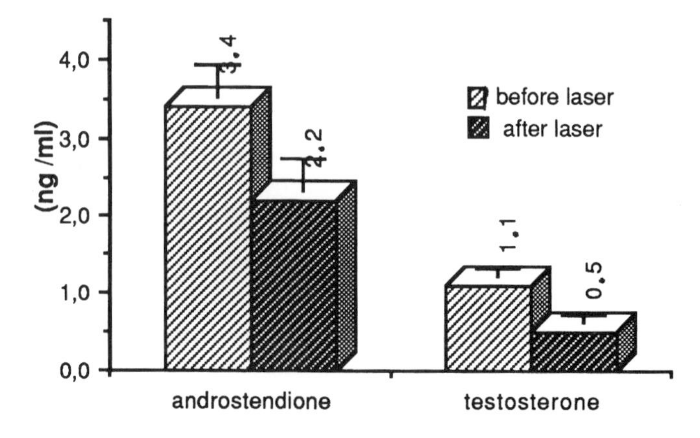

Figure 13. Serum androstendione and testosterone concentrations (mean $\pm$ SD) of 11 patients before and 2 days after non-contact Nd-YAG laser coagulation of the ovary.

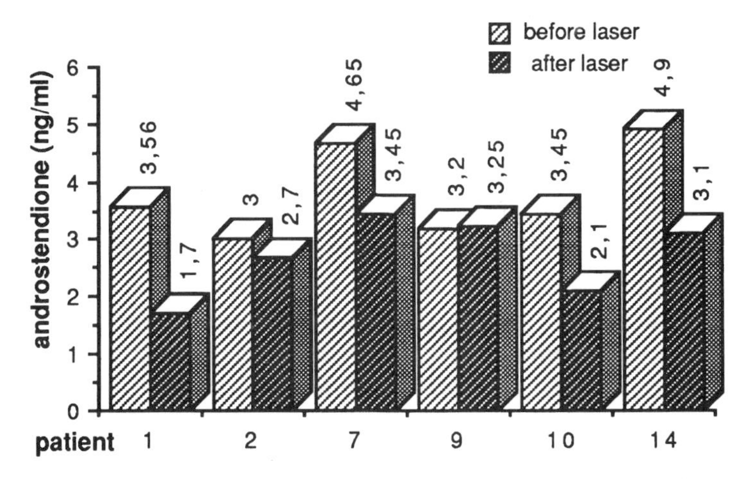

Figure 14. Serum androstendione concentrations before and after CO_2 laser vaporization (six patients with significantly elevated values preoperatively).

Figure 14 illustrates the decrease of androstendione and testosterone after CO_2 laser vaporization in six patients with significantly elevated androgen levels. The individual variation in reduction may be explained by variable androgen concentrations in the follicular fluid. Interestingly high pregnancy rates were found in our study among patients with significantly elevated androgen levels in the follicular fluid. (Table 3). This may confirm the hypothesis that only drainage of the follicles with high androgen levels is necessary to alter ovarian function.

Table 3. Androgen concentration (median) of follicular fluid in patients with and without postoperative pregnancy.

	Patients conceiving	Patients not conceiving
Right ovary		
Androstendione (ng/ml)	34.00	24.00
Testosterone (ng/ml)	36.00	20.00
Left ovary		
Androstendione (ng/ml)	29.15	20.40
Testosterone (ng/ml)	34.00	13.17

Gonadotrophins

It is well documented that secretion of excessive amounts of androgen leads to an increase of pituitary sensitivity to gonadotrophin releasing hormone (GnRH) and has a positive feedback on anterior pituitary LH secretion. Therefore, the normal cyclic patterns of FSH and LH are typically absent in patients with PCOD: there is a disproportionately high secretion of LH with consistently low FSH secretion (Hutchinson and De Cherney, 1987). The significant reduction in basal LH secretion has been associated with a decrease in circulating androstendione and testosterone after ovarian electrocautery (Aakvaag and Gjønnæss, 1985; Gjønnæss and Norman, 1987; Greenblatt and Casper, 1987; Sumioki, 1988). Sumioki (1988) found a marked reduction in the mean LH level (mean ± SEM: 33.7 ± 3.74–20.0 ± 2.49 mIU/ml; $p < 0.01$) 4 days after the multiple punch resection of the ovaries.

Though Greenblatt and Casper (1987) demonstrated a less dramatic decrease of LH in comparison with the effect on androgen levels after electrocautery, the rise of FSH values contributed to a decrease of the abnormally elevated LH:FSH ratio.

In the series presented by Aakvaag and Gjønnæss (1985), postoperative serum LH levels were different in women who ovulated shortly after ovarian electrocautery than those who did not. There was an increase of the LH level the day after electrocautery in the 'early ovulator' group with a significant subsequent decrease during following days. This postoperative LH increase is explained by Gjønnæss and Norman (1987) as the result of a reduced negative feedback due to the fall of androgens.

Hypothalamo-pituitary axis

The disparity between LH and FSH secretion seems to be caused by the greater inhibitory effect of oestrone E_1 and oestradiol E_2 on FSH than on LH. In addition, a heightened pituitary sensitivity to GnRH and probably also an elevated GnRH secretion has been described. The pituitary

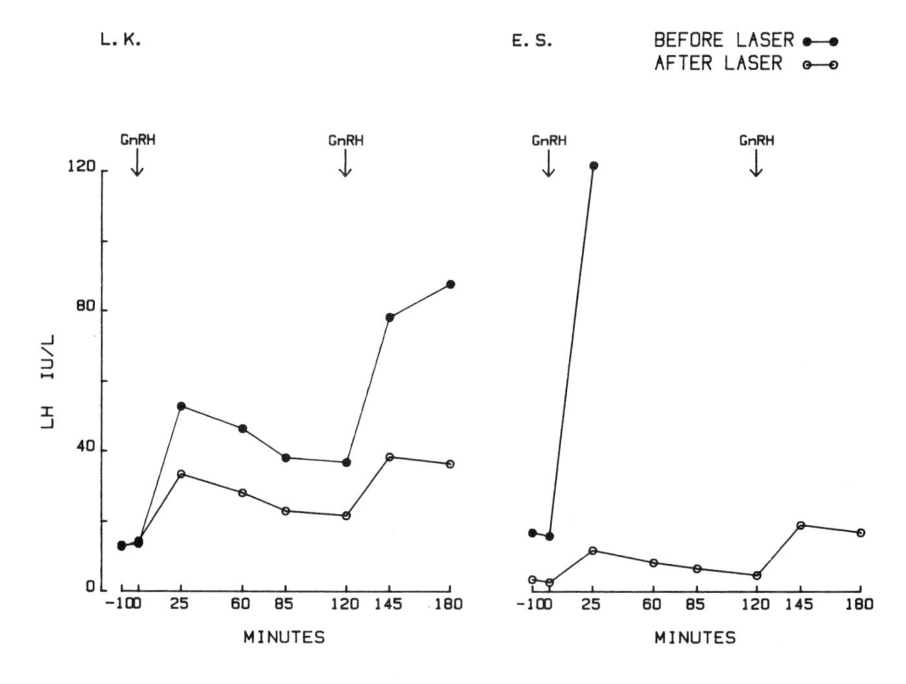

Figure 15. Patterns of GnRH tests before and after Nd-YAG laser coagulation in two patients.

responses to exogenous GnRH injection in patients with PCOD are characterized by high LH response with a relatively low FSH response.

Sumioki (1988) examined the patterns of response to GnRH the day before operation, 3 or 4 days after the operation, and 6 weeks after operation. The net increase of LH at 30 minutes after the GnRH injection was 224.7 ± 56.3 mIU/ml 133.0 ± 46.5 mIU/ml, and 40.3 ± 12.7 mIU/ml, respectively.

In our study all patients showed a decrease of the pituitary response of variable degree (Figure 15) after Nd-YAG laser coagulation of the ovaries. This marked reduction of pituitary sensitivity was not confirmed by Gjønnæss and Norman (1987). They found an enhanced response of FSH and LH to GnRH stimulation in 16 patients after electrocautery of the ovaries.

Patterns of pulsatile GnRH secretion

Gonadotrophins are released in a pulsatile fashion. In patients with PCOD the amplitude and/or the frequency of LH pulses are substantially increased (Rebar et al, 1976).

Sumioki (1988) demonstrated the reduction of a preoperative exaggerated LH pulsation by laparoscopic punch resection. Though there was a significant decrease of the pulse amplitude, the pulse frequency did not change after the operation.

In our series this effect could not be confirmed after Nd-YAG laser

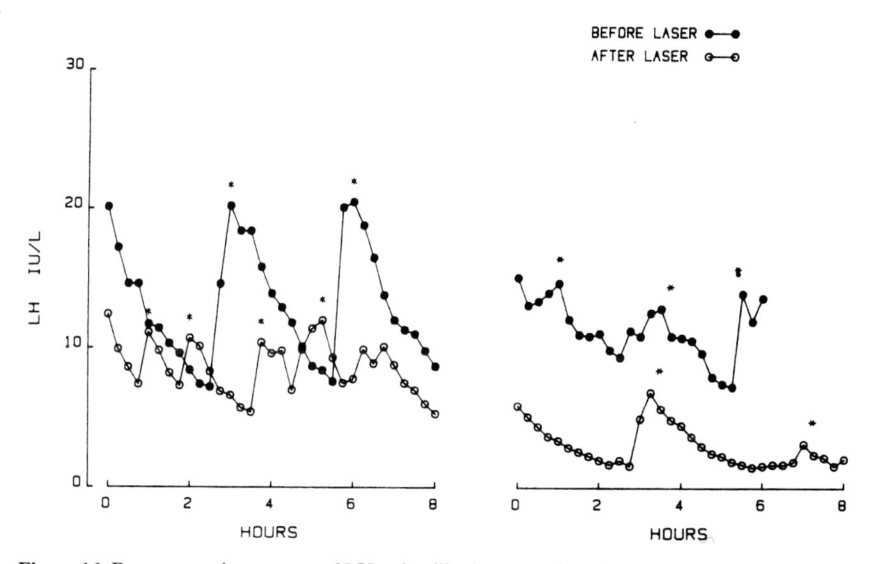

Figure 16. Representative pattern of LH pulsatility in two patients before and after non-contact Nd-YAG laser treatment (same patients as in Figure 15).

treatment. There was no consistent change in the pattern of pulsatility in five patients being followed-up after treatment until now. Figure 16 illustrates two different patterns of LH pulsatility in two patients preoperatively and their reaction postoperatively. There was a marked reduction of mean LH levels in both patients, and of LH pulse amplitude in patient L.K. However, pulse frequency increased in patient L.K. and decreased in patient E.S.

Ultrasound findings after therapy

Presence of multiple small cystic structures and an increase in ovarian stroma are ultrasound criteria for the indentification of polycystic ovaries. Ultrasound studies demonstrate a significant decrease in ovarian size after contact Nd-YAG laser coagulation (Grochmal, 1988). In contrast CO_2 laser vaporization does not reduce significantly ovarian size, as confirmed by animal studies (Keckstein et al, 1988a).

Postoperative adhesions

In general there are less adhesions after laparoscopy in comparison with laparotomy. However, bleeding or extensive zones of necrosis cause postoperative adhesions, which have been demonstrated in animal experiments (Riedel, 1986).

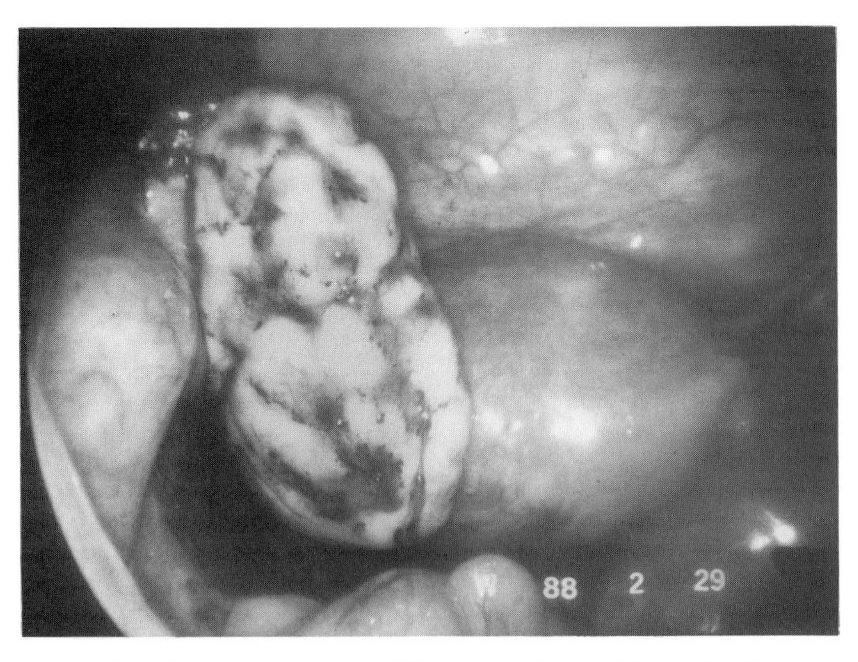

Figure 17. Second-look laparoscopy after CO_2 laser vaporization of the ovaries. The ovarian surface shows dotted like scars (residuals of the carbonized debris) and small vascularized areas.

There are only a few investigations on the incidence of adhesions after laparoscopic treatment of PCOD (Portuondo et al, 1984; Van der Weiden and Alberda, 1987). Adhesions were found in 12–15% of patients after CO_2 laser vaporization, and 3% of patients after Nd-YAG contact application, as reported by Grochmal (1988).

In our series 7 patients were evaluated by second-look laparoscopy or laparotomy (caesarian section) after CO_2 laser vaporization (Figure 17). In three cases, filmy adhesions covering parts of the ovary were seen. These pelvic adhesions may be attributed to the residual carbonized debris after vaporization and to the poor haemostatic properties of the CO_2 laser. We did not see any adhesions in four out of 11 patients treated with the Nd-YAG laser. These results reconfirm our findings evaluated in a study, comparing various techniques of vaporization or coagulation in rabbits (Keckstein et al, 1988a).

Complications

With the exception of the postoperative adhesions already discussed no other complications have been reported.

SUMMARY

Laparoscopic techniques show a number of advantages in comparison with the classic ovarian wedge resection for the treatment of PCOD. An equally high ovulation rate is achieved with less trauma, and fewer postoperative adhesions result in a higher pregnancy rate. The procedure may be done on an outpatient basis with reduced operative and recovery time.

No clear advantages have so far been shown to exist for any of the available techniques, i.e. laparoscopic biopsy, electrocautery, and the four laser systems (CO_2, Nd-YAG, argon, KTP). It appears, however, that the laser techniques will be the methods of choice for the future. They combine optimal precision of operation handling with maximal safety and excellent bleeding control.

With laparoscopic biopsy traumatic bleedings may occur, which can occasionally be difficult to control. With electrocautery, burns due to the uncontrolled effect of electric current have been described. Optimal application of the laser techniques requires extensive personnel training and experience. The laser equipment requires considerable capital expenditure of the order of £20 000–70 000.

The exact mechanism by which induction of ovulation and regular cycles are induced is yet unknown. Alteration of the ovarian surface including the underlying tissue particularly the atretic follicles leads to a significant postoperative change of the pathophysiological mechanism. The following factors are postulated to be responsible for postoperative ovulation:

1. The drainage of the follicular fluid which contains high androgen levels results in an acute reduction of the intraovarian androgen level.

2. With coagulation and/or vaporization of the atretic follicles androgen production is significantly limited.
3. This localized reduction of androgen decreases their inhibitory effect on follicular maturation.
4. Lowered androgen levels result in diminished peripheral conversion of androgen to oestrogen and descreased positive feedback on LH production.
5. The secondary reduction of ovarian inhibin permits a rise of FSH secretion which results in a normal LH:FSH ratio.

Acknowledgements

The author is grateful for the assistance of Dr V. Schneider, Mrs White and Mrs Francy in the preparation of this manuscript.

REFERENCES

Aakvaag A & Gjønnæss H (1985) Hormonal response to electrocautery of the ovary in patients with polycystic ovarian disease. *British Journal of Obstetrics and Gynaecology* **92:** 1258–1264.

Buttram VJ & Vaquero C (1975) Post-ovarian wedge resection adhesive disease. *Fertility and Sterility* **26:** 874–876.

Campo S, Garcea N, Caruso A & Siccardi P (1983) Effect of celioscopic ovarian resection in patients with polycystic ovaries. *Gynecologic and Obstetric Investigation* **15:** 213–222.

Daniell J & Miller W (1989) Polycystic ovaries treated by laparoscopic laser vaporization. *Fertility and Sterility* **51:** 232–236.

Fleming R, Haxton M, Hamilton M et al (1985) Successful treatment of infertile women with oligomenorrhoea using a combination of LHRH agonist and exogenous gonadotrophins. *British Journal of Obstetrics and Gynaecology* **92:** 369–379.

Franks S, Sagle M, Mason H & Kiddy D (1987) Use of LHRH agonists in the treatment of anovulation in women with polycystic ovary syndrome. *Hormone Research* **28:** 164–168.

Gjønnæss H (1984) Polycystic ovarian syndrome treated by ovarian electrocautery through the laparoscope. *Fertility and Sterility* **41:** 20–24.

Gjønnæss H & Norman N (1987) Endocrine effects of the ovarian electrocautery in patients with polycystic ovarian disease. *British Journal of Obstetrics and Gynaecology* **94:** 779–783.

Greenblatt E & Casper R (1987) Endocrine changes after laparoscopic ovarian cautery in polycystic ovarian syndrome. *American Journal of Obstetrics and Gynecology* **156:** 279–285.

Grochmal S (1988) Contact Nd:Yag superior to CO_2 for treatment of ovarian disease. *Laser Practice Report* **3:** 1S–2S.

Huber J, Hosman J & Spona J (1989) Endoskopisch vorgenommene Laserincision des polycystischen Ovars. *Geburtshilfe und Frauenheilkunde* **49:** 37–40.

Hutchinson W & De Cherney A (1987) Pathogenesis and treatment of polycystic ovary disease. *International Journal of Fertility* **32:** 421–430.

Judd H, Rigg L, Anderson & Yen S (1976) The effects of ovarian wedge resection on circulating gonadotrophin and ovarian steriod levels in patients with polycystic ovary syndrome. *Journal of Clinical Endocrinology and Metabolism* **43:** 347–355.

Katz M, Carr P, Cohan B & Millar R (1978) Hormonal effects of wedge resection of polycystic ovaries. *Obstetrics and Gynecology* **41:** 437–444.

Keckstein J, Finger A & Steiner R (1988a) Laser application in contact and noncontact procedures; sapphire tips in comparison to ‘bare-fiber’, argon laser in comparison to Nd:YAG laser (in German). *Laser in medicine and surgery* **4:** 158–162.

Keckstein J, Tuttlies F & Steiner R (1988b) Lasereffekt am ovar: CO_2 versus Nd:YAG versus argon. *Proceedings of 4.Jahrestagung der deutschen Gesellschaft für Lasermedizin e.V.*, in press.

Kirschner M, Zucker I & Jespersen D (1976) Idiopathic hirsutism—an ovarian abnormality. *New England Journal of Medicine* **294:** 637–640.

Mori T, Fujita Y, Hihnobu K et al (1982) Significance of atretic follicles as the site of androgen production in polycystic ovaries. *Journal of Endocrinological Investigation* **5:** 209–215.

Portuondo J, Melchor J, Neyro J & Alegre A (1984) Periovarian adhesions following ovarian wedge resection or laparoscopic biopsy. *Endoscopy* **16:** 143–145.

Rebar R, Judd H, Yen S et al (1976) Charactarization of the inappropriate gonadotropin secretion in polycystic ovary syndrome. *Journal of Clinical Investigation* **57:** 1320–1329.

Riedel H (1986) Die Anwendung verschiedener Koagulationstechniken zur Eileitersterilisation und ihre Bedeutung für das Auftreten von ovariellen Ausfallserscheinungen. *Habilitationsschrift*, Kiel.

Semm K & Mettler L (1980) Technical progress in pelvic surgery via operative laparoscopy. *American Journal of Obstetrics and Gynecology* **138:** 121–127.

Stein I & Leventhal M (1935) Amenorrhea associated with bilateral polycystic ovaries. *American Journal of Obstetrics and Gynecology* **29:** 181–191.

Sumioki H (1988) The effect of laparoscopic multiple punch resection of the ovary on hypothalamo-pituitary axis in polycystic ovary syndrome. *Fertility and Sterility* **50:** 567–572.

Van der Weiden R & Alberda A (1987) Laparoscopic ovarian electrocautery in patients with polycystic ovarian disease reistant to clomiphen citrate. *Surgical Endoscopy* **1:** 217–219.

Yen S (1980) The polycystic ovary syndrome. *Clinical Endocrinology* **12:** 177–208.

Yuzpe A & Rioux J (1975) The value of laparoscopic ovarian biopsy. *The Journal of Reproductive Medicine* **15:** 432–442.

8

Laparoscopic treatment of ectopic pregnancy

WILLIAM R. MEYER
ALAN H. DECHERNEY

THE DIAGNOSIS OF UNRUPTURED ECTOPIC PREGNANCY

New questions concerning the treatment of ectopic pregnancy have surfaced as more sensitive diagnostic techniques have arisen. Recent modalities including transvaginal ultrasound, serum progesterone levels and advances in biochemical monitoring of β human chorionic gonadotrophin (HCG) are presently redefining the originally proposed discriminatory zone.

Vaginal sonography allows detection of an ectopic pregnancy one week earlier than the abdominal route. Transvaginal sonography can now identify an intrauterine sac, on average, at a serum βHCG concentration of 1398 mIU/ml (First Standard Preparation) (Fossum et al, 1988), whereas previously a threshold level of 6500 mIU/ml (FSP) was used in conjunction with the transabdominal sonograph. The absence of an intrauterine sac with this titre was associated with an ectopic pregnancy in 87% of cases (Romero et al, 1985).

The value of progesterone levels in the detection of ectopic pregnancy is under investigation. Yeko et al (1987), in a recent retrospective study of 70 women, concluded that a progesterone level less than 15 ng/ml was predictive of either a non-viable or ectopic pregnancy. Similarly in another study by Matthews et al (1986) of 29 women with ectopic pregnancy the progesterone level never exceeded 12.9 ng/ml. The twenty women in this report with intrauterine pregnancies had a mean progesterone level of 30.9 ± 6.9 ng/ml. It appears that transvaginal sonography and progesterone levels may become valuable adjuncts to serum HCG values measured by rapid radio-immuno assays, allowing earlier diagnosis of ectopic pregnancy, perhaps allowing intervention prior to tubal rupture.

CONSERVATIVE TREATMENT OF ECTOPIC PREGNANCY

Interventional approaches by laparotomy including salpingostomy may soon be regarded as 'radical' if not obsolete, as surgery evolves to a more 'conservative' endoscopic approach. Presently laparoscopy is widely accepted as the gold standard for the diagnosis of ectopic pregnancy.

However technical advances in instrumentation have allowed the surgeon opportunity to use the laparoscope as a mode of therapy as well as a means of diagnosis. Unfortunately, as described by Gonzalez and Wayman (1981) and Samuelson and Sjovall (1972), even diagnostic laparoscopy lacks complete sensitivity in the detection of ectopic pregnancy. This necessitates persistent attention to certain precautions, guidelines, and follow-up when laparoscopy is used as a therapeutic tool for treatment. This chapter will discuss the indications, techniques, results and follow-up of endoscopically treated ectopic pregnancies.

INDICATIONS AND CONTRAINDICATIONS

Previous restrictive criteria in the treatment of ectopic pregnancy have relaxed as endoscopic experience has been gained. However haemodynamic instability still remains an absolute and obvious contraindication to a laparoscopic approach. Presently haematoperitoneum, tubal rupture, excessive tubal diameter, pelvic adhesive disease, and concurrent medical diseases such as hiatus hernia are less often reasons to avoid laparoscopy. DeCherney et al (1981) initially excluded laparoscopic intervention if the contralateral adnexa appeared abnormal. Conservative laparoscopic treatment had been previously reserved only for unruptured ampullary or infundibular pregnancies with a diameter less than 3 cm and in cases without a haematoperitoneum. This was a result of complications from immediate and delayed haemorrhage along with the inability to deliver larger gestational contents associated with ectopics exceeding this size restriction. However, operative experience and new instrumentation often allows attempts at laparoscopic treatment in cases where it was previously not technically possible.

CHOICE OF OPERATIVE TECHNIQUE

Six basic laparoscopic techniques are available for managing ectopic pregnancy the choice of methods depending on the future fertility desires of the patient and the extent of disease. These are (i) mechanical aspiration, (ii) fimbrial expression (milking) (iii) coagulative destruction, (iv) salpingostomy, (v) segmental resection, and (vi) salpingectomy. Rapid induction general anaesthesia is recommended for all of the techniques described.

Mechanical aspiration and fimbrial expression

Tubal abortions may be atraumatically removed from the fimbriated distal end of the oviduct. However extension of this technique to involve infundibular aspiration or tubal 'milking' is mentioned only to condemn it. Bruhat et al (1980) describes aspiration in 17 patients in which three women subsequently underwent incomplete delivery of the ectopic, two remained infertile and two had repeat ectopics. In the milking technique the tube proximal to the ectopic is grasped and then progressively compressed distally towards the fimbriated end to extrude out the products of conception. As noted by Timonen and Niemimen (1967), the procedure produces excessive tubal mucosal damage resulting in higher subsequent ectopic pregnancy rates.

Coagulative destruction

Coagulative obliteration of the ectopic pregnancy using bipolar forceps (for example Kleppinger) or thermocoagulation is useful when conservative therapy is not a prerequisite or the ectopic gestation lies within the isthmic portion of the tube. The inherent failure of lack of histological confirmation of the products of conception is an obvious drawback of this procedure.

Linear salpingostomy

As with laparotomy, endoscopic linear salpingostomy may be performed allowing either primary closure, or closure by means of secondary intention. Stromme (1953) described the first salpingotomy closure at the time of laparotomy. Some gynaecologists have advocated primary closure with sutures for several reasons (Semm, 1987). These include haemostatic insurability, reduction of adhesion formation by the prevention of exposure of raw serosal surface area and the prevention of peritoneal–tubal fistula formation. Suturing through the laparoscope requires additional training and familiarity with pelviscopy, but is not an unsurmountable task after pelviscopic instruction.

Those supporting salpingostomy argue that serosal closure with salpingotomy may induce tissue ischaemia promoting adhesion formation. The obvious foreign body reaction to suture material may also contribute to adhesion formation. Salpingotomy may also limit proper serosal drainage, increase the chances of incomplete trophoblastic removal and increase the chances of postoperative haemorrhage (Kelly et al, 1979; Richards, 1984). Initially linear salpingostomies were accomplished by Israel (1951) in cases of pelvic inflammatory disease. When used in animals no evidence of a visible scar and complete fusion of incision edges was noted 8 weeks postoperatively. Most convincing were clinical studies in which salpingotomy or salpingostomy were performed in women with an ectopic in the last remaining fallopian tube. Oelsner et al (1986) reported elevated (43%) ectopic rates associated with salpingotomy at laparotomy in women with only one oviduct remaining. This is in sharp contrast to a report by DeCherney et al (1982) of a low (20%) repeat ectopic rate and successful (53%) intrauterine pregnancy rate after salpingostomy in the sole oviduct. Regardless of technique used, Nelson et al (1986) reported no significant differences in pregnancy rates, nidation indices, or adhesion-free tubes when the two procedures were directly compared in the rabbit model.

Histologically, ampullary gestational contents characteristically lie extraluminally. Eighty five percent of 84 ampullary tubal ectopic pregnancies recently described histologically by Senterman (1988) had an intact muscularis layer. This indicates that tubal closure is not mandatory for maintenance of tubal patency.

Preparation of the incision site

Prior to performing the linear salpingostomy incision, approximately 5 ml of vasopressin (Pitressin: Parke-Davis, Morris Plains, New Jersey) in a concentration of 0.05 to 1.0 units/ml of a saline containing solution is injected into the antimesenteric serosal bulge. Injection is performed with either a puncture cannula or a 22-gauge spinal needle. The latter is introduced separately into the peritoneal cavity. Mesosalpingeal injection has been suggested but direct intravascular instillation must be avoided. Although a theoretical concern, delayed postoperative haemorrhage from the use of vasoconstrictors is uncommon. Successful prostaglandin ($PGF_{2\alpha}$) tubal and corpus luteal injection without succeeding salpingostomy has been reported by Lindblom et al (1987) in nine women. Unfortunately post-therapy tubal patency rates were not described. Thermocoagulation prior to linear salpingostomy seems to obviate the need for vasopressin injection (Semm, 1987). Pelvic adhesions should be left alone until after the procedure if their positioning allows greater tubal access and stability; features which might enhance operative performance and technique. Adhesions should be lysed after completion of the salpingostomy unless they hinder access to the antimesenteric border of the tube.

Choice of surgical tool for incision

Various modalities can be used to perform the linear salpingostomy incision including scissors, electrocautery or the carbon dioxide (CO_2), argon or potassium titanyl phosphate (KTP) laser. Unipolar current is generally thought to be the most dangerous method of performing the salpingostomy incision. Since the patient becomes an integral party of the electrical circuit, tissue damage up to 5 cm has been reported (Martin and Diamond, 1986). A unipolar hook or knife electrode with low voltage (40–80 W) is recommended to reduce complications. Bipolar coagulation when applied by paddles may be cumbersome, therefore, application by a bipolar coagulator button may be more reasonable. This method limits tissue damage to 2–5 mm. The use of the thermocoagulator negates electrical tissue damage with only 2–3 mm of lateral tissue damage, a direct result of tissue heating.

The laser's inherent properties of precision and accuracy is gaining it popularity as a means of creating a linear salpingostomy. The CO_2 laser works by vaporization with tissue damage limited to a depth of 0.1–0.2 mm. Martin and Diamond (1986) note that extended thermal damage is due to tissue heating and is related to tissue type, power density, and duration of vaporization. Rapid vaporization manoeuvres limit thermal spread to 200–400 μm. A slower vaporization process doubles the extent of injury. The CO_2 laser's limited depth of injury allows one to perform a more superficial linear salpingostomy in an attempt to avoid endosalpingeal injury. Johns and Nardie (1986) reported successful salpingostomies with the CO_2 laser under continuous mode with power densities of 4000 W/cm^2 and beam diameters of 0.5 mm. Power densities are approximated by the following equation:

$$\text{Power density} = \frac{100 \times (\text{total beam power in watts})}{(\text{effective beam diameter in mm})^2}$$

Power densities greater than 4800 W/cm^2 in the continuous mode and greater than 2375 W/cm^2 in the pulse mode are needed to limit circumferential tissue damage (Taylor et al, 1986).

In contrast to the CO_2 laser's initial depth of penetration of 0.1–0.2 mm the argon laser penetrates 0.4–0.8 mm. Inherent lateral dispersion of the argon laser beam may offer the surgeon increased haemostasis during the procedure. Unfortunately these haemostatic advantages are overshadowed by increased chances of tubal luminal damage. Presently the comparative relative efficacies of the differing modes of performing linear salpingostomy are untested.

Operative details

The preferable antimesenteric incisional length performed for linear salpingostomy is approximately two thirds the length of the tubal bulge.

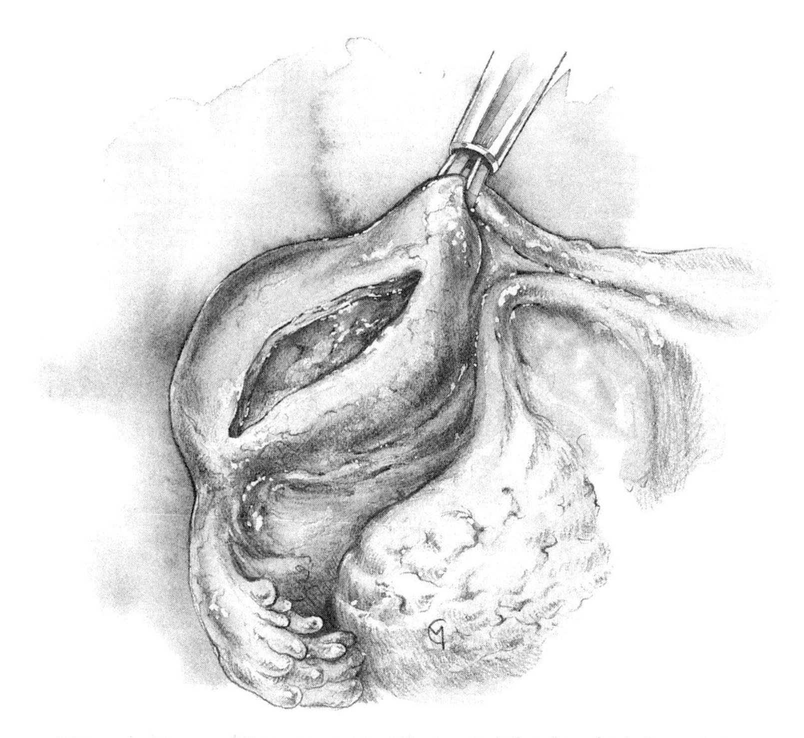

Figure 1. Linear salpingostomy on antimesenteric border of tubal pregnancy.

After the tubal incision is completed, contents often extrude spontaneously. This is most likely a result of the increased extrinsic pressure from the pneumoperitoneum. Excessive bleeding may be controlled by either defocusing the laser beam or using the bipolar cautery to coagulate bleeders on the serosal surface or the feeder vessels in the broad ligament. Interestingly bleeding during endoscopic procedures seems reduced in comparison to similar conditions during laparotomy (Semm, 1987) (Figure 1).

Extruded products of conception are most easily removed with atraumatic biopsy forceps or large spoon forceps (Figure 2). To the inexperienced eye excess trophoblastic tissue always seems residual in the tubal cavity. Attempts at aggressive and total removal of this necrotic tissue is often plagued by excessive bleeding, frequently requiring salpingectomy, so attempts at its removal are not advocated.

Semm (1987) suggests copious irrigation and aspiration with a lactated Ringer's solution over and inside the tube, pelvic and upper abdominal cavity not only to allow greater appraisal of haemostasis, but to prevent adhesive disease and afford a shorter recovery time. Blood allowed to remain in the cul-de-sac increases postoperative discomfort and may promote adhesion formation.

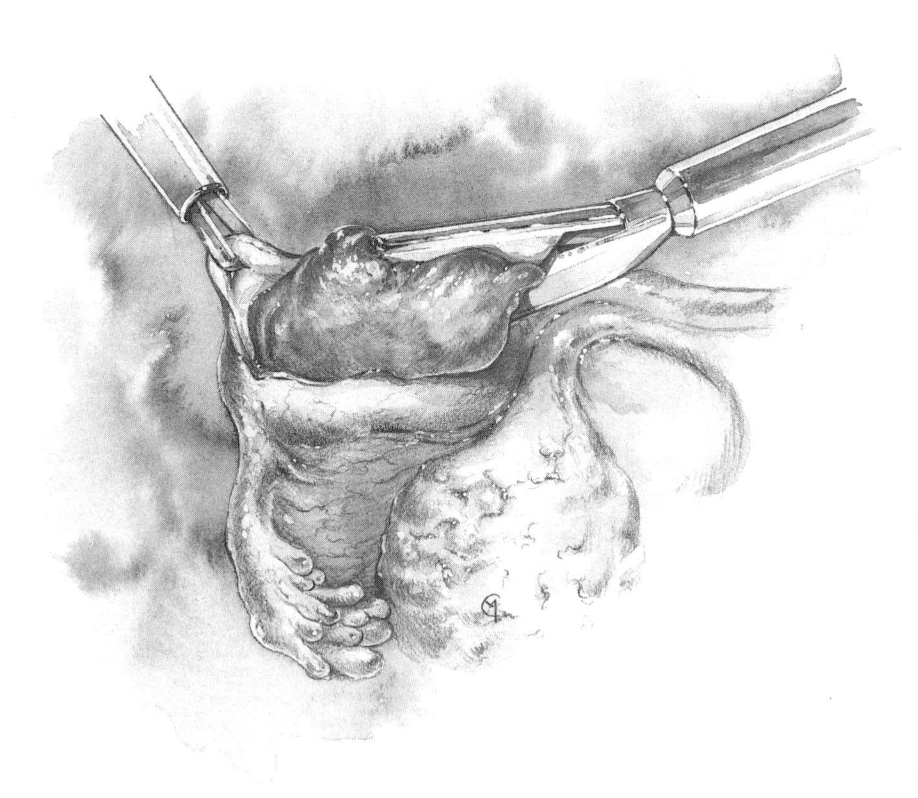

Figure 2. Removal of extruded products of conception from salpingostomy incision.

Salpingectomy—partial and complete

While salpingectomy and partial salpingectomy are technically similar, they are performed under differing surgical situations. Both procedures are generally performed more expediently than salpingostomy.

Partial salpingectomy, or conservative mid-tube resection, is performed for failed salpingostomy, tubal rupture with persistent bleeding and in the conservative treatment of isthmic ectopic gestations. In isthmic pregnancies disruption of the tubal wall is usually so extensive as to exclude the possibility of linear salpingostomy. However it should be noted that at the time of laparotomy one report by Smith et al (1987) demonstrated comparative efficacy of linear salpingostomy to microsurgical anastomosis in cases of isthmic tubal pregnancies. As illustrated in Figures 3a and b, bipolar forceps and laparoscopic scissors may be introduced successively to coagulate and cut the mesosalpinx with eventual segmental resection. In animal studies the denervation which probably accompanies this surgical procedure does not have a significant impact on tubal function (Winston et al, 1974). The endoloop presutured technique and electric snare technique can also be used for this procedure. During endoloop use the tube is often elevated by forceps through the third puncture site. The endoloop is introduced through the suprapubic puncture. Two loops are placed distal to the ectopic pregnancy. Scissors are used for the final transection (see Figure 4). Complete salpingectomy is only an extension of this described technique. Transection of the fimbria ovaricum often facilitates separation from the ovary and total incorporation of the oviduct.

Tubal extraction from the peritoneal cavity may be performed by various means. Ampullostomy is sometimes performed prior to salpingectomy to decrease the quantity of tissue initially extracted. Removal through the operating channel of the right angle laparoscope is usually all that is needed. Removal of the second puncture trochar prior to extraction with long clamps or polyp forceps may allow a great volume of tissue to be removed. The use of morcellating devices for extraction avoids the previous infrequent need for posterior colpotomy or minilaparotomy. Preferentially after tissue extraction, adhesions may be lysed. Intraoperative visualization is of little value in predicting tubal patency rates. Hysterosalpingography several months later remains the best diagnostic tool for tubal patency (Mitchell et al, 1987).

Perioperative adjuvants and follow-up

The value of perioperative antibiotics and anti-inflammatory agents, instillation of high molecular weight solutions at closure, and second-look laparoscopy remains unsettled. Prophylactic tetracycline and less often 100 ml of 32% dextran 70 are used in our laparoscopic cases. An interrupted dissolvable suture is used for subdermal closure. Incorporation of the fascia in the subdermal closure in puncture sites exceeding 10 mm is recommended. To ensure complete removal of trophoblast it is important to measure HCG concentrations serially until they become negative. Laparo-

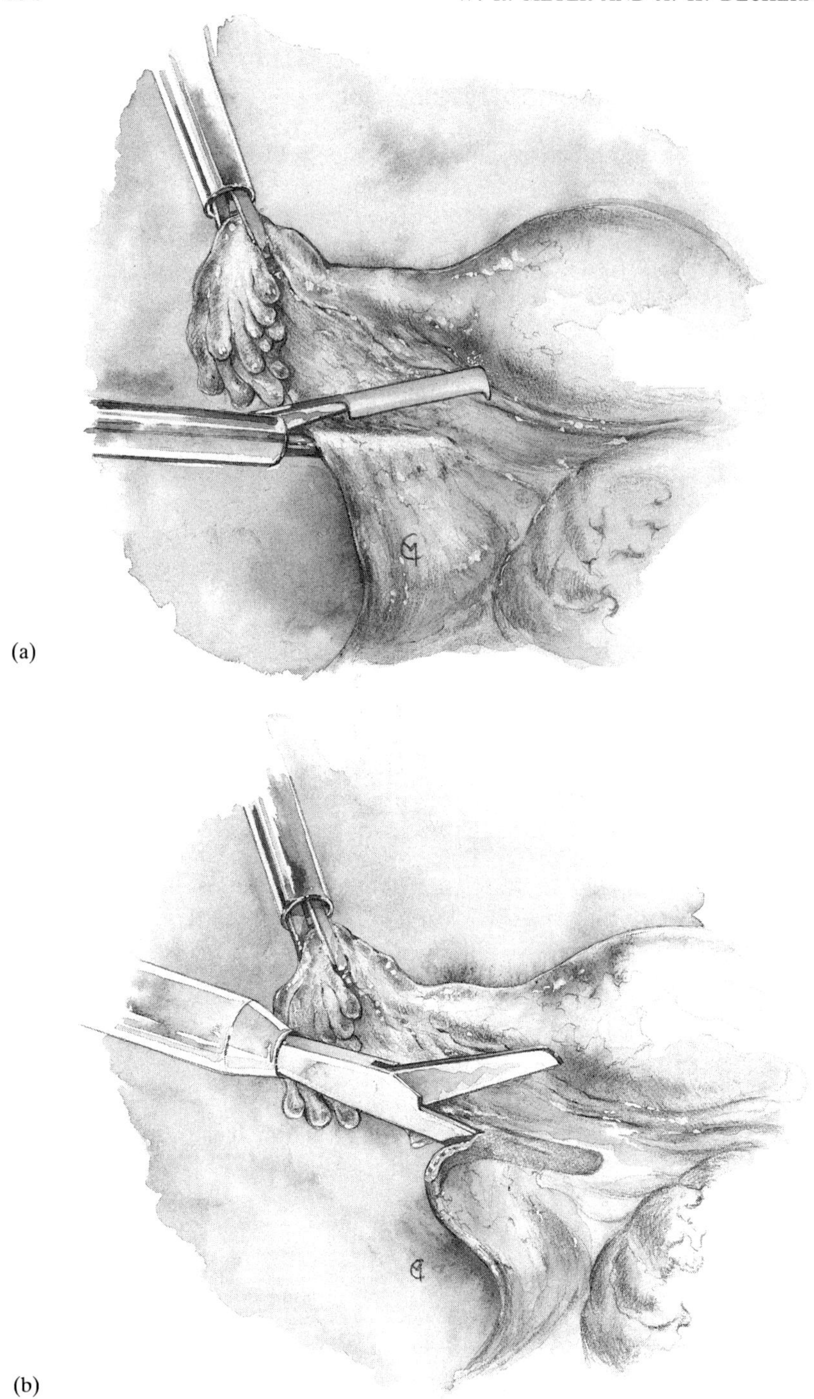

Figure 3. Coagulation/cutting of mesosalpinx with (a) laparoscopic forceps and (b) scissors with segmental resection or complete salpingectomy.

scopy at 8–10 days post-procedure has been shown by Trimbos-Kemper et al (1985) in 188 patients to decrease subsequent adhesion formation and the percentage of repeat ectopic gestations. Decidualization, inflammation and haemorrhagic tubal debris may still falsely lower expected tubal patency rates if second-look laparoscopy is performed within this time frame.

SUMMARY

Over the last decade and a half the success and safety of endoscopic surgery for ectopic pregnancy has been established. Shapiro and Adler (1973) reported laparoscopic salpingectomy using electrocoagulation followed by excision. Soderstrom (1981) followed with the snare technique of salpingectomy. Valle and Lifchez (1983) reported tubal patency rates approaching

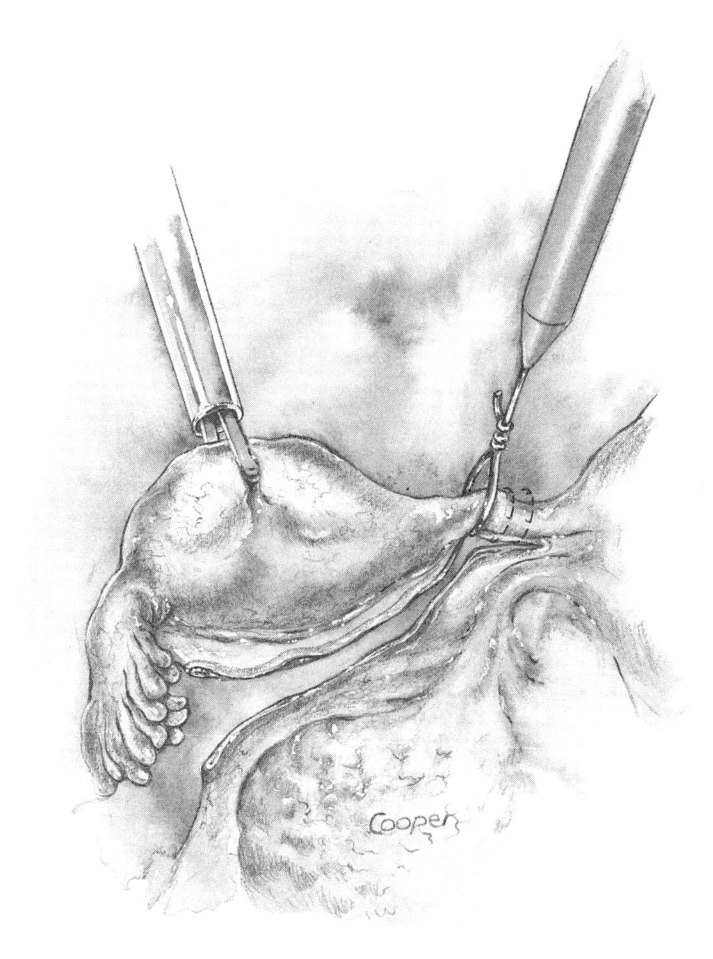

Figure 4. Endoloop placement around ectopic pregnancy using three-puncture technique.

and attaining 100% following salpingostomy in the sole oviduct during laparotomy encouraged continued laparoscopic approach. DeCherney (1981) described linear salpingostomy via a cutting current in 18 women with an intrauterine pregnancy rate of 50% 1 year afterwards. No spontaneous abortions or repeat ectopics were reported. Pouly et al (1986) described laparoscopic salpingostomy in 321 women with a resultant 64% intrauterine pregnancy and 22% repeat ectopic rate.

These studies support the realization that previous surgical approaches per laparotomy for ectopic pregnancy may be achieved endoscopically, but intraoperative and postoperative complications have occurred. As noted by Kelly et al (1979) and Richards (1984) these consist mainly of persistent or delayed haemorrhage along with continued trophoblastic growth. Haemorrhage is most often a result of failed salpingostomy in larger ectopics. Continued trophoblastic development requiring repeat surgical exploration due to incomplete removal of tissue has been reported by Pouly (1986) in as many as 5% of cases. This rare but reported consequence signals the importance of following quantitative HCG concentrations into the negative range. Occasionally HCG levels remain elevated more than 30 days postoperatively with eventual resolution; Cartwright et al (1986) claim that tubal patency rates appear to be unaffected by this prolonged clearance of tissue.

Despite infrequent morbidity, laparoscopic treatment of ectopic pregnancy, in comparison to laparotomy, significantly shortens hospital stays, operating time, convalescence and postoperative analgesic requirements (Brumsted et al, 1988). Endoscopic surgery also reduces postoperative formation of pelvic adhesions (Fayez and Schneider, 1987). As familiarity and technical expertise with endoscopy continues to increase, exploratory laparotomy may be considered too radical an approach to ectopic pregnancy treatment regardless of the procedure performed.

REFERENCES

Bruhat MA, Manhes H, Mage G et al (1980) Treatment of ectopic pregnancy by means of laparoscopy. *Fertility and Sterility* **33:** 411–414.

Brumsted J, Kessler C, Gibson C et al (1988) A comparison of laparoscopy and laparotomy for the treatment of ectopic pregnancy. *Obstetrics and Gynecology* **71:** 889–892.

Budowich M, Johnson TR Jr, Genadry R et al (1980) The histopathology of the developing tubal ectopic pregnancy. *Fertility and Sterility* **34:** 169–171.

Cartwright PS, Herbert CM & Maxson WS (1986) Operative laparoscopy for the management of tubal pregnancy. *Journal of Reproductive Medicine* **31:** 589–591.

DeCherney AH & Diamond MP (1987) Laparoscopic salpingostomy for ectopic pregnancy. *Obstetrics and Gynecology* **70:** 948–950.

DeCherney AH & Maheux R (1983) Modern management of tubal pregnancy. *Current Problems in Obstetrics and Gynecology* **6:** 1–38.

DeCherney AH, Romero R & Naftolin F (1981) Surgical management of unruptured ectopic pregnancy. *Fertility and Sterility* **35:** 21–24.

DeCherney AH, Maheaux R & Naftolin F (1982) Salpingostomy for ectopic pregnancy in the sole patent oviduct: reproductive outcome. *Fertility and Sterility* **37:** 619–622.

Diamond MP & DeCherney AH (1987) Surgical techniques in the management of ectopic pregnancy. *Clinical Obstetrics and Gynecology*, pp 200–209.

Dubuisson JB, Aubriot FX & Cardone V (1987) Laparoscopic salpingectomy for tubal pregnancy. *Fertility and Sterility* **47:** 225–228.
Fayez JA & Schneider PJ (1987) Prevention of pelvic adhesion formation by different modalities of treatment. *American Journal of Obstetrics and Gynecology* **157:** 1184–1188.
Fossum GT, Davajan V & Kletzky O (1988) Early detection of pregnancy with transvaginal ultrasound. *Fertility and Sterility* **49:** 788–791.
Gonzalez FJ & Wayman M (1981) Ectopic Pregnancy. A retrospective study of 501 consecutive patients. *Diagnosis in Gynecology and Obstetrics* **3:** 181–186.
Israel SL (1951) Total linear salpingostomy. Clinical and experimental observations. *Fertility and Sterility* **2:** 505–513.
Johns DA & Nardie RP (1986) Management of unruptured ectopic pregnancy with laparoscopic carbon dioxide laser. *Fertility and Sterility* **46:** 703–705.
Johnson TRB, Sanborn JR, Wagner KS et al (1980) Gonadotropin surveillance following conservative surgery for ectopic pregnancy. *Fertility and Sterility* **33:** 207–208.
Kadar N, DeVore G & Romero R (1981) Discriminatory hCG zone: its use in the sonographic evaluation for ectopic pregnancy. *Obstetrics and Gynecology* **58:** 156–161.
Kamrava MN, Taymor ML, Berger MJ et al (1983) Disappearance of human chorionic gonadotropin following removal of ectopic pregnancy. *Obstetrics and Gynecology* **62:** 486–488.
Kelly RW, Martin SA & Strickler RC (1979) Delayed hemorrhage in conservative surgery for ectopic pregnancy. *American Journal of Obstetrics and Gynecology* **133:** 225.
Lindblom B, Hahlin M, Kaufelt B et al (1987) Local prostaglandin $F_{2\alpha}$ injection for termination of ectopic pregnancy. *Lancet* **i:** 776–777.
Martin DC & Diamond MP (1986) Operative laparoscopy: The role of the CO_2 laser. In *Intra-Abdominal Laser Surgery*, pp 105–136. Memphis: Resurge Press.
Matthews CP, Coulson PB & Wild RA (1986) Serum progesterone levels as an aid in the diagnosis of ectopic pregnancy. *Obstetrics and Gynecology* **30:** 148–154.
Mitchell DE, McSwain HF, McCarthy JA et al (1987) Hysterosalpingographic evaluation of tubal patency after ectopic pregnancy. *American Journal of Obstetrics and Gynecology* **157:** 618–621.
Nelson LM, Margara RA & Winston RML (1986) Primary and secondary closure of ampullary salpingotomy compared in the rabbit. *Fertility and Sterility* **45:** 292–295.
Oelsner G, Rabinovitch O, Movad J et al (1986) Reproductive outcome after microsurgical treatment of tubal pregnancy in women with a single fallopian tube. *Journal of Reproductive Medicine* **31:** 483–486.
Richards BC (1984) Persistent trophoblast following conservative operations for ectopic pregnancy. *American Journal of Obstetrics and Gynecology* **150:** 100.
Romero R, Kadar N, Jeanty P et al (1985) The diagnosis of ectopic pregnancy: the value of the HCG discriminatory zone. *Obstetrics and Gynecology* **66:** 357–360.
Samuelson S & Sjovall A (1972) Laparoscopy in suspected ectopic pregnancy. *Acta Obstetrica Gynecologica Scandinavica* **51:** 31–35.
Semm K (1987) *Operative Manual for Endoscopic Abdominal Surgery*, pp 189–194. London: Friedrich.
Senterman M, Jibodh R & Tulandi T (1988) Histopathologic study of ampullary and isthmic tubal ectopic pregnancy. *American Journal of Obstetrics and Gynecology* **159:** 939–941.
Shapiro HI & Adler DLN (1973) Excision of an ectopic pregnancy through the laparoscope. *American Journal of Obstetrics and Gynecology* **117:** 290–291.
Smith HO, Toledo AA & Thompson JD (1987) Conservative surgical management of isthmic ectopic pregnancies. *American Journal of Obstetrics and Gynecology* **157:** 604–608.
Stromme WB (1953) Salpingotomy for tubal pregnancy. *Obstetrics and Gynecology* **1:** 472–475.
Taylor MV, Martin DC, Poston W et al (1986) Effect of power density and carbonization of residual tissue coagulation using the continuous wave carbon dioxide laser. *Colposcopy and Gynecologic Laser Surgery* **2:** 169–175.
Timonen S & Nieminen U (1967) Tubal pregnancy, choice of operative method of treatment. *Acta Obstetrica Gynecologica Scandinavica* **46:** 327–339.
Trimbos-Kemper TCM, Trimbos JB & van Hall EV (1985) Adhesion formation after tubal surgery: Results of the eight-day laparoscopy in 188 patients. *Fertility and Sterility* **43:** 395–400.
Valle JA & Lifchez AS (1983) Reproductive outcome following conservative surgery for tubal

pregnancy in women with a single fallopian tube. *Fertility and Sterility* **39:** 316–320.
Winston RML, McClure M & Browne JC (1974) Pregnancy following autograft transplantation of the fallopian tube and ovary in the rabbit. *Lancet* **ii:** 494–495.
Yeko TR, Gorril MJ, Hughes LN et al (1987) Timely diagnosis of early ectopic pregnancy using a single blood progesterone measurement. *Fertility and Sterility* **48:** 1048–1050.

9

Double-optic laparoscopy

Salpingoscopy, ovarian cystoscopy and endo-ovarian surgery with the argon laser

I. A. BROSENS
P. J. PUTTEMANS

The place of laparoscopy in the investigation of infertility is now well established. Double optic laparoscopy is a new technique which extends the endoscopic accessibility of laparoscopy and increases its diagnostic efficiency. Salpingoscopy allows direct examination of the mucosa in the ampullary segment of the fallopian tube. Ovarian cystoscopy allows exploration of ovarian cystic structures with benign, functional or endometrial characteristics. In addition, a new approach of atraumatic endo-ovarian surgery has been developed using the argon laser to treat large ovarian endometriomas in situ.

SALPINGOSCOPY

Until recently there was no endoscopic means of examining the tubal mucosa and it had to be assumed that normal findings at hysterosalpingography (HSG) and laparoscopy equated with tubal normality. Examination of tubal mucosa at the time of tubal surgery has been introduced by microsurgeons using either microbiopsies (Brosens and Vasquez, 1976; Vasquez et al, 1980, 1983), the operating microscope (Boer-Meisel et al, 1986), or an endoscope (Henry-Suchet et al, 1985). More recently salpingoscopy during laparoscopy has been developed with the use of either a flexible or a rigid telescope.

Techniques

Cornier (1985) developed the flexible salpingoscope by using a 3.4 mm flexible bronchoscope in combination with an operating laparoscope. The fimbriae are grasped with an atraumatic forceps and the telescope is inserted into the tube. The insufflating channel is connected with a saline drip. The telescope is advanced very gently under laparoscopic control as far as the isthmoampullary junction. The hand movements to insert the telescope must be very gentle to avoid damage of the mucosa. While the saline drip distends the lumen the tubal mucosa is inspected by moving the telescope back and forward.

The rigid salpingoscope as developed by Brosens et al (1987a) consists of three parts: the sheath, the obturator and the 2.6 mm telescope. This endoscope is 4 cm longer than the sheath (Figure 1). The sheath is 3 mm in diameter and has a connection for a saline drip. An atraumatic forceps with a rounded end, introduced through a second suprapubic incision, is used to grasp and align the ampullary segment to the axis of the laparoscope. The sheath with the obturator is passed down the operating channel of the laparoscope, the fimbrial opening is identified and the sheath is introduced

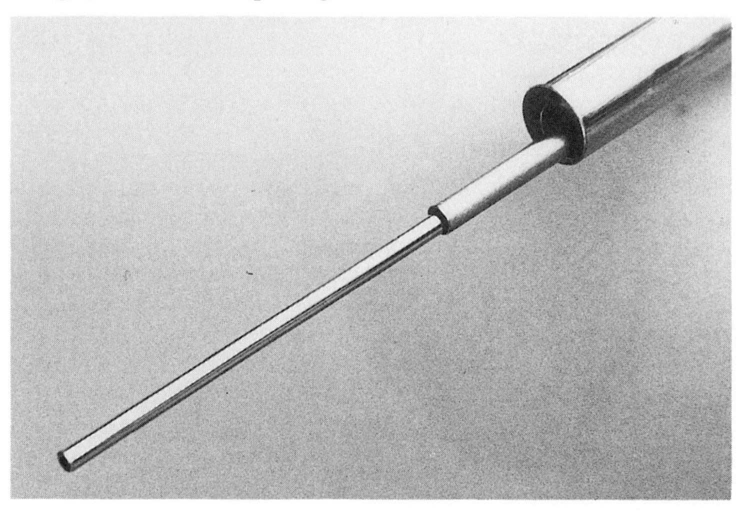

Figure 1. The salpingoscope inside its sheath placed in the operative channel of the laparoscope; the fallopian tube is atraumatically clamped around the sheath and a slow saline drip distends the lumen; the telescope is then gently advanced up to 4–5 cm within the ampulla.

into the tubal infundibulum. The blunt obturator is used to aid introduction into the tube. In most cases the endoscope can be inserted into the tube without difficulty. The saline drip should run freely before the introduction and is helpful in identifying the tubal ostium by the floating of the fimbriae. The grasping forceps with its rounded end is then used to clamp the tube around the sheath at the level of the infundibulum, right behind the fimbriae. The obturator is now replaced by the telescope. A slow saline drip distends the tube and under direct vision the telescope is slowly and gently advanced into the ampulla. The mucosal folds can be inspected while they float in the saline. This rigid salpingoscope gives a clearer and brighter image with a wider field of view and is less expensive than the flexible salpingoscope. In patients with peritubal adhesions or hydrosalpinges the tube must first be mobilized by endoscopic surgery using conventional instruments or laser. A hydrosalpinx is opened by a small incision at the site where the scar of the occlusion can be identified.

Findings

Normal structure

In the ampulla there are four to five major longitudinal folds with several accessory folds arising from them on each side (Figure 2). Between the major folds there are four or five minor folds (Figure 3). As one can imagine these folds have a delicate structure with a fine vascular network (Figure 4). At the level of the isthmoampullary junction, the major folds level off to four or five small rounded folds which continue into the narrow, isthmic segment. At first the fluid in the ampullary segment may be turbid with flocculent material, particularly when salpingoscopy is performed around the time of menstruation or following hysteroscopy.

In some cases the ampullary folds have a more irregular structure with sometimes finger-like extensions. In the so-called 'convoluted infantile' tube (Moore-White, 1960) the lumen is very distensible with flattened and separated folds and an extremely thin and transparent tubal wall (Figure 5). This abnormality has been related to herniation of the mucosa which may be due to a hypoplasia or aplasia of the ampullary myosalpinx. It can involve segments of different size or even the entire ampulla. These fallopian tubes may create the impression of a hydrosalpinx at HSG, due to the extensive filling with contrast medium. However, this finding is unlikely to be a cause of infertility as bilateral tortuous tubes have been found to occur in patients with proven fertility.

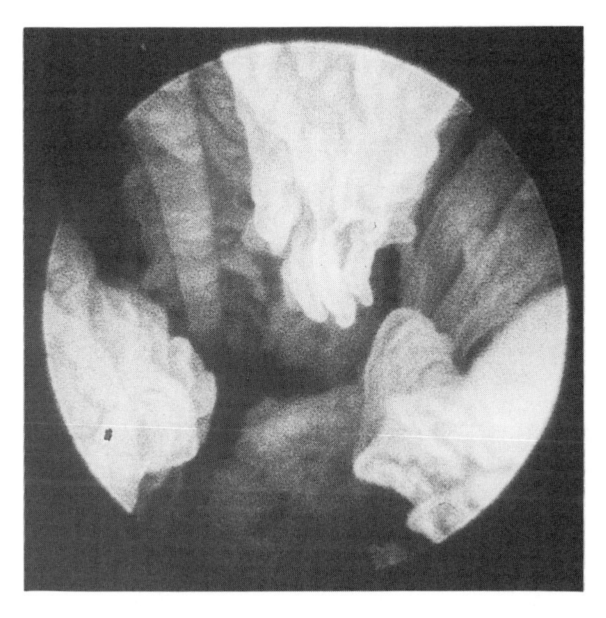

Figure 2. Three normal major folds with several secondary mucosal folds on top of each, and some minor folds running in between.

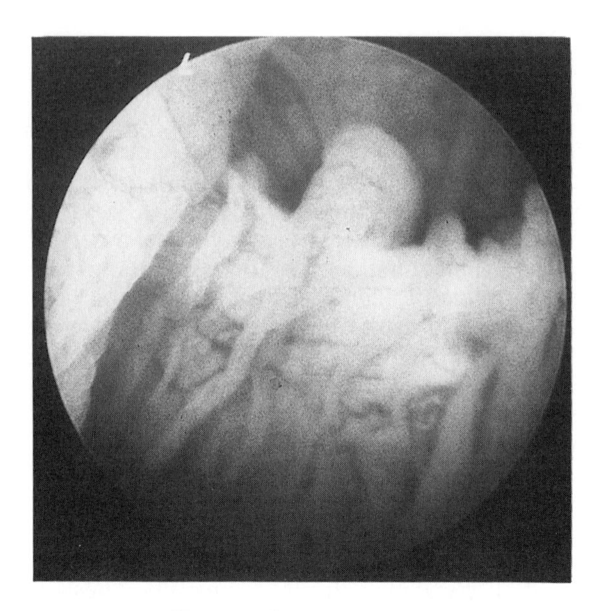

Figure 3. Close-up of several normal minor folds.

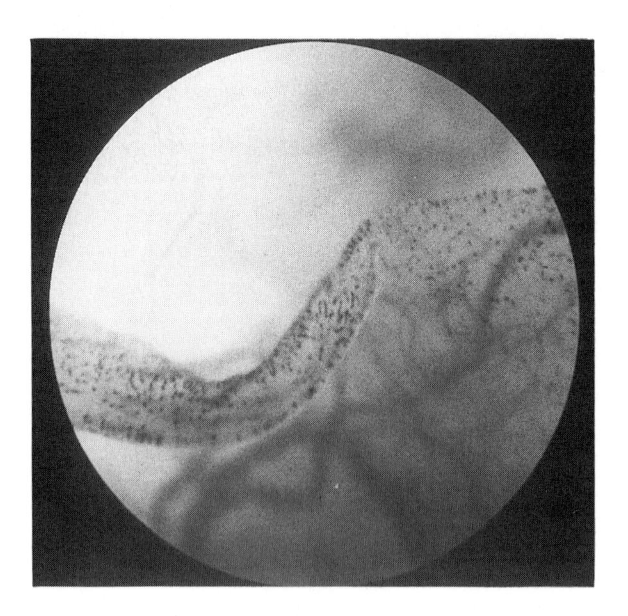

Figure 4. Detail of the delicate vascularization of the ampullary mucosal folds.

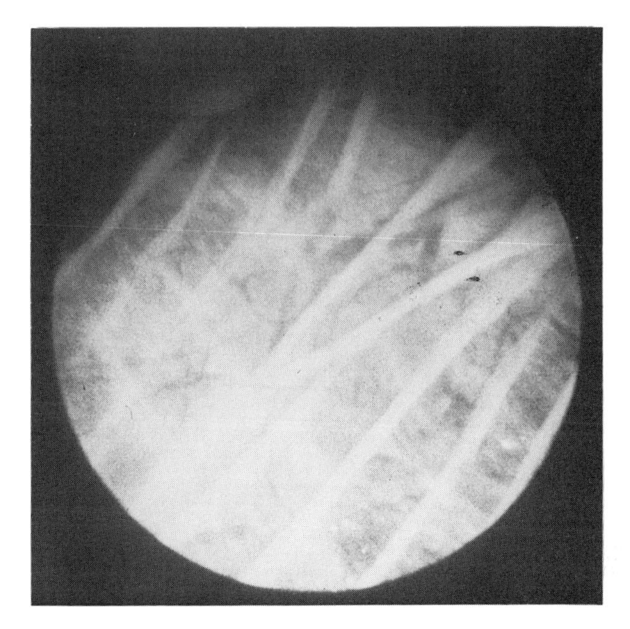

Figure 5. Pseudohydrosalpinx: HSG suggested hydrosalpinx formation, but at laparoscopy the tube is patent and the fimbriae look normal; the ampullary lumen, however, is very distended with an excessive separation of folds and an extremely thin and translucid tubal wall.

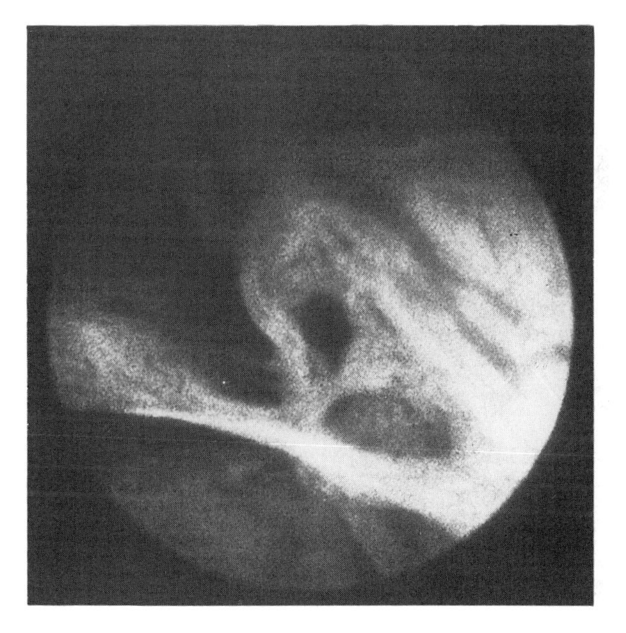

Figure 6. Focal adhesions between folds are easily demonstrated in this hydrosalpinx at the time of diagnostic laparoscopy.

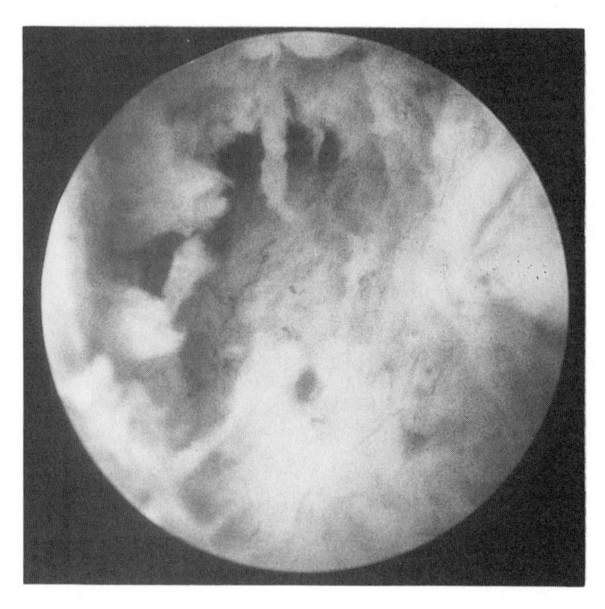

Figure 7. Extensive lesions with agglutination of folds and severe adhesion formation create a web-like appearance in this thick-walled hydrosalpinx.

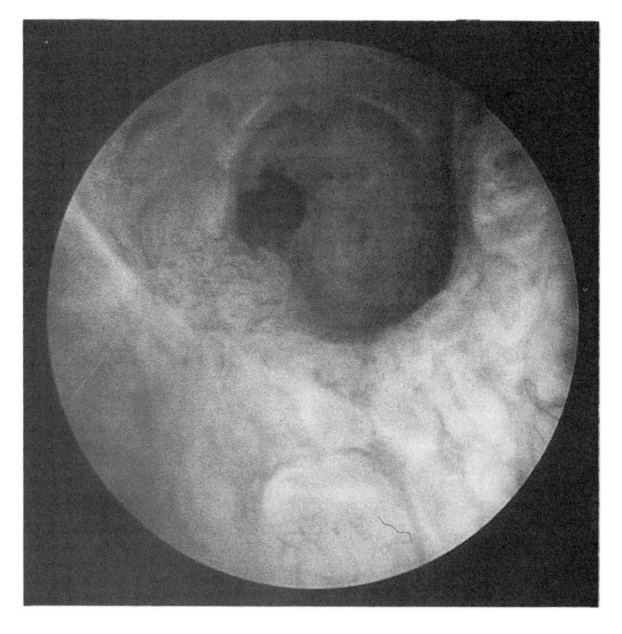

Figure 8. Complete destruction of the mucosal layer in this ampulla: the lumen appears as a naked hollow tube with some fold remnants at 8 o'clock.

Lesions

Adhesions between the ampullary folds can be filmy and avascular and adhere between otherwise normal folds (Figure 6). Severe adhesions are thick and vascularized and the fold structure is distorted (Figure 7). These adhesions can occur focally although usually they extend over the entire length of the ampullary segment. A complete loss of the mucosal folds can occur and make the tube appear as a rigid, hollow channel with some occasional remnants of folds (Figure 8). A simple classification (Table 1) enables us to compare patients and make retrospective and prospective studies.

Table 1. Salpingoscopy: endoscopy of the ampulla—classification of lesions.

Grade 1	Normal fold pattern
Grade 2	Separation and flattening of folds
Grade 3	Focal lesions, e.g. small adhesions
Grade 4	Extensive adhesive or destructive lesions
Grade 5	Complete loss of folds

Cannulation of accessory canals can occur. Folds are totally absent in these canals which are likely to represent patent remnants of the wolffian duct system. They should be differentiated from diseased fallopian tubes by the complete absence of a fold texture. A dye test may be helpful to locate the abdominal tubal ostium exactly. Vascular abnormalities such as small venectasies can be seen in the folds. Their significance is not known. The presence of an increased vascularization and haemorrhagic spots suggests chronic inflammation.

Complications and difficulties

Complications from salpingoscopy can occur but they are infrequent and mild. The tubal grasping and holding forceps may damage the serosa on the fimbriae and cause minor bleeding. The telescope can perforate the tubal wall when it is advanced blindly or if the movements of the telescope are rough or clumsy. However, with gentle handling of the instruments and the fallopian tube these complications are rare and there should be no significant mucosal trauma from salpingoscopy.

Clinical value

Salpingoscopy allows detailed examination of the tubal mucosa and is a logical extension of the endoscopic examination of the female genital tract. In infertile patients with normal findings at HSG and laparoscopy unsuspected lesions of the tubal mucosa are detected in 5%. In patients with postsurgical pelvic adhesions but with patent fallopian tubes only salpingoscopy allows exclusion of the presence of intratubal adhesions for certain. Also, when a tubocornual block is diagnosed salpingoscopy is the only technique to evaluate the patency and the quality of the mucosa of the ampullary segment.

In hydrosalpinx the findings at HSG and laparoscopy are frequently inadequate and dubious (Puttemans et al, 1987). Mucosal lesions not detected at HSG or laparoscopy were revealed at salpingoscopy in 52% of patients. On the other hand, adhesions were absent in 43% of patients who were suspected of having a defective fold pattern from HSG (Table 2). A prospective study of salpingoscopy in hydrosalpinges (De Bruyne et al, 1989) showed a 59% pregnancy rate in patients without intratubal adhesions. Salpingoscopy is apparently superior to HSG and laparoscopy. Therefore it should also be useful in the selection of patients for gamete intrafallopian transfer (GIFT) by excluding unsuspected tubal lesions.

Table 2. Correlation between findings at hysterosalpingography (HSG) and salpingoscopy in hydrosalpinges.

	Salpingoscopy						
	Folds preserved		Abnormal fold pattern				
Information from HSG	Grade 1	Grade 2	Grade 3	Grade 4	Grade 5	Total	Conformity
Normal fold pattern	5	6	7	2	3	23	48%
Abnormal or defective fold pattern	3	6	3	4	5	21	57%
No visualization	1	1	0	4	1	7	0%
Total	9	13	10	10	9	51	

Conclusion: HSG was false negative in 52%, false positive in 43% and of no use in 14%.

Salpingoscopy can also be useful in patients with ectopic pregnancy. The salpingoscope can be introduced into the fallopian tube with an unruptured tubal pregnancy to evaluate the presence and extent of lesions and to locate the ampullary lumen. In fact every effort should be made to avoid incision of the tubal lumen itself to prevent iatrogenic adhesion formation which may further enhance the risk of recurrent tubal pregnancy. In addition it is particularly important to evaluate the quality of the contralateral fallopian tube. The normal outer (i.e. laparoscopic) appearance of a tube is absolutely *no* guarantee of an intact mucosa. Further prospective studies are needed to assess the value of salpingoscopy in the estimation of the risk of ectopic pregnancy.

The question remains whether intratubal surgery, e.g. with an argon laser or small scissors, has any value. Although technically quite feasible in cases with small focal adhesions between mucosal folds, one must emphasize that these adhesions are the visible signature of probably irreversible microscopic damage, such as adhesions, deciliation, etc. As for the use of the argon laser inside the fallopian tube, the scattering coefficient and depth of penetration are probably too high, so the laser beam may damage the adjacent mucosa or the tubal wall itself by secondary thermal necrosis.

OVARIAN CYSTOSCOPY OR ENDO-OVARIOSCOPY

Ovarian cystic structures occur frequently during reproductive life. Ultrasound and laparoscopy are useful tools to assess their benign characteristics, but are inadequate for exact diagnosis. Whenever it is impossible to differentiate between functional, endometrial and true neoplastic cysts surgery may be indicated. However, conservative ovarian surgery is the most frequent cause of adhesive pseudocystic disease of the ovary for which a second pelvic procedure may have to be performed. Conditions such as the ovarian cyst in pelvic endometriosis or the recurrent postoperative cyst in the young patient frequently present diagnostic and therapeutic dilemmas to the gynaecologist. Ovarian cystoscopy is proposed as a new tool for endo-ovarian exploration and in selected cases atraumatic endo-ovarian surgery of these cystic structures can be performed with the use of the argon laser.

Instrumentation and technique

The double-optic laparoscope for ovarian cystoscopy is a combination of an operating laparoscope and a 2.6 mm rigid endoscope located in a 5 mm sheath which in turn is introduced through the operating channel of the laparoscope (Karl Storz GmbH, Tüttlingen, West Germany). The sheath has a 1 mm channel which allows passage of small flexible instruments such as a biopsy forceps or laser fibres and an infusion (Figure 9).

Ovarian cystoscopy is performed when ultrasound and laparoscopy indicate benign characteristics of the ovarian tumour and conservative ovarian surgery is considered. The cyst is first punctured and its content aspirated for cytological examination. The sheath with the saline drip is introduced through the puncture hole. Under continuous flow of the saline

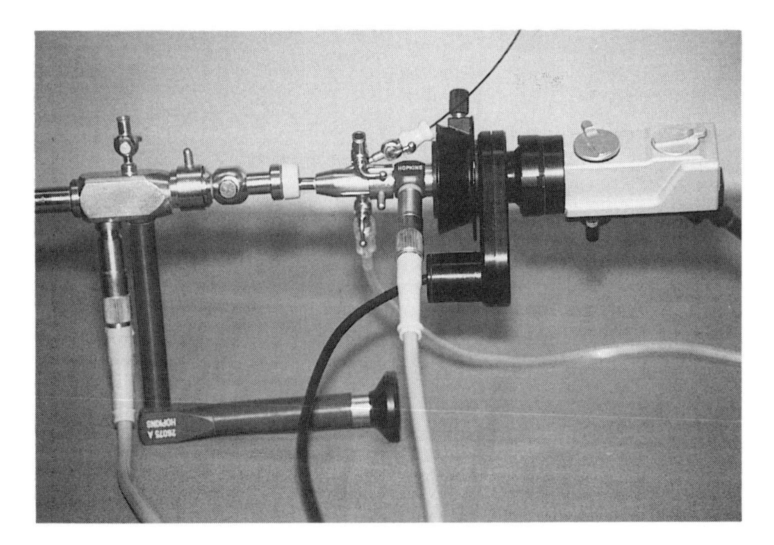

Figure 9. Double optic laparoscopy: the ovarioscope is introduced into the laparoscope and both the argon laser shutter and a CCD camera are mounted on its eyepiece; with a saline infusion and the laser fibre in place the system is ready to perform endo-ovarian argon laser surgery.

drip the cyst is distended and the inner wall can be inspected. Biopsies are easily obtained from selected areas. 'Chocolate cysts' are first aspirated and flushed abundantly with saline until the fluid becomes clear. As it is another double-optic technique, constant surveillance of the entire ovary (e.g. during endo-ovarian surgery) is possible through the laparoscope.

Diagnostic criteria

Benign cystic ovarian tumours include a range of non-neoplastic cysts (persistent follicular cyst, cystic corpus luteum, germinal inclusion), endometrial and true neoplastic cysts (serous, mucinous and dermoids). Ovarian cystoscopy is only performed after careful evaluation of the characteristics of the ovarian tumour, using clinical examination, real time scanning, tumour markers and eventually laparoscopic inspection itself (Table 3). The technique has been applied in patients when the ovarian tumour presented the characteristics of either a dysfunctional or an endometrial cyst. The term 'chocolate cyst' of the ovary is descriptive and lends itself readily to misinterpretation if one notices only the chocolate-coloured haemorrhagic content. A somewhat similar content may be found in some follicular or lutein haematomas and also the fluid content of a cystadenoma may be chocolate-coloured because of haemorrhagic admixture (Novak and Woodruff, 1974). The technique must not be used in patients with a suspected malignant tumour until a spill-proof system is developed.

Table 3. Evaluation of criteria for ovarian cystoscopy.

History
Age
Pelvic imaging
Ultrasound
CT scan
Tumour markers
CA-125
Laparoscopy
Inspection
Transillumination
Fine needle aspiration

Endoscopy of ovarian cystic structures reveals characteristics such as luteinization, pigmentation, different patterns of vascularization which are useful in identifying the type of cyst. In addition to the aspiration cytology, biopsies are obtained from selected areas for histopathology. The *follicular cyst* is characterized by a smooth, undulating surface of the wall overlying a fine and regular network of small vessels. The *corpus luteum cyst* is identified by the presence of luteinized areas which sometimes have an annular pattern. The vascular network in the wall shows areas of extravasation and early organization within which fibrin fibres can be seen.

The *ovarian endometrioma* is characterized by an irregular vascularization and a mosaic pattern of siderophagic pigmentation. There is no superficial network of fine vascularization, but in some areas congested vessels are prominent. The vessels protruding on the surface in the endometrial cyst frequently have an haemorrhagic appearance. Bleeding from these congested vessels rather than endometrial shedding is likely to contribute to the formation of the endometrioma. Indeed, ovarian endometrial implants tend to be fibrotic and show a weak morphological response during the menstrual cycle and hormone therapy (Brosens et al, 1987b). Endometriotic implants and their associated fibrosis and retraction appear to interfere with the venous plexus particularly at the hilus of the ovary and irritation of these congested veins rather than endometrial shedding may cause chronic bleeding. If this hypothesis is correct, selective coagulation of these congested vessels rather than complete resection of the fibrotic capsule may be sufficient for the treatment of the endometrial ovarian cyst.

The structure of endometriotic lesions depends upon the localization and it is probable that the evolution of the lesion is regulated in accordance with local conditions. Endometriosis may develop on the surface of the ovary or in a rare case cover completely the inner surface of a small cavity in the ovary such as a corpus fibrosum. Such free-growing lesions are 'flourishing' growths and are closely reminiscent of the eutopic endometrium in their histological structure. Cyclic changes in the blood vasculature of free-growing endometriosis fully correspond with cyclic changes in the endometrial vasculature, including extravasation and shedding as in menstrual bleeding. In most cases however, the cystic ovarian endometrioma is an enclosed lesion in which the cavity is covered with fibrotic tissue. In this fibrotic pseudowall we may or may not find poorly differentiated glandular epithelium sparsely surrounded by stroma. The cyclic changes of these enclosed lesions are less significant than those in the former group. Late secretory changes and menstrual bleeding are absent in enclosed lesions (Nieminen, 1962).

Endo-ovarian laser surgery

Endo-ovarian laser surgery of endometrial ovarian cysts has been performed with the use of the argon laser (HGM, Medical Laser Systems Inc, Salt Lake City, Utah, US). This laser uses argon gas as the laser medium and produces a blue–green light representing a composite of approximately ten different wavelengths, the most pronounced being at 488 and 515 nm. This laser light is colour-dependent which means that it is preferentially absorbed by pigments of its complementary colour, red (e.g. haemoglobin), or by black pigments, which contain all colours (e.g. melanin). Unlike the carbon dioxide laser, argon laser light is not absorbed by water, explaining its use both in ophthalmology and inside the ovary, where saline is used as a distension medium. In unpigmented tissue scattering of laser light is the primary form of heat production. Since absorption and scatter both contribute to the energy conversion of light into heat in either pigmented or unpigmented tissue, higher power densities are usually required for argon lasers to coagulate and/or vaporize human tissue. In gynaecology, therefore, the use of a 20 watt model is recommended. Depth of penetration ranges between 0.4 and 0.8 mm, so the potential for damage to adjacent tissue is far less a problem than for instance with a Nd-YAG laser (depth of penetration up to 4.2 mm). Carried through optical fibres that are available in different sizes, the argon laser beam is guided to the target site. Set-up of this laser through the operative channel of an endoscope is therefore very easy. Since the beam from a fibre is divergent (7°), no backstops are needed and power density is at its maximum at the tip of the fibre. This explains that incisional power can be obtained by touching the target with the fibre tip. In the non-contact mode the distance between the target and the fibre tip determines the tissue effect—rapid or slow vaporization, coagulation (protein denaturation without ablation), or just surface heating. In this mode carbonization and smoke production are negligible. To avoid retinal or camera damage, a special shutter of a precise wavelength is used, covering the endoscope's optical channel only when the laser is activated. This changes the colour but not the visibility of the operating field. Table 4 compares the basic laser physics of three medical lasers (the KTP 532 laser, a frequency doubled Nd-YAG laser, has approximately the same characteristics as the argon laser); Figure 10 illustrates the setting procedure of an argon laser.

Table 4. Comparison of laser physics of CO_2, argon and Nd-YAG lasers.

Laser physics	CO_2	Argon	Nd-YAG
Wavelength	10.600 nm	488/515 nm	1064/1318 nm
Colour dependence	None	Yes	Yes
Main tissue effect	Vaporization	Coagulation	Coagulation
Depth of penetration	0.1 mm	0.4–0.8 mm	0.6–4.2 mm
Forward scattering	None	Slight	Moderate
Absorption in water	Total	None	None
Carbonization	+++	+	±
Smoke production	+++	+	±
Passed through	Mirrors	Fibres	Fibres
Beam alignment	+++	−	−
Surgical technique	No-touch	No-touch and direct contact	No-touch and direct contact (sapphire tips)

As for endo-ovarian surgery with the argon laser, a 300 or 600 μm fibre is introduced through the channel of the sheath into the cystic cavity. The absorption spectrum of the argon laser makes it an efficient instrument for coagulation of the superficial vessels and the haemorrhagic foci we already mentioned. The depth of coagulation is easily controlled by adjusting the power density (power output between 8 and 12 watts) and the duration of coagulation (mostly in the continuous mode). While the cyst is distended under continuous flow of a saline drip the superficial haemorrhagic vessels protruding on the inner surface are coagulated. The wall can also be coagulated to a depth of 1–2 mm. The 6 month follow-up study of a first series of 11 patients treated by this technique showed no recurrence of the ovarian endometrioma.

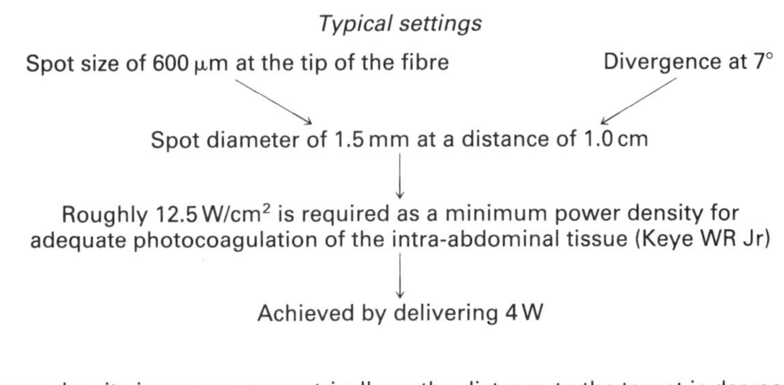

Power density increases geometrically as the distance to the target is decreased

↓

Delivering 1 W, at the tip, yields a density of approximately 350 W/cm^2

Initial tissue response should be assessed at a conservative power setting and pulse duration, typically 2.5 W (indirect method) and 0.5 s pulsed duration. Increases in power and duration should be made in small increments until a suitable setting is reached, e.g.:

Lesion	Typical power	Mode
Endometriotic implant	5–10 W	Continuous
Uterosacral ligament	7.5–11 W	Continuous

Figure 10. The procedure for setting an argon laser.

SUMMARY

Salpingoscopy gives detailed visual information on the mucosal pattern of the tubal ampulla as far as the isthmoampullary junction. With experience it takes 10 minutes to perform salpingoscopy on both sides and with an additional dye test a most complete evaluation of tubal morphology and patency can be obtained during routine diagnostic laparoscopy. Comparative studies proved the technique to be superior to HSG and the laparoscopic inspection of the tubal serosa and of the fimbriae. In some instances, like a tubocornual block, only salpingoscopy can provide additional information. Eventually, with the current techniques of operative laparoscopy salpingoscopic inspection of a phimosis or even a hydrosalpinx can be performed quite easily and these findings help us in the clinical management of patients requiring either microsurgical cuff-salpingostomy (giving a more realistic chance of a spontaneous pregnancy every month) or in vitro fertilization (avoiding laparotomy). Salpingoscopy also guides us in the selection of patients for a GIFT procedure and probably provides a better estimation of the risk of ectopic pregnancy.

Ovarian cystoscopy can be applied for accurate diagnosis of non-malignant ovarian cysts at the time of laparoscopy. The wall of the cyst is inspected in detail and selective biopsies are obtained. Unnecessary surgery for non-neoplastic tumours can be avoided and endometrial and cystic tumours can be treated in situ using an argon laser with minimal surgical damage to the ovarian capsule. This laser technique is under further investigation to evaluate its place in the diagnosis and conservative surgical treatment of benign ovarian cysts occurring during reproductive life.

REFERENCES

Boer-Meisel ME, Te Velde ER, Habbema JDF & Kardaun JWPF (1986) Predicting the pregnancy outcome in patients treated for hydrosalpinges: a prospective study. *Fertility and Sterility* **45:** 23–29.

Brosens IA & Vasquez G (1976) Fimbrial microbiopsy. *Journal of Reproductive Medicine* **16:** 171–178.

Brosens I, Boeckx W, Delattin Ph, Puttemans P & Vasquez G (1987a) Salpingoscopy: a new preoperative diagnostic tool in tubal infertility? *British Journal of Obstetrics and Gynaecology* **94:** 722–728.

Brosens IA, Verleyen A & Cornillie FJ (1987b) The morphological effect of a short-term medical therapy of endometriosis. *American Journal of Obstetrics and Gynecology* **157:** 1215–1221.

Cormier E (1985) l'Ampulloscopic per-coelioscopique. *Journal de Gynecologic, Obstétrique et Biologic Reproductive* **14:** 459–466.

De Bruyne F, Puttemans P, Boeckx W & Brosens IA (1989) The clinical value of salpingoscopy in tubal infertility. *Fertility and Sterility* **51:** 339–340.

Henry-Suchet J, Loffredo V, Tesquier L & Pez J (1985) Endoscopy of the tube (= tuboscopy): its prognostic value for tuboplasties. *Acta Europea Fertilitatis* **16:** 139–145.

Moore-White M (1960) Evaluation of tubal plastic operations. *International Journal of Fertility* **5:** 237–250.

Nieminen U (1962) Studies on the vascular pattern of ectopic endometrium with special reference to cyclic changes. *Acta Obstetricia et Gynecologica Scandinavica* **41**(supplement 3): (academic dissertation).

Novak ER & Woodruff JD (1974) Pelvic Endometriosis. In Novak ER & Woodruff JD (eds) *Novak's Gynecologic and Obstetric Pathology*, p 508. Philadelphia: WB Saunders.

Puttemans P, Brosens I, Delattin Ph, Vasquez G & Boeckx W (1987) Salpingoscopy versus hysterosalpingography in hydrosalpinges. *Human Reproduction* **2:** 535–540.

Vasquez G, Boeckx W, Winston RML & Brosens IA (1980) Human tubal mucosa and reconstructive microsurgery. In Crossignani PG & Rubin BL (eds) *Microsurgery in Female Infertility*, pp 41–56. London: Academic Press.

Vasquez G, Winston RML, Boeckx W, Gordts S & Brosens IA (1983) The epithelium of human hydrosalpinges: a light optical and scanning electron microscopic study. *British Journal of Obstetrics and Gynaecology* **90:** 764–770.

10

Laparoscopic female sterilization

G. M. FILSHIE

HISTORICAL OVERVIEW

Laparoscopic female sterilization has revolutionized modern family planning services and its use makes it the most important permanent method amongst all contraceptive acceptors: an estimated 140 million women throughout the world are sterilized. How did this revolution occur? Laparoscopy was first reported by Kelling in Hamburg in 1901 (Kelling, 1923) when he used a Nitze (Nitze, 1893) cystoscope to visualize the abdominal cavity of a dog. Jacobeus from Sweden, who in 1910 conceived the phrase laparoscopy (Jacobeus, 1911), was credited as the first to use the technique for looking into the abdomen of humans.

Following these two pioneers many clinicians used laparoscopy for diagnostic purposes, both in gynaecology and in general surgery. Zollikofer (1924) from Switzerland (who used carbon dioxide for the first time to produce a pneumoperitoneum) and Kalk in Germany (1929) both reviewed a large number of cases of liver disease (Kalk, 1929). The use of the laparoscope to facilitate female sterilization was first recorded by Ruddock (1934, 1937). Later Anderson (1937), from the United States of America, developed the first purpose-built electrode for tubal fulguration and he predicted that these procedures 'would soon become recognised standard techniques'. Subsequently Powers and Barnes (1941) wrote an article devoted entirely to laparoscopic tubal fulguration techniques. Instrumentation was fairly crude and hazards were ever present and little attention was paid to these methods for nearly 20 years.

Two important innovations led to the method becoming accepted and popular. First was the introduction of the cold light source by Fourestier Galdu and Vulmiere in 1952. The hot direct light bulb at the end of the modified cystoscope was changed for an external supply of light transmitted along a quartz rod cable to the abdomen. The dangers of the hot light bulb disappeared. The second important technological advance was the Hopkins rod lens system (Hopkins, 1976) which was incorporated into the laparoscope. This improved the angle of vision, the depth of field and clarity of image.

With the improved technology the use of the laparoscope for diagnostic, as well as therapeutic, purposes was greatly enhanced. Raoul Palmer (1960,

1962), also known as the founder of 'modern' laparoscopy published extensively on the use of laparoscopy in gynaecology and he popularized tubal cautery in France. He described the use of the Palmer forceps which are still used today. Similarly, Hans Frangenheim (1964) popularized laparoscopy and tubal cautery in Germany. Patrick Steptoe was the British pioneer (Steptoe, 1965), eventually going on to write the first monograph in the English language on laparoscopy (Steptoe, 1967). Publications on the subject in the United States followed later. Cohen (1967) and Clifford Wheeless (1972), were responsible for popularizing tubal cautery in the United States. As tubal cautery became widespread the dangers of the system emerged (Thompson and Wheeless, 1973) and this prompted Jacques Rioux from Quebec to develop a bipolar system for cautery (Rioux and Cloutier, 1974). Richard Kleppinger from the United States also recognized the problems of unipolar cautery and he developed his own operative forceps for the same procedure (Kleppinger, 1977). Hans Hirsh from Germany also developed forceps (Hirsh and Roos, 1974). Semm, also from Germany, developed a thermal coagulation technique (endocoagulation) which limited the local temperature to approximately 140C which improved further the safety of electrocautery (Semm, 1973).

In order to eliminate completely all dangers from electrocautery a number of mechanical methods emerged, which included the Yoon ring (Yoon and King, 1975), the Hulka-Clemens clip (Hulka et al, 1973), the Filshie clip (Filshie et al, 1981), the Bleier clip (Bleier, 1973), the Tupla clip (Babenerd and Flehr, 1978) and the Weck clip (Wheeless, 1974). The end result of these new methods of laparoscopic female sterilization was that the procedure could be performed simply and safely as a day-case procedure. It is not surprising that Anderson's prophecy made in 1937 has become a reality.

LAPAROSCOPIC INSTRUMENTATION FOR FEMALE STERILIZATION

The type of laparoscope depends much on whether a double-puncture or single-puncture technique is employed.

Double-puncture laparoscopes

The double-puncture technique was the original method: any operative procedure was affected by a second-puncture down which the operative instruments were inserted. Fundamentally any laparoscope may be used to visualize the pelvic organs. The 10 mm diameter laparoscope was the standard for many years. However, as lenses improved laparoscopes of 7 mm and 5 mm diameter emerged which gave similar views to the previous 10 mm laparoscopes and in many cases replaced them.

Laparoscopes smaller than 5 mm diameter are less robust, although they can be maintained with careful handling. Examples of smaller laparoscopes included the 'emergency' laparoscope from Storz (4 mm) and the 2.7 mm laparoscope from Thackray. Most laparoscopes for double-puncture technique have a straight angle at the end (0°), although angled laparoscopes (e.g. 30°) are eminently suitable for diagnostic procedures. They can also be used for operative procedures and their use depends on availability or personal preference.

Single-puncture laparoscopes

A single-puncture laparoscope has an optical channel to view the pelvic organs, a light channel to conduct the light fibres to illuminate the pelvic organs and an operating channel for the passage of the appropriate operative instruments. They tend to be larger than the double-puncture laparoscopes.

When diathermy was popular a 5 or 6 mm operating channel was generally necessary. The advent of rings and clips inevitably increased the diameter of the appropriate trocar and cannula. The applicator for the Falope ring (the Laprocater) is approximately 13 mm in diameter. The Wolf operating laparoscope and the Storz Universal operating laparoscope are just over 12 mm in diameter and their operating channels are 8 mm and 7.4 mm respectively.

Insufflators

Carbon dioxide (CO_2) is the standard gas for insufflation. It is absorbed quickly and it does not support combustion. It is therefore mandatory for tubal cautery, particularly for unipolar cautery. Nitrous oxide may also be used and it is particularly useful for cases performed under local anaesthesia: CO_2 causes more abdominal pain than nitrous oxide, probably because of the alteration of the pH of the peritoneal fluid. A small number of patients are unusually sensitive to the introduction of CO_2. Female sterilization is now a quick procedure and requires insufflation of only 1.5–2.5 litres of gas. The standard insufflation rate is 1 litre per minute, but this can be increased by a fast-flow control which increases this rate to 3 litres per minute. Maintenance of the flow throughout the procedure is approximately 0.2 litres per minute.

Where large numbers of sterilizations are performed, as in India, the rate of insufflation may be substantially increased to speed up the individual procedures. In developing countries, particularly if mechanical methods are employed, ordinary air is used for insufflation. This may be administered by any means, one of the popular ones being the use of a converted fish tank aerator. Care must always be taken, however, to ensure that the air is not insufflated anywhere except the peritoneal cavity. A standard Veress needle is still ideal for insufflation. A longer needle is also available for patients who are excessively obese. In mass sterilization programmes the Veress needle is omitted, the operating trocar and cannula being introduced into the abdominal cavity to begin with, and insufflation performed down the gas channel of the cannula (Dingfelder, 1977). This technique seems somewhat dangerous. However, when the surgeon is experienced in this procedure it appears to be a satisfactory method of insufflation. When transabdominal insufflation fails due to excessive obesity, insufflation may be successfully achieved by inserting the Veress needle through the cervix and up through the uterine fundus (Sanders and Filshie, 1974). Alternatively the needle may be placed through the posterior fornix (Van Lith et al, 1983).

Uterine manipulators

To help visualize the fallopian tubes the uterus may be manipulated into anteversion and elevated. This can be achieved by a number of specifically designed instruments, e.g. The Hulka uterine elevator (both pregnant and non-pregnant), Soonawalla, and the Wadia elevator (De Grandi). However, if none of these are available a Spackman cannula may be used. If an assistant is available, a uterine sound or a 4–6 mm Hegar dilator may be inserted into the uterine cavity to achieve the same effect. If a Trendelenberg position is adopted and an anteverted uterus is present, the fallopian tubes can easily be visualized making uterine manipulation unnecessary. Any patient with a retroverted uterus, however, will inevitably require uterine elevation to ensure satisfactory visualization of the fallopian tubes. Uterine elevation should always be practised when learning to perform female sterilization.

METHODS OF LAPAROSCOPIC FEMALE STERILIZATION

Electrocautery

Unipolar diathermy

Formerly an extensively used technique, this is now only rarely employed (Editorial, 1980). Its use is virtually prohibited in Canada and Europe as many medical insurance agencies will not cover the mishaps resulting from this method. With unipolar diathermy a substantial pneumoperitoneum of 5–6 litres of CO_2 is recommended by Steptoe (1967). The fallopian tube is grasped by Palmer biopsy forceps and the electric current applied to three separate places along the isthmic part of the fallopian tube. The tube becomes first pale and then dessicated. Cauterizing the cornual portion of the tube appears to increase the rate of fistula formation and subsequent ectopic pregnancies (Stock, 1984). The high frequency current should only be administered in short bursts; the temperature produced locally may be in the order of 300–400C. The hot tubes must not be allowed to lie adjacent to bowel or other abdominal structures as a thermal injury might ensue. Smoke generated during a diathermy procedure may obscure the view, also increasing the possibility of inadvertent thermal injuries to visceral structures. Faulty equipment may cause burns to the anterior abdominal wall and sparks may be observed during the passage of the current. Burns may be noted at distant sites not accessible by the forceps, e.g. the inferior mesenteric artery. These distant burns may occur by freak accumulation of electrical energy. It is this last complication which has prompted the use of bipolar cautery.

Bipolar cautery

Bipolar cautery forceps were devised by Rioux and Kleppinger to eliminate distant and inadvertent thermal injury. Local injury, however, may still occur, since the temperature of the cauterized tube is as high as that with unipolar cautery. Once again it is important to cauterize all layers of the fallopian tube on and near to the isthmus. An important cautionary note is that each pair of bipolar forceps has to match up exactly with the electrocautery machine for which it was designed. Mismatch of forceps and electrocautery units has been responsible for incomplete cautery of the fallopian tube causing a number of 'outbreaks' of unsuccessful procedures with disastrous results.

Thermal coagulation

This method was introduced by Semm to minimize even further the dangers of electrocautery. The method involves the electrical heating of a filament in the forceps to between 120 and 140C. The electricity is of low voltage (6 V) and high wattage. The forceps should be applied to the fallopian tube for 20 seconds at a time in three different places adjacent to one another. Semm recommends transection of the tube.

Laser vaporization and photocoagulation

With the advent of laser techniques tubes have been divided by laser vaporization. Long-term follow-up studies have not yet been completed, but it is likely to be found that the CO_2 laser transects the fallopian tube so cleanly that fistula formation may be encouraged, thus promoting an increased incidence of ectopic pregnancies and a high incidence of tubal re-canalization. Indeed, the very properties that make the CO_2 laser an ideal tool for fertility mitigate against its use when a permanent tubal blockage is desired. The Nd : YAG laser with its deeper tissue penetration has a certain potential but it is difficult to justify such expensive methods when cheaper and safer physical methods are universally available.

Mechanical methods of female sterilization (Figure 1)

The Falope ring

The Falope ring was devised and described by Imbae Yoon in 1972. The ring is made from silicone rubber and is impregnated with 5% barium sulphate. The outer diameter is 3.1 mm, the inner diameter 1.1 mm and the thickness 2.2 mm. The ring may be applied by either a single- or double-puncture technique. Usually both the rings may be loaded on to the applicator at the same time. The fallopian tube is grasped in the mid-isthmic portion and is pulled into the applicator lumen. During this manoeuvre the applicator is slightly advanced. A ring is then pushed over the knuckle of the tube and the procedure is repeated on the opposite side. The Falope ring destroys 2–3 cm

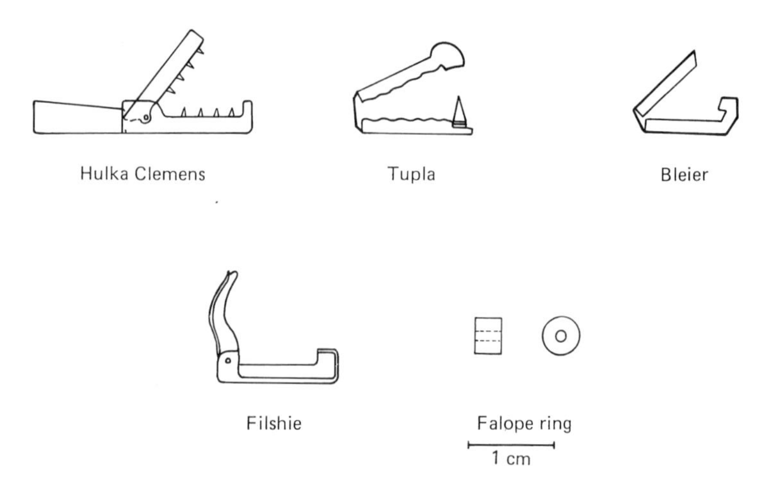

Figure 1. Mechanical methods of tubal occlusion.

of tube. Technical difficulties include transection of the fallopian tube while drawing it up into the lumen of the applicator. If the tube is large a milking process should be adopted which involves squeezing the oedema fluid out of the fallopian tube as it is slowly drawn into the lumen of the applicator. If the tube is too large or fibrotic another method of sterilization should be employed.

Hulka-Clemens clip

This clip was devised by Hulka and Clemens in 1972. It comprises two jaws of Lexan (polycarbonate) with a stainless steel hinge pin and a gold-plated stainless steel spring which is pushed over the two jaws to press them together. The clips are 3 mm wide and 15 mm long. They may be applied by the double- or single-puncture technique, but the latter has a higher failure rate. The clip should be applied at right angles across the isthmic portion of the fallopian tube. The constant pressure of the spring ensures avascular necrosis of the fallopian tube between the jaws in the majority of cases. The clip causes minimal tubal damage (3–4 mm on each side) and is associated with a low morbidity rate.

Filshie clip

This clip is made from an outer layer of titanium lined on the inner surface with silicone rubber. There is a hinge at one end and a latch at the other. When the tube is compressed, the rubber exerts external pressure on the tube to maintain occlusion. There is never any dead space between the jaws of the clip to allow for re-canalization. The clip is 1.3 cm long and 4 mm wide and may be applied by double- or single-puncture technique. The original applicator was 8 mm in diameter and the new model is 7.4 mm in diameter.

There are three single puncture applicators—8 mm, 7.4 mm (especially designed for the Storz Universal operating laparoscope) and 6 mm in diameter. The latter has to be assembled into the laparoscope prior to use. The clip should be placed over the isthmic portion of the tube 1–3 cm from the cornu. Special care should be taken to check that the whole tube is occluded.

Bleier clip

This is made entirely of plastic and has an integral hinge mechanism on one end and a snapping latch at the other. Small gaps at either end may occur after application of the clip to the tube and this has led to an unacceptable number of spontaneous recanalizations (Adelman, 1984).

The Weck clip

This was one of the original clips used for female sterilization. The gap between the jaws however allows an unacceptably high rate of recanalization—a gap of 0.33 mm is all that is necessary to allow recanalization. The failure rate of the Weck clip is in the order of 1–4% which is generally considered unacceptable (Hayashi, 1972).

Tupla clip

This clip is also made out of plastic. It has a projection at the lower mouth of the clip which initially pierces the mesosalpinx to become latched firmly into an aperture of the upper jaw.

ANAESTHETICS FOR LAPAROSCOPIC STERILIZATION

Female sterilization may be performed under general or local anaesthesia.

General anaesthetic

When general anaesthesia is employed, only a short-acting agent is usually necessary. Intubation after administering a short-acting muscle relaxant is popular, although there is no statistical difference in morbidity when intubation methods are compared with non-intubation methods (Chamberlain and Brown, 1972). Respiratory arrest may occur if the abdomen becomes over distended with gas or if the Trendelenburg angle is too steep (over 35°).

Local anaesthetic

This is an under-used method, but gaining in popularity. It is used extensively in the developing world because of its simplicity and safety. Its use for clips and rings is well documented (Fishburne et al, 1974; Filshie et al, 1981;

Paterson, 1982; Mackenzie et al, 1987). If a double-puncture technique is contemplated 10 ml of local anaesthetic (1% lignocaine and 1:200 000 adrenaline) is injected immediately below the umbilicus and 10 ml just above the pubic hair line in the midline. The injection should infiltrate all layers of the abdomen down to the peritoneum. When the abdomen is punctured by the instruments, the patient is asked to distend her abdomen. This moves the anterior abdominal wall away from the vital structures beneath and confers an added safety factor to the Veress needle. One millilitre of 4% lignocaine may be dropped on to each fallopian tube to minimalize local discomfort during the sterilization procedure. The tubes may be cauterized, clipped or ringed. Nitrous oxide is less uncomfortable to the awake patient.

As general anaesthetic has been attributable for at least one third of all the deaths associated with sterilization, local anaesthetic should be offered to the patient as an alternative.

FAILURE OF STERILIZATION METHODS

The failure rates of each method varies considerably from series to series; there are a number of excellent reviews available which document the spectrum of results (Shepard, 1974; Bhiwandiwala et al, 1982; Frances and Darroch, 1982; Newton, 1984; Chick et al, 1985). The efficacy rates quoted here are average figures.

Electrocautery

Unipolar coagulation

The failure rate varies from 0.35 (Yuzpe et al, 1977) to 22 (Hughes and Liston, 1975) per thousand cases. Large studies however demonstrate a failure rate in the region of 2.6–3.7 per thousand. There appears to be a higher failure rate when coagulation is followed by tubal transection (Phillips et al, 1977).

Bipolar cautery

The failure rate should be the same for bipolar as for unipolar. When the operation is correctly performed a failure rate of 1.1 per thousand may be achieved (Yuzpe et al, 1977). Higher failure rates have been recorded when faulty equipment has been employed.

Thermal coagulation

The failure rate is between 0.21 (Semm, 1983) and 0.4 (Van Lith et al, 1983) per thousand women months. Although Semm quotes 1%, Yoon quotes a failure rate of 5 per thousand which is similar to other authors; it may however be as high as 16 per thousand (Yoon et al, 1977; Yoon and Poliakof, 1979; Newton, 1984).

Mechanical methods

The Hulka-Clemens clip

Failure rates appear to vary according to experience, Lieberman (Lieberman et al, 1978; Lieberman, 1983) reports a failure rate of less than 5 per thousand on average, although long-term failure rates of up to 3.7% have been recorded (Griffin and Mandsager, 1987).

The Filshie clip

The reported failure rate of the mark IV clip was 4.9 per thousand (Filshie et al, 1981); Mark VI, which incorporates a hinge, is between 0.9 and 2.7 per thousand (Chick et al, 1985; Filshie, 1987).

The Bleier and Tupla clips

Large long-term follow-up studies are not available for these methods, but some studies have shown that the failure rate of the Bleier clip is up to 8.2% of cases, which has detracted from its use (Adelman, 1984; Lee and Rubin, 1984).

The Weck clip

This clip has a failure rate of approximately 1% (Najar, 1972), but failure rates of up to 6.4% have been recorded—too high for the equipment to be used generally (Hsu et al, 1973).

Ectopic pregnancies relating to failures

Whenever tubal damage occurs tubal pregnancies ensue. The pathophysiological causes of an ectopic pregnancy in these circumstances may vary (Stock, 1984):

1. A direct tuboperitoneal fistula may arise from the proximal stump of the tube following salpingectomy, diathermy or following use of clips or rings.
2. A fistula may form in association with the occurrence of endosalpingosis following tubal ligation.
3. A tubo-tubal fistula may occur causing an ectopic pregnancy to lodge in the abnormal area along the tubo-tubal fistula.

Ectopic pregnancies (Tatum and Schmidt, 1977; McClousland, 1980; Bhiwandiwala et al, 1982) are highest when electrocautery methods are employed (50–60% of all failures). Mechanical methods have the lowest ectopic failure rate (about 4% of all failures) (Bhiwandiwala et al, 1982; Doll, 1988).

MORBIDITY

Laparoscopic sterilization is a sophisticated technique which, when performed by a skilled surgeon using well-serviced instruments, is associated with a very low morbidity; operations are usually day-case procedures. Typical morbidity of infection or haemorrhage at the site of the laparoscopic trocar wounds are rare—less than 1% of patients. This compares very favourably with the general morbidity following vasectomy (Frances and Kovacs, 1983), which is in the order of 3%. When obesity or pathology exist, morbidity is increased. Fat tubes, adhesions, cysts or a retroverified uterus increases intraoperative morbidity and also increases its failure rate (Loffer and Pent, 1976; Bhiwandiwala et al, 1982).

Anaesthesia

Complications of anaesthesia include cardiorespiratory arrest often due to overdose of anaesthetic agents. Cardiac arrhythmias may occur due to the absorption of CO_2 into the circulation (Marshall et al, 1972; Lewis and Aasad, 1974). When local anaesthesia is employed, lignocaine toxicity may produce bradycardia and cardiac arrest. Intravenous sedation should always be light as an overdose can also produce cardiorespiratory arrest from hypoventilation, particularly when valium and pethidine are used. Atropine is an important adjunct to prevent cardiac arrhythmias and bradycardia.

Laparoscopy

Hypercapnia and carbon dioxide embolus are rare complications which can be minimized by instilling only 1–2 litres of CO_2 into the abdominal cavity and checking first that the installation is in the right place by performing the saline test. This involves injecting 5 ml of saline down the Veress needle with a syringe, then aspirating. If no reflux occurs then the saline is in the peritoneal cavity (Berci and Cuschieri, 1986).

Over-distension of the abdomen and too steep a Trendelenberg position increases substantially the adverse effect, particularly on the heart and lungs, and therefore should be avoided.

Although punctures of the blood vessels or visceral structures by the Veress needle or trocar and cannula are infrequent they continue to cause substantial morbidity when they arise. Puncturing of the bowel when adherent to the anterial abdominal wall can always occur if the puncture is a blind technique. Semm has described a sight-controlled peritoneal puncture if previous abdominal surgery has been employed, and this should minimize this hazard (Semm, 1988).

This accident may be noticed immediately by the surgeon, particularly by the faeculent smell of gas which may leak from the Veress needle. Sometimes the interior of the viscera (e.g. bowel or stomach) may be visualized down the laparoscope. Occasionally the laparoscope and cannula may totally penetrate through the bowel and injury may not be immediately recognized. A check for bowel puncture should always be made by viewing down the laparoscope during its withdrawal from the peritoneal cavity; the bowel lumen may then be noticed. To avoid such injuries the open laparoscopic technique devised by Harith Hasoon should be employed.

The uterus may be perforated either by the uterine manipulator or a dilator (Bhiwandiwala et al, 1982). Care must therefore always be exercised during this procedure and equipment should be available to deal with ongoing bleeding although, unless it is coming from a gravid uterus, the bleeding usually ceases after a few minutes.

Electrocautery

Thermal injury may involve the anterior abdominal wall or abdominal visceral structures. The bowel is the most frequent structure to be damaged but bladder, ureter and major blood vessels can also be injured. Damage to distant sites such as the mesenteric artery may be associated with the use of unipolar diathermy. Bowel perforation or infarction leads to the serious complication of faeculent peritonitis, which is associated with the loss of life in nearly 50% of cases (Thompson and Wheeless, 1973).

Mechanical methods

Yoon rings

Transection of the fallopian tubes occurs in approximately 3% of cases. Extra rings may need to be applied to control haemorrhage. A change of method may be required if these fail and cautery or endocoagulation equipment should be available if needed. Peritubal adhesions or fat tubes may prohibit the use of rings. Difficulties with equipment occur in a small number of cases (0.01%) (Bhiwandiwala et al, 1982).

Clips

Clips must completely occlude the tubes; if one does not do the job, a second clip should be applied. Many surgeons, including Hulka, now place two Hulka clips adjacent to one another on the tube. Extra clips need to be applied in 6% of cases employing Filshie clips, and 10% with Hulka clips. Equipment and application difficulties are encountered with 10% of Filshie clips and 27% of Hulka clips (Toplis and Newman, 1988). If two clips or rings are placed within a short length of tube a hydrosalpinx may occur between them.

MORTALITY

Laparoscopic female sterilization, like any other procedure, has a certain amount of mortality associated with it. The exact incidence of death is difficult to obtain as the procedures are performed in many different settings. Any problems which arise following the operation may be referred to surgical departments, often at a time or place distant from the one where the original procedure was performed. Information on mortality is available from the Laparoscopic Survey (Chamberlain and Brown, 1978), conducted by the Royal College of Obstetricians and Gynaecologists. Further information is obtained from the Association of Gynaecological Laparoscopists (AAGL) (Phillips et al, 1977), and Centre for Disease Control (CDC) in the United States (Strauss et al, 1984; Peterson et al, 1983).

The Royal College of Obstetricians and Gynaecologists' survey demonstrated a mortality of 10.2 per hundred thousand compared with 2.5 per hundred thousand from the AAGL; it is, however, generally accepted that the RCOG report is more accurate since information from the AAGL may have favoured under-reporting because of the medicolegal situation in the United States.

Causes of death have been documented by Peterson and colleagues and also by the Association of Voluntary Surgical Contraception. The main courses of death are as follows:

Deaths related to anaesthesia

Deaths relating to anaesthesia still represent the largest subgroup (40%). Too much anaesthesia resulting in hypoventilation and cardiorespiratory arrest is the most common cause. Cardiorespiratory arrest may still occur with the administration of too much epidural or spinal anaesthesia. Other associated causes are aspiration, pneumonia, airway obstruction, hypotension and meningitis.

Bowel injury

Bowel injury is still responsible for a large number of deaths and this may or may not be associated with laparoscopy. Because laparoscopy is a blind technique the bowel may be damaged by the Veress needle or the trocar. Approximately half of the bowel injuries are caused in this way.

The bowel may also be injured as a direct result of electrocautery, particularly with unipolar diathermy. The bowel may receive a thermal injury which may not be recognized at the time of surgery. The thermal injury results in dehiscence usually 3 days following the procedure and this results in faeculent peritonitis, which has a high mortality. Open laparoscopy reduces, but does not eliminate, this problem (Hasson, 1979). Bowel injury accounts for approximately 25% of all laparoscopic deaths.

Infection

Infection in the absence of bowel damage is a relatively rare cause of death following laparoscopy. It is often associated with pre-existing pelvic inflammatory disease or with an intrauterine contraceptive device (Wright, 1974). The administration of antibiotics is recommended in these circumstances.

Haemorrhage

Intra-abdominal haemorrhage is still an important cause of mortality (approximately 20%). Vessels may be punctured by the Veress needle or by the trocar and cannula. The aorta and vena cava are accessible, particularly if the Veress needle and trocar and cannula are inserted at right angles to the incision. The internal iliac artery and vein is also vulnerable, particularly if the instruments are placed laterally, or if the scalpel blade for the skin incision penetrates too deeply.

Gas embolism

Gas embolism is a rare cause of maternal mortality and may be associated with instilling CO_2 into the areola tissue of the anterior abdominal wall. Occasionally the Veress needle may be injected into a vein in the omentum, but this can be avoided by the saline drip test.

Incidental causes

Myocardial infarcts, pulmonary embolism, anaphylactic shock and cerebral infarcts have all been recorded; fortunately, however, these are relatively rare (Peterson et al, 1983).

In spite of this somewhat bewildering list of complications laparoscopic female sterilization performed carefully by a well-trained laparoscopist using physical methods for tubal occlusion remains an extremely safe procedure with a high rate of patient acceptance.

REFERENCES

Adelman R (1984) High Failure Rate Of A Plastic Tubal (Bleier) Clip. *Obstetrics and Gynecology* **64:** 721–723.

Anderson ET (1937) Peritoneoscopy. *American Journal of Surgery* **35:** 136–139.

Babenerd J & Flehr I (1978) Erfahrungen mit dem Tupla-Clip zur Tubensterilisation per laparascopiam. *Geburtshilfe und Frauenheilk* **38:** 299.

Bauchpunktionen. *Deutsche Medizinische Wochenschrift* **41:** 1480–1481.

Berci G & Cuschieri A (1986) *Practical Laparoscopy*. London: Baillière Tindall.

Bhiwandiwala PP et al (1982) A comparison of different laparoscopic sterilization occlusion techniques in 24 439 procedures. *American Journal of Obstetrics and Gynecology* **144:** 319.

Bleier W (1973) *Tubensterilisation mit einem Polyacetalclip*. London: Planned Parenthood Foundation.

Chamberlain G & Brown JC (eds) (1978) *Gynaecological Laparoscopy—The report of the Working Party of the Confidential Enquiry into Gynaecological Laparoscopy*. London: Royal College of Obstetricians and Gynaecologists.

Chick PM, Frances M & Paterson PJ (1985) A comprehensive review of female sterilisation—tubal occlusion methods. *Clinical Reproduction and Fertility* **3:** 81–97.

Dingfelder JR (1977) Direct trocar insertion without prior pneumoperitoneum. In Phillips JM & Downey CA (eds.) *Endoscopy in Gynecology*, pp 49–53. American Association of Gynecologic Laparoscopists.

Doll HC (1988) *Canadian Sterilisation Survey*. AVSC Annual Report.

Editorial (1980) Female sterilisation: No more tubal coagulation. *British Medical Journal* **280:** 1037.

Filshie GM (1987) Current Status Of The Filshie Clip. *XIth Asian & Oceanic Congress of Obstetrics & Gynecology*, p 280 (abstract).
Filshie GM, Casey D, Pogmore JR et al (1981) The titanium/silicone rubber clip for female sterilisation. *British Journal of Obstetrics and Gynaecology* **88:** 655–662.
Fishburne JI, Omran HK, Hulka JF, Mercer JP & Edelman DA (1974) Laparoscopic clip tubal sterilisation under local anaesthetic. *Fertility and Sterility* **25:** 762.
Frances M & Darroch RK (1982) *Contraceptive sterilisation—a comparative review*. MSc Australian National University, Canberra.
Frances M & Kovacs GT (1983) A comprehensive review of the sequelae of male sterilisation. *Contraception* **28:** 455–474.
Frangenheim H (1964) Die tuben sterilisation unter sicht mit dem laparoscope. *Gerbutsh. Frasenheilk* **24:** 470–473.
Griffin WT & Mandsager NT (1987) Spring clip sterilisation: long-term follow-up. *Southern Medical Journal* **80:** 301–304.
Hayashi M (1972) Tubal Sterilisation with clips. Proceedings of the conference, Cherry Hill, New Jersey, October 28–31, 1969. pp 201–203. Springfield, Illinois: Charles C. Thomas.
Hirsch HA & Roos E (1974) Laparoskopische Tubensterilisation mit einer neuen Bikoagulationszange. *Geburtshilfe und Frauenheilkunde* **34:** 340.
Hopkins HH (1976) Optical principles of the endoscope. In Berci G (ed.) *Endoscopy*, pp 3–27. New York: Appleton-Century-Crofts.
Hsu HC, Wang SL & Chen AC (1973) Oviductal sterilisation with tantalum clips. *Journal of Obstetrics and Gynecology of the Republic of China* **12:** 1–9.
Hughes G & Liston WA (1975) Comparison between Laparoscopic Sterilization and Tubal Ligation. *British Medical Journal* **3:** 637–639.
Hulka JF, Fishburne JI, Mercer JP et al (1973) Laparoscopic sterilization with a spring clip: A report on the first fifty cases. *American Journal of Obstetrics and Gynecology* **116:** 715.
Jacobeus HC (1911) Kurze Ubersicht uber meine Erfahrungen mit der Laparoskopie. *Munchener Medizinische Wochenschrift* **58:** 2017–2019.
Kalk H (1929) Erfahrungen mit der Laparoskopie. *Zeitschrift Klinische Medizinische* **111:** 303–348.
Kalk H & Bruhl W (1951) *Leitfaden der Laparoskopie*. Stuttgart: Thieme.
Kelling G (1923) Zur Colioskopie. *Archives Klinische Chirurgie* **126:** 226–229.
Kleppinger RK (1977) Ancillary uses of bipolar forceps. *Journal of Reproductive Medicine* **18:** 254.
Kleppinger RK (1977) Laparoscopy at a community hospital: An analysis of 4,300 cases. *Journal of Reproductive Medicine* **19:** 353.
Lee NC & Rubin GI (1984) Report of a high pregnancy rate after sterilisation with the Bleier clip. *Southern Medical Journal* **77:** 5.
Lewis GBH & Prasad K (1974) Sodium bicarbonate treatment of ventricular arrhythmias during laparoscopy. *Anesthesiology* **41:** 41–416.
Lieberman B (1983) The Hulka Clemens clip. In van Lith DAF, Keith LG & van Hall EV (eds) *New Trends in Female Sterilisation*, pp 105–114. Chicago, London: Year Book Medical.
Lieberman BA, Gordon AG & Bostock JF (1978) Menstrual patterns after laparoscopic sterilisation using a spring loaded clip. *British Journal of Obstetrics and Gynecology* **85:** 376.
Loffer FD & Pent D (1976) Laparoscopy in obese patients. *American Journal of Obstetrics and Gynecology* **125:** 104.
Marshall RL, Jebson PJR, Davie IT & Scott DB (1972) Circulatory effects of carbon dioxide insufflation of the peritoneal cavity for laparoscopy. *British Journal of Anaesthesiology* **44:** 680–684.
McCausland A (1982) Endosalpingosis ('endosalpingoblastosis') following ectopic pregnancy. *American Journal of Obstetrics and Gynecology* **143:** 12–22.
McClousland A (1980) High rate of ectopic pregnancy following laparoscopic tubal coagulation failures. *American Journal of Obstetrics and Gynecology* **136:** 97.
Mackenzie IZ, Turner E, O'Sullivan GM & Guillebaud J (1987) Two hundred out-patient laparoscopic clip sterilizations using local anaesthesia. *British Journal of Obstetrics and Gynaecology* **94:** 449–453.
Najar AG (1972) Culdoscopy as an aid to family planning. In Duncan GW, Falb RD, Speidel JJ

(eds) *Female Sterilisation: Prognosis for Simplified Outpatient Procedures*. New York: Academic Press.
Newton JR (1984) Contraception Update. In Newton JR (ed.) *Clinics in Obstetrics and Gynaecology* **11**(3): 603–640.
Nitze M (1893) Zur Photography der menschlichen Harnrohre. *Berl. med. Wschr.* **31:** 744.
Palmer R (1960) Discussion of modern methods of salpingostomy. *Proceedings of the Royal Society of Medicine* **53:** 357–359.
Palmer R (1962) Essaie de sterilisation tubaire coelioscopique par electrocoagulation isthmique. *R. C. Soc. Franc. Gynecol.* **5:** 3.
Paterson P (1982) Laparoscopic sterilisation with the Filshie clip under local anaesthesia. *Medical Journal of Australia* **2:** 476–477.
Peterson HB, De Stefano F, Rubin GL et al (1983) Deaths attributable to tubal sterilisation in the United States 1977 to 1981. *American Journal of Obstetrics and Gynaecology* **146:** 131–136.
Phillips J, Keith D, Hulka B et al (1977) Survey of laparoscopy: 1971–1975. In Phillips JM (ed.) *Laparoscopy*, pp 342–352. Baltimore: Williams & Wilkins.
Phillips J, Hulka B, Hulka J, Keith D & Keith L (1977) American Association of Gynecologic Laparoscopists' 1976 Membership Survey. *Journal of Reproductive Medicine* **21:** 3–6.
Power FH & Barnes AC (1941) Sterilization by means of peritoneoscopic tubal fulguration. *American Journal of Obstetrics and Gynecology* **41:** 1038.
Rioux JE & Cloutier D (1974) Bipolar cautery for sterilization by laparoscopy. *Journal of Reproductive Medicine* **13:** 6.
Rock JA, Parmley TH & King TM (1981) Endometriosis and the development of tuboperitoneal fistulas after tubal ligation. *Fertility and Sterility* **35:** 16–20.
Ruddock JC (1934) Peritoneoscopy. *West. J. Surg. Obstet. Gynec.* **42:** 392–394.
Ruddock JC (1937) Peritoneoscopy. *Surgery, Gynecology and Obstetrics* **65:** 523–539.
Sanders RR & Filshie GM (1974) Transfundal induction of pneumoperitoneum prior to laparoscopy. *Journal of Obstetrics and Gynaecology of the British Commonwealth* **8**(10): 829–830.
Semm K (1973) Thermal coagulation for sterilization. *Endoscopy* **5:** 218.
Semm K (1983) Endocoagulation A Nearly 99% Effective Method of Tubal Sterilization. In Phillips J (ed.) *Endoscopic Female Sterilisation: A Comparison of Methods*, pp 89–104. Downey, California: American Association Of Gynecologic Laparoscopists.
Semm K (1988) Sight controlled peritoneum puncture for surgical pelviscopy. *Geburschilfe Frauenheilkunde* **48:** 436–439.
Shepard MK (1974) Female contraceptive sterilization. *Obstetrical and Gynecology Survey* **12:** 291.
Steptoe PC (1965) Gynaecological endoscopy, laparoscopy & culdoscopy. *Journal of Obstetrics and Gynaecology of the British Commonwealth* **72:** 535–543.
Steptoe PC (1967) *Laparoscopy in Gynecology*. Edinburgh: E & S Livingstone.
Stock RJ (1984) Ectopic pregnancy subsequent to sterilisation; histologic evaluation and clinical implications. *Fertility and Sterility* **42:** 211–215.
Strauss LT, Huezo CM, Krames DG et al (1984) Sterilization-Associated deaths: A Global Survey. *International Journal of Gynaecology and Obstetrics* **22:** 67–75.
Tatum HJ & Schmidt FH (1977) Contraceptive and sterilisation practices and extra uterine pregnancy: a realistic perspective. *Fertility and Sterility* **28:** 407.
Thompson BH & Wheeless CR Jr (1973) Gastrointestinal complications of laparoscopic sterilization. *Obstetrics and Gynecology* **41:** 669.
Toplis PJ & Newman RB (1988) Laparoscopic sterilisation—a comparison of Hulka-Clemens and Filshie Clips. *British Journal of Family Planning* **14:** 43–45.
Van Lith DAF, van Schie KJ, Beetchuizen W & Binstock M (1983) Coagulation by the Semm and the Wolf techniques. In van Lith DAF, Keith LG & van Hall EV (eds) *New Trends in Female Sterilization*, pp 61–82. Chicago, London: Year Book Medical.
Wheeless CR Jr (1972) The status of out-patient sterilisation by laparoscopy: improved techniques and review of 1000 cases. *Obstetrics and Gynecology* **39:** 635.
Wheeless CR (1974) Laparoscopically applied hemoclips for tubal sterilisation. *Obstetrics and Gynecology* **44:** 752–755.
Wright FC (1974) Tuboovarian abscess associated with laparoscopic tubal cauterization and the intrauterine contraceptive device. *American Journal of Obstetrics and Gynecology* **119:** 1133.

Yoon I & King TM (1975) A preliminary and intermediate report on a new laparoscopic tubal ring procedure. *Journal of Reproductive Medicine* **15:** 54.

Yoon I & Poliakof SR (1979) Laparoscopic tubal ligation: a follow-up report on the Yoon Falope ring methodology. *Journal of Reproductive Medicine* **23:** 76.

Yoon I, King TM & Parmley TH (1977) A two-year experience with the Falope ring sterilization procedure. *American Journal of Obstetrics and Gynecology* **127:** 109–112.

Yuzpe AA, Rioux JE, Loffer FP & Pent D (1977) Laparoscopic tubal sterilisation by the burn-only technique. *Obstetrics and Gynecology* **49:** 106.

Zollikofer R (1924) Zur Laparoskopie. *Schweizerische Medizinische Wochenschrift* **54:** 264–265.

11

Documentation in laparoscopic surgery

KEES WAMSTEKER

Human nature obviously incorporates the drive to record and use documentation for communication and the transfer of information. Drawings from ancient times are able to inform us of customs of life and diseases of past cultures. Imaging and its documentation has also always been an essential expedient in diagnosis, education and communication in medicine. Ancient medical drawings and paintings reproduced external findings in diseased humans and post mortem anatomical dissections.

Modern technology enables physicians to actually 'view' inside human bodies using electromagnetic (EM) radiation of different wavelengths. Some of the non-visible parts of the EM spectrum are used as a carrier for imaging techniques like scintigraphy, radiography and magnetic resonance imaging (MRI). No one will deny the need to record the images produced with these techniques.

The retina of the human eye can only detect electromagnetic radiation with a wavelength between 400 and 800 nm (visible light). Thus, only a very small part of the EM radiation can be seen by humans and hence be used for endoscopy, which should be considered as just an optical or electronic extension of the human eye (Noordveld et al, 1987). As we are not accustomed to recording everything we see (except for holiday photography) the threshold to document routine endoscopic procedures has been high for a long time (Table 1). While multidisciplinary imaging systems with non-visible electromagnetic carriers today almost all have built-in documentation possibilities, endoscopic documentation still requires supplementary equipment, so that written operative reports are still the first choice for documentation in laparoscopy. Modern instrumentation and electronics,

Table 1. Attitude towards documentation in different imaging techniques.

Carrier radiation	Technique	Visualization	Threshold to documentation
Gamma	Scintigraphy	Indirect	Low
Röntgen	Radiology	Indirect	Low
Visible light	*Endoscopy*	*Direct*	*High*
Infrared	Thermography	Indirect	Low
High frequency	MRI	Indirect	Low
Ultrasound (non EM)	Ultrasonography	Indirect	Low

however, have simplified tremendously the means of obtaining image records in endoscopy at constant high quality and it is beyond doubt that pictures with good quality say much more than long written reports.

Documentation in endoscopy is just as essential as it is in radiology and MRI, especially in diagnostic and surgical laparoscopy. Visual image documentation is of the utmost importance when comparing results before and after treatment and with different techniques, in explaining the indication for open or endoscopic surgery, in teaching and in patient education.

METHODS OF DOCUMENTATION

Cerebral

The human brain with the eyes is one of the most superb imaging and image recording systems for laparoscopy. The only problem is that it is not capable of producing hard copies or transmitting images to others. Besides, storage in one's memory is not always reliable with the passage of time! For that reason other methods have to be used to record endoscopic findings of surgical techniques.

Written

The most widely used method of documentation in laparoscopy is the written operative report. Depending on the time available for description and the capabilities of the surgeon, the report can be very informative and complete or poor and almost useless for others. Advantages of written reports are that the documentation material is always available and does not require any specific skill. However, a written report can never compete with one good quality photograph.

Drawings

Drawing materials are also always available. Quite often combinations of drawings and written reports are much more informative than just plain text. Some three-dimensional effects can be suggested, and trans-sections can be produced, although in laparoscopy they will only represent imaginary images. The famous drawings of Frank Netter are the best example of the informative value of high quality drawings, however the value of drawings is highly dependent on personal artistry and available time.

Diagrams

The time required to prepare a 'visual' report can be reduced with preprinted diagrams of the organs to be described. This system is often used in laparoscopic reports, but the diagrams seem to encourage quick sketching and details are frequently omitted. Besides, the majority are only two-dimensional and do not easily allow three-dimensional effects.

Although these techniques are the most widely used, they can rarely rival the results achieved with photography, film, video recording and optical disc recording, all of which require supplementary equipment.

Photography

High quality photographic slide documentation provides optimal full colour hard copy records of laparoscopic images. Special equipment is always necessary and has to be in perfect condition for good results. One disadvantage of slide photography is that instant hard copy documentation, immediately after the procedure, is not possible, and it requires a good system of patient identification, storage and retrieval. Instant hard copy photography is possible with an instant endocamera and the sensitive Polaroid film type 779 (Figure 1), but the quality of endoscopic image reproduction is often quite poor.

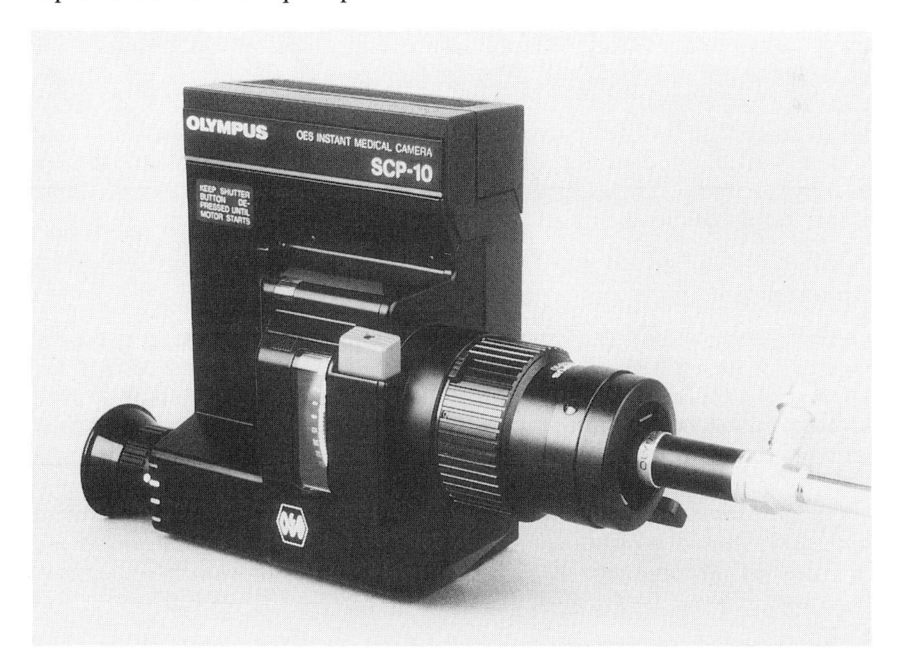

Figure 1. Instant endocamera for Polaroid film photography.

Film

The highest quality reproduction of real-time laparoscopic procedures is best achieved using 16 mm film. Suitable cameras are the Arriflex, Bolex and Beaulieu. Only the latter has automatic optical light measuring through the lens, but the Arriflex and the Bolex give a better image in the viewfinder (Semm, 1987). These cameras are, however, very expensive and very heavy, requiring a special support system. Editing and reproduction also requires special equipment, which is not always easily available.

Film recording does not provide one with the possibility of producing instant still image reproduction such as is offered with video printing devices. With the rapid improvements of the quality of videotape recordings with small lightweight cameras the importance of the classic 16 mm movie is fast decreasing.

Video recording

Video imaging and documentation is practically a standard procedure in laparoscopy today. The development of miniature electronic cameras at a reasonable cost started a tremendous growth in interest in the application of video in gynaecological endoscopy. The combination of high-power light sources and the increased sensitivity of 'chip' cameras enables the surgeon to perform laparoscopic video procedures with very little discomfort. The ability of operators to follow the actual procedure closely is vitally important in increasing their efficiency. Any specific part of the procedure can be recorded immediately and via a video printer a still picture can be produced instantaneously for the patient's records. Depending on the recording system used, equipment for reproduction of video tapes is available almost everywhere today. Difficulties only arise as a result of different international video standards (see below).

Optical disc

Optical laser video disc documentation equipment provides excellent quality for digitalized, electronic still picture storage and may be of great importance for endoscopic documentation in the future, possibly even replacing endoscopic photography. The image can be displayed on a video monitor or a hard copy reproduction can be made with an image printing device.

One advantage of this method of recording is the very easy computerized filing and retrieval possibilities. Pictures of earlier findings or procedures can be recalled instantaneously. The equipment is still rather expensive, however, and not always available in PAL (European) version.

The two most important image documentation techniques today, photography and video, and their application in laparoscopy and laparoscopic surgery are discussed in more detail below.

APPLICATIONS OF IMAGE DOCUMENTATION

Image documentation in laparoscopy and laparoscopic surgery can be applied in different ways:

1. Diagnosis (hard copy reproduction for patient records).
2. Treatment evaluation (before and after laparoscopic surgery).

3. Follow-up (endometriosis, adhesions and cancer).
4. Scientific education.
5. Patient education.
6. Communication with other physicians.

Thus, patients, and fellow workers, are completely dependent on the ability of investigators to reproduce accurately their findings. In multidisciplinary cases, as in the staging of malignant disease, these can be of vital importance for treatment. Similarly, accurate documentation is vital if patients undergo diagnostic laparoscopic procedures, which indicate the need for endoscopic surgery by another surgeon, possibly in a different speciality. Quite often written and/or drawn reports are inadequate, sometimes necessitating additional investigations.

PHOTOGRAPHY AND VIDEO DOCUMENTATION IN ENDOSCOPY: THE IMAGING CHAIN

The complete imaging and documentation system in laparoscopic photography and video recording can be considered as an imaging chain, from light source to film or videotape (Figure 2). The end result relies upon the

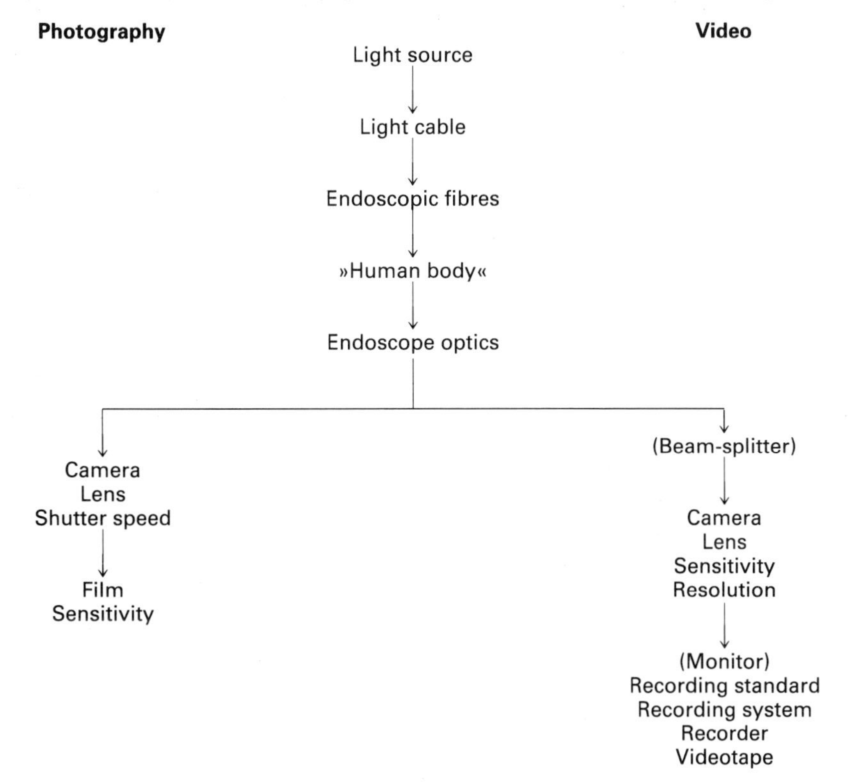

Figure 2. The imaging chain in photography and video documentation in endoscopy.

quality of each individual component of the chain. Each connection in the chain reduces the quality, non-fitting connections being extremely detrimental to the process.

In photography five technical parts with five different connections (optical, magnetic and/or electronic) have to be in good order to complete the chain through the human body to documentation (Figure 2). Video recording can require six or seven technical parts with seven or eight connections. Because of the relative complexity of these systems the separate parts need to be compatible to reach the optimal end-result. As industrial equipment often does not fit well with components from other brands, the matching of different brands should be investigated thoroughly before buying equipment.

PHOTOGRAPHY

Photographic documentation has to match its purpose. For patient records an instant hard copy photograph is ideal. Unfortunately the Polaroid system, which should fit this purpose perfectly, rarely produces photographs of acceptable quality. The image size is too small and the film sensitivity is not adequate to match the conditions required for gynaecological endoscopy. The Polaroid camera connected with video freeze-frame facilities gives much better results, but should be considered as an alternative technique to video printing.

For presentation and publication the best results are obtained with mirror reflex cameras and professional 35 mm films. For non-colour, hard-copy reproduction a professional, high resolution, black and white, plain film can also be used.

Equipment

Light source

Four different types of light source can be used for laparoscopic photography:

1. Separate flash generator. A flash tube is mounted directly between the laparoscope and the light cable. The shutter speed of the camera should not exceed 1/30 s. The camera is connected to the flash generator by a synchronizing cable. A separate examining light source is required. The intensity of the flash light is quite sufficient for good quality photography.

2. Automatic flash and examining light sources (Figure 3). Modern light sources for photography have automatic light, film speed and/or endoscope diameter measurement facilities in connection with the camera. A separate light source for examination is built-in, or the flashlight tube is used for examination at a lower intensity. Their performance in laparoscopic photography is very good.

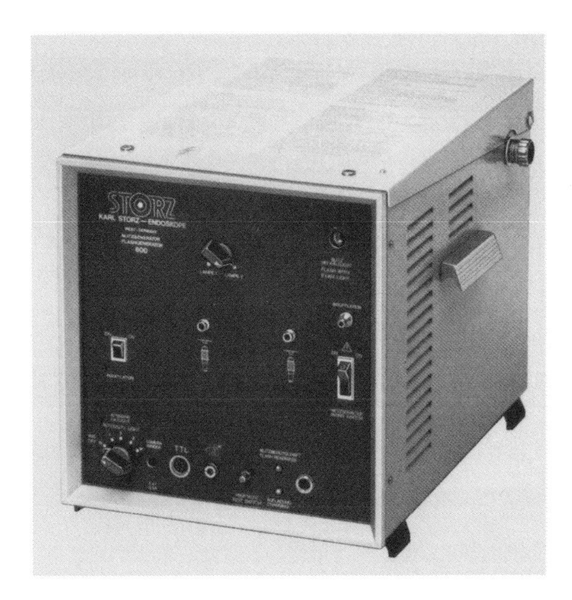

Figure 3. Automatic flash light source for visualization and photography.

3. Video light source (Figure 4). With an automatic camera (Olympus OM-2) a video light source can be used for photography with the camera set in the automatic position. The shutter speed of the camera is set by the photosensitive device in the camera. For laparoscopy the capacity of the light source should be ≥300 W. A synchronizing cable is not required. The photographic quality depends on the object–lens distance (light intensity), resulting in automatic setting of the shutter speed.

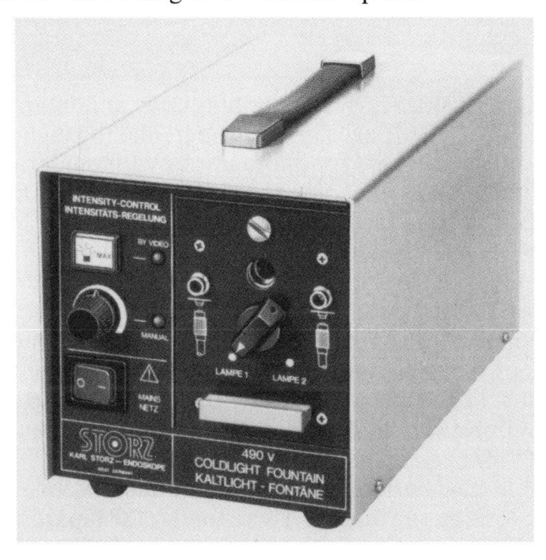

Figure 4. Video light source with automatic light intensity adaptation.

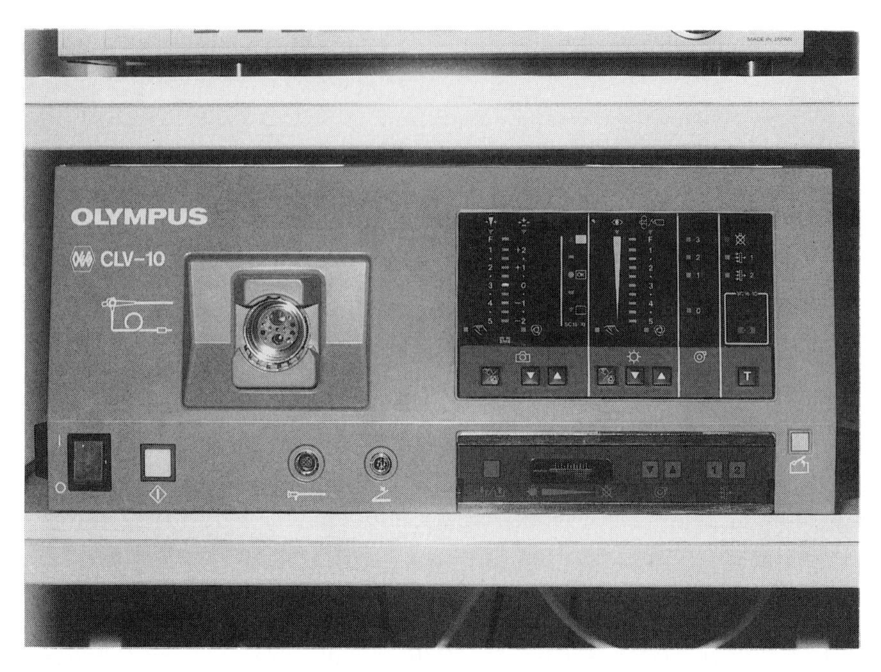

Figure 5. Integrated light source for laparoscopy, automatic photography and video imaging with autobrightness adjustment.

4. Integrated examining, photo and video light sources (Figure 5). Examining light, automatic flash generator and xenon video source (300–450 W) are integrated in larger and more expensive universal light source units.

Light cable

Two types of light cables are available: fibreoptic and fluid. Light is transmitted through fibreglass threads in the former, and through a fluid medium in the latter. Both can be used for photography with modern high-intensity light sources. Fluid cables are somewhat less flexible than fibre cables and can be bent less, but have increased light transmission.

Olympus cables have condenser lenses built into the fibre cables in order to improve the focus of the light at the light source–light cable and the light cable–laparoscope connections, which produces a higher light intensity (5 mm cable diameter for laparoscopy). Fibreoptic light cables are available with diameters of 3.5, 4.8 and 5 mm. The diameter of fluid cables is 3 or 5 mm. Fibreoptic light cables should be checked regularly for ruptures, because broken fibres significantly reduce light transmission. Leaking fluid cables are worthless.

The light cable can be integrated with the laparoscope to reduce the number of light-losing connections. These integrated laparoscopes are more expensive, however, and must always be used in sterile conditions, which raises the threshold for routine photographic documentation.

Laparoscope

Laparoscopes to be used for photography should have a diameter of at least 10 mm to obtain the best results. With smaller diameters an integrated light cable should be used.

Photographic camera

For laparoscopic photography a 35 mm single-lens mirror reflex camera (TTL, 'through-the-lens') is best (Figure 6). The usual ground-glass focusing screen should be replaced by a clear glass screen. Standardized adaptors between camera and laparoscope are available. For external flash generators a non-automatic camera body can be used. Some automatic flash generators require an automatic camera body (light measurement in the camera body), while others will cope with a non-automatic body (light measurement in the lens) (Figure 7). Accessory equipment for cameras includes: motor drive winder for film advance and record data-back for superimposing different items of information.

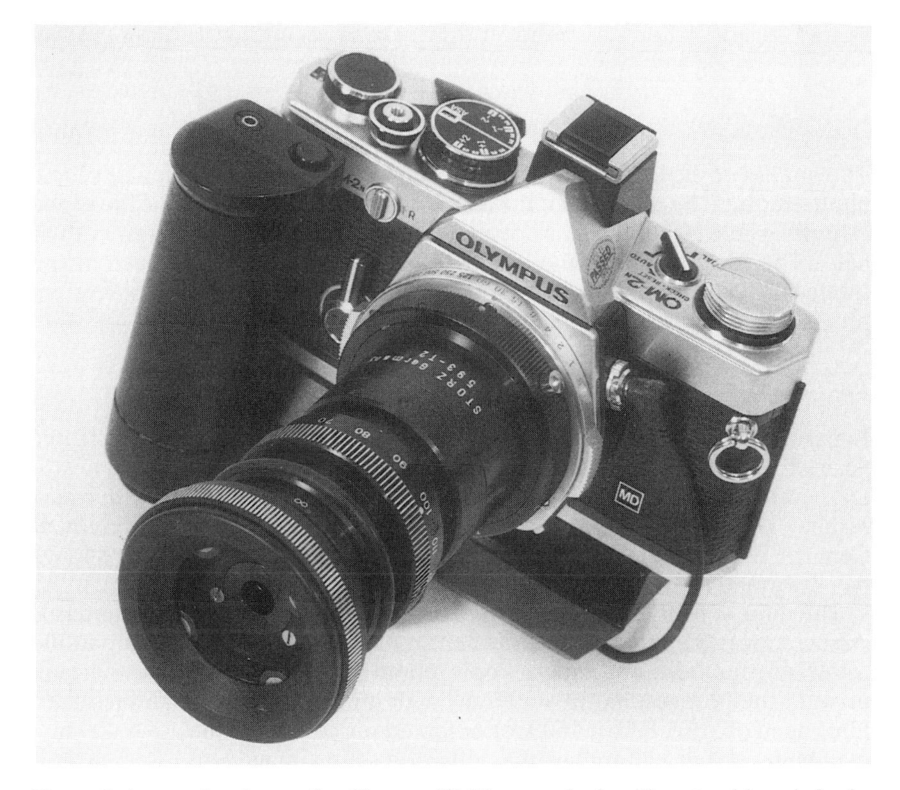

Figure 6. Automatic mirror reflex Olympus OM-2 camera body with motor drive winder for film advance, record data-back and Storz ($f = 70$–140 mm) zoom lens.

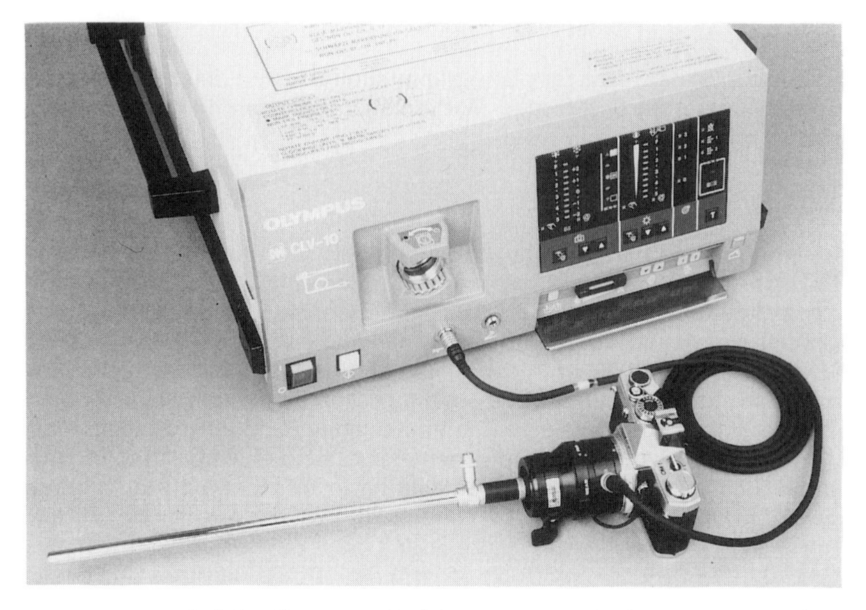

Figure 7. Automatic light adjustment with light measurement in the camera lens and non-automatic Olympus OM-1 mirror reflex camera body.

Lens

The quality of the lens is one of the most important features in laparoscopic photography. The aperture of the lens is calibrated in F-stops. The lower the F-number, the larger the lens opening (more light), but the less the depth of field. The focal length of the lens (*f* in mm) determines how much of the frame of the 35 mm film is exposed (Marlow, 1989). Some manufacturers provide zoom lenses with a focal length of 70–140 mm (Figure 6).

Film

Laparoscopic photography requires colour-slide films balanced for electronic flash, the so-called 'daylight' film, emphasizing the blue-light spectrum with temperatures between 5000 and 6100 K. Professional film gives the best results. These films however should be stored at ≤13°C and be removed from the refrigerator 1 hour before use. For good results processing should be performed as soon as possible after use (Marlow, 1983).

The film sensitivity is designated by the ASA (American Standards Association), DIN (German equivalent) or more recently ISO (comparable to ASA) number. For laparoscopic photography ASA 200 or 400 will provide the best results. In situations with low light intensity an increased film speed of ASA 800 or 1600, or enforced procession of the ASA 400 film may be used, but will reduce the definition of the image.

It is very important in laparoscopic photography to take many pictures so that only the best few can be chosen for filing.

VIDEO IMAGING AND DOCUMENTATION

With the introduction of the small single tube cameras and the more recent miniature electronic 'chip' cameras, the possibilities for video imaging and recording in endoscopy have been extended enormously. With very little discomfort to the surgeon the laparoscopic images can be displayed on a monitor and recorded simultaneously in high quality on any desired video recording system.

Video standards

Unfortunately the video world is divided mainly into three incompatible parts, determined by their norm-standards (Gisolf, 1987):

1. The *PAL* standard (phase alternating line), used in Western Europe (except for France), most countries in the Far East, most African countries, Australia and New Zealand.
2. The *NTSC* standard (National Television Standards Committee), also referred to as 'never the same colour', because of its colour instability, used in Northern America, Japan, some South American and Asian countries.
3. The *SECAM* standard (Séquentiel Couleur a Mémoire), used mainly in France and Eastern Europe and also in some African and Asian countries.

In Brazil yet another standard is used called PAL-M and still less important standards, such as SECAM-Ost and NTSC-M, are being used in different countries all over the world.

Most professional equipment in Europe can be used for either PAL or SECAM and recently video players and monitors are also available which are suitable for NTSC. For translation of videotapes from PAL to NTSC, or vice versa, special norm-translation equipment is always necessary.

The most important differences between PAL and NTSC are different colour coding and different number of image lines—PAL/SECAM, 625 lines; NTSC, 525 lines. Another difference is that PAL is more expensive, but has a higher stability and a true colour reproduction, while NTSC has colour instability due to atmospheric interferences and other disturbances. Using videotape recordings in different countries requires knowledge of the used video standard and, if applicable, norm-translation into the appropriate standard.

Video systems

It is not solely the different, incompatible video standards which complicate international video communication and exchange. The various recording systems and tape formats are also totally incompatible. Unfortunately the technical developments move towards greater variety and thus greater confusion.

Professional quality required 1- or 2-inch tapewidth for a long time, but

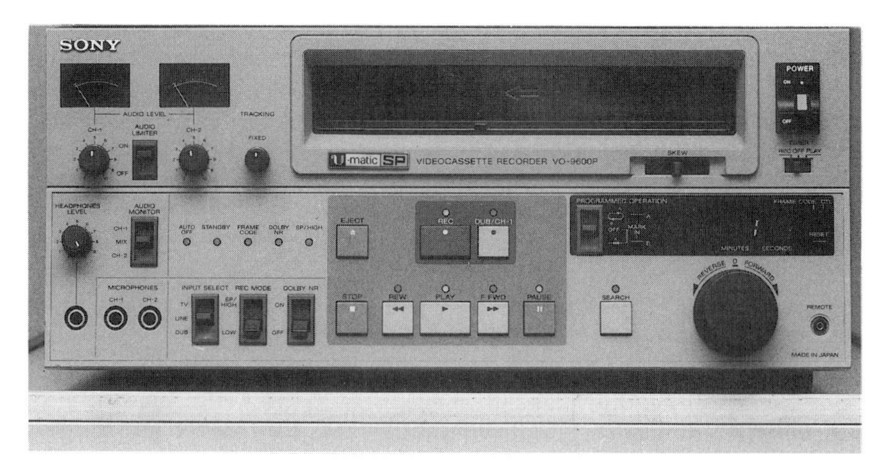

Figure 8. Sony VO-9600P U-matic high-band and low-band video recorder.

for several years now 0.75-inch U-matic tapes, in the so called 'high-band' recording fashion, are accepted as the professional (or broadcast) system. Although U-matic high-band (also called BVU) uses the same tape as U-matic 'low-band', which is the most widely used for medical purposes, they are incompatible. The latest Sony recorders however can accept both U-matic high-band and low-band (Sony VO-9600P recorder (Figure 8) and Sony VP-9000P player). Editing U-matic high-band tapes will inevitably be more expensive than U-matic low-band tape editing.

Another system, accepted relatively recently as professional (or broadcast), is the Betacam-system, which takes a 0.5-inch Betamax cassette tape, but again it is not compatible with the Betamax recorder. A comparable professional 0.5-inch VHS counterpart is the M2 format. A (semi)professional system will be available soon in 0.5-inch VHS: the Super-VHS (S-VHS) recorders and tapes with a higher horizontal resolution of 400 lines (standard VHS approximately 250 lines).

To combat this chaos in video standards and systems it is essential to understand the principles behind choice of materials. For video recording in laparoscopic endoscopy 0.75-inch U-matic high-band provides the best quality at reasonable costs. At least 0.75-inch U-matic low-band (and in the future maybe 0.5-inch S-VHS) should be used for recordings that need to be edited. For routine use standard 0.5-inch VHS is acceptable. If editing is required the VHS tape should be upgraded to 0.75-inch U-matic high-band or even 1 inch and edited in this format. After editing, the mastertape can be translated to VHS again but there will inevitably be loss of quality due to second generation reproduction. Editing in the normal VHS format will give unacceptable loss of quality. Not enough is known yet about the new 8 mm format (V8) to comment on its use in laparoscopic documentation and its editing capabilities. An overview of the different video systems is presented in Table 2.

Table 2. Tape formats and video systems.

Format	System	Quality
1 inch	A-, B-, C-Format	Professional/broadcast
0.75 inch	U-Matic high-band/BVU	Professional/broadcast
	U-Matic low-band	Semi-professional
0.5 inch	Betacam	Professional/broadcast
	M-Format	Professional/broadcast
	Super-VHS	Semi-professional
	VHS	Consumer
	(Betamax)	Consumer
	(V2000)	Consumer
8 mm	Video 8	Consumer

Equipment

Light source

Light sources for video imaging and documentation in laparoscopy are xenon or halogen and should have a capacity of at least 300 W. Colour temperature has to be in the range of 5000–6100 K (daylight). Most companies, which sell video cameras, have special light sources for video with automatic light control in combination with the video camera, which regulates brightness according to the video signal and prevents blooming of very bright areas of the image (see Figures 4 and 5). In situations where the light source is just 'reading' the brightness of the video signal and no special connection is required, except for a coaxial cable, it can be used with different video cameras. The brightness is directly related to the object–lens distance.

Light cables

The light cables used for laparoscopic video documentation are the same as the ones used for photography.

Laparoscope

The best results with video laparoscopy are obtained with a telescope of at least 10 mm diameter. The lower limit for good performance appears to be 9 mm. Brightness will be increased if the camera is attached directly to the telescope, omitting the use of a beam-splitter.

Beam-splitter

The video camera can be attached directly with a special adaptor to the laparoscope, a method by some authors referred to as video endoscopy, in which case the complete procedure is performed from the image on the monitor. If the surgeon prefers to have the direct view of the laparoscope, a beam-splitter lens with adaptor has to be attached between the telescope

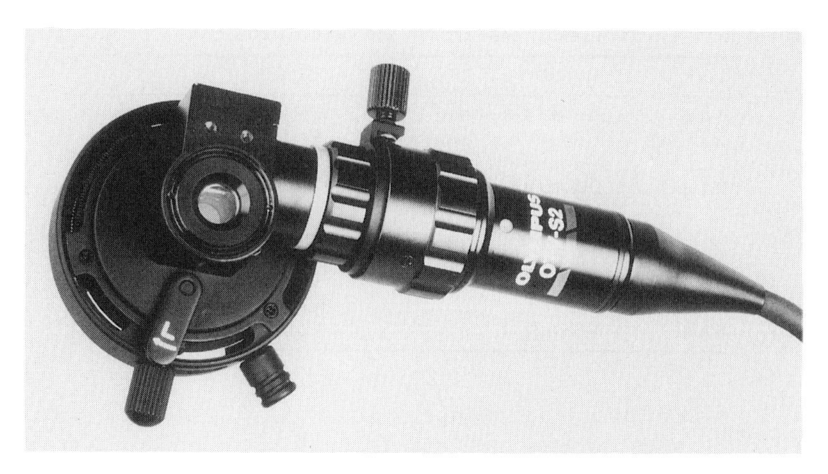

Figure 9. Beam-splitter attached to CCD Olympus OTV-S2 video camera.

and the camera (Figure 9), which inevitably reduces the brightness of the video image. The telescope must be able to rotate freely inside the beam-splitter adaptor to prevent the video image from whirling around on the display monitor.

Video camera

Video imaging and documentation in laparoscopy has reached its third generation with the miniature electronic chip camera. The first generation consisted of a professional three-colour tube camera, still providing the highest quality image and used for broadcasting and commercial purposes. The disadvantage of these cameras is that they are relatively large and heavy, and have to be connected with an endoscope via an articulated optical arm, widely used as a teaching device in gynaecological endoscopy. This optical arm, however, considerably reduces the brightness of the image and limits the surgeon in his movements. In addition, the rotation of the image on the display, caused by the moving of the joints, has to be corrected continuously by an assistant.

The second generation endoscopy camera consisted of a single-colour tube, the 0.5-inch Newvicon camera. These cameras had a good picture quality, a relatively good colour reproduction and were much smaller and less heavy, than the three-tube cameras. This camera could be attached directly to the telescope or with a beam-splitter.

An important breakthrough in the use of video in endoscopy came with the third generation video camera: the so-called CCD (charge-coupled device) or chip camera.

CCD video camera. The CCD was invented in 1969 by WS Boyle and GE Smith. Video cameras with a CCD were first used in astronomy in the mid-1970s. It is referred to as a 'chip' because of its basic form as a small silicon wafer.

The CCD is an integrated circuit image sensor and depends on the sensitivity of silicon to light. Light striking a silicon device decreases the electrical resistance of the silicon and generates current carriers. The photosensitive silicon elements store and transfer information as packets of electrical charge, which can be amplified. Individual picture elements are called pixels and the number of pixels determines the sensitivity and resolution (Sivak, 1986).

The way the electrical charges are moved on the device is called charge-coupling. Colour is identified by different red, green and blue pixels (CCD video cameras), or by an RGB sequencing system, each pixel performing red, green and blue imaging roles in sequence (electronic, flexible CCD video endoscopes) (Cooper, 1987).

CCD video cameras are very small and lightweight, have a high sensitivity and relatively high resolution and can be immersed in disinfectant solutions. The cameras are connected with a cable to a camera control unit (CCU), which regulates light adjustment (via light source), (auto or manual) colour adjustment and (auto) white balance. Most modern cameras have auto-gain control, which can compensate for the reflections of very bright sites of the image.

The most important CCD video cameras for endoscopy available in Europe are:

1. Olympus OTV-S2 (Figures 9 and 10): camera head weight, 25 g; auto-gain control; auto-brightness control with Olympus light sources Twinlight, CLV-10 (see Figure 5) and CLV-F10; auto-colour correction; auto-white balance.
2. Storz endovision 535 and endopocket 536 (Figure 11): weight 120 g (including adaptor); auto-gain control; auto-light adjustment with Storz light source 490 BV (see Figure 4); Colorama colour control at camera head; no white balance required.
3. Storz endovision 534: weight 120 g (including adaptor); zoom lens ($f = 18$–34 mm); auto-gain control; automatic light adjustment with Storz light source 490 BV; automatic white balance.
4. Wisap endo CCD view: weight of camera head 70 g; automatic white balance.

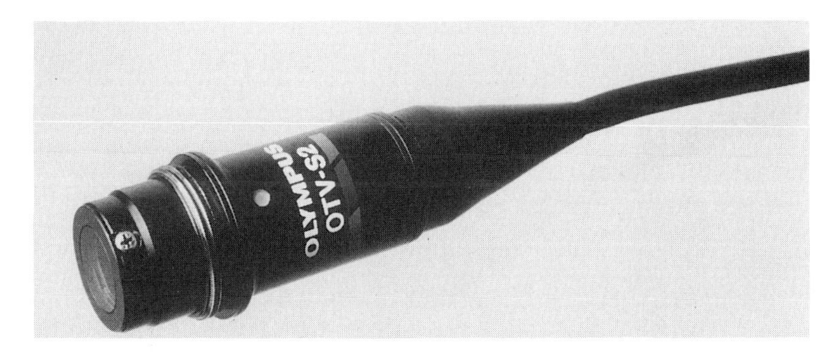

Figure 10. Olympus OTV-S2 CCD video camera for endoscopy.

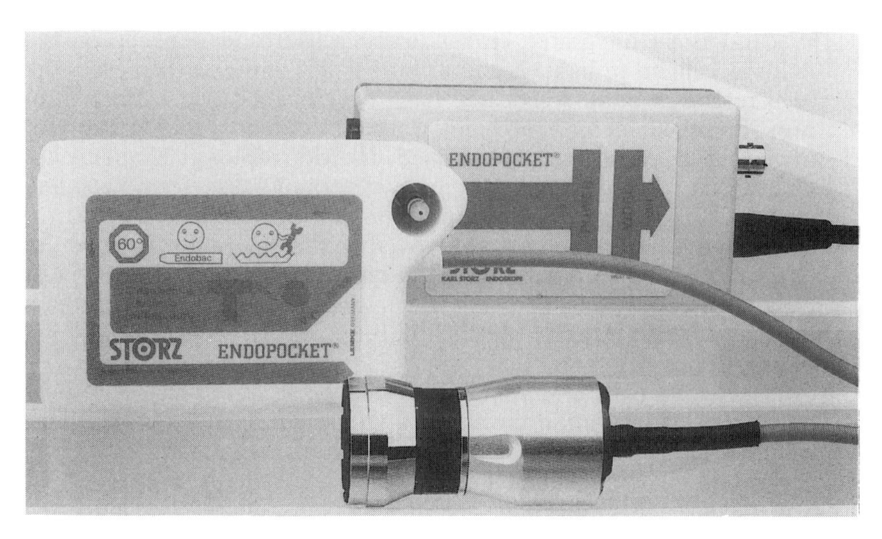

Figure 11. Storz Endopocket 536 CCD video camera with control unit and power supply.

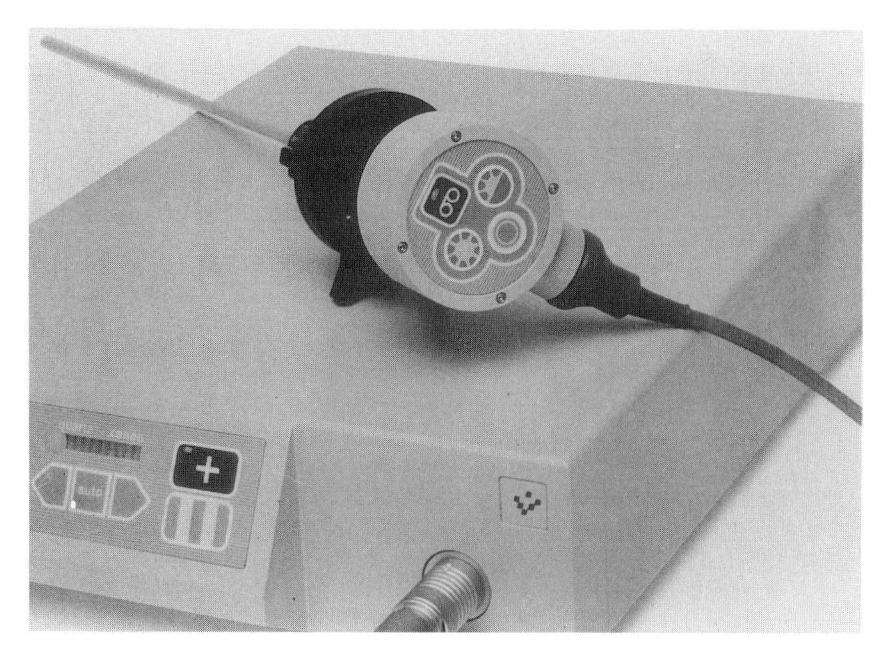

Figure 12. Vistek VIS-3000 CCD video camera with light adjustment, video 'boost' and recorder start/pause switch on camera head.

5. Wolf endocam 5370: weight of camera head 90 g; auto-gain control; automatic light adjustment with Wolf light source Auto-TCP 5108; auto-colour correction; no white balance required.
6. Medical Dynamics HPS 5930: no blooming; colour correction; manual light adjustment; video recorder pause/start control on camera head.
7. MP Video MC-6: weight of camera head 91 g; auto-gain control; manual light adjustment (can be connected with auto-light source).
8. Vistek VIS-3000: auto-gain control; video 'boost' switch located on camera head, providing for increased colour saturation in low light or high contrast situations; Vistek light source control located on camera head; auto-white balance; video recorder pause/start switch on camera head (Figure 12).

Some automatic video light sources recommended for specific cameras can be combined with other cameras, without loosing the automatic brightness control function (see 'Light source' section).

Video endoscope

Some confusion exists as to what should be considered a video endoscope. Strictly speaking, the name video endoscope should be reserved for any endoscope that only allows viewing of the image from a video display and has no possibility for direct viewing of the image through the endoscope. Endoscopes currently considered video endoscopes are:

1. Electronic flexible endoscopes with the CCD chip built-in at the tip of the endoscope (electronic image transmission).
2. Endoscopes without ocular and the CCD chip built-in or immediately attached at the eye piece end of the endoscope, at the original site of the ocular (optical and electronic image transmission).

If a video camera is attached, without a beam-splitter, directly to the ocular of an optical endoscope and the image is viewed only from the display, this may be called video endoscopy (which does not necessarily mean a video endoscope is being used). Videoendoscopy is a *method*, while the name video endoscope refers to an *instrument*.

Monitor

High quality professional RGB monitors should be used (Figure 13). They must be equipped with the same norm-standard as used in the video imaging system. Most modern professional monitors are multinorm and can be used with PAL, NTSC and SECAM standards. Some companies recommend their own special monitors, although they do not necessarily provide specific advantages over other makes.

Recorder

As stated above, a good quality recording system for laparoscopy is 0.75-inch U-matic low-band (and look out for 0.5-inch Super-VHS in the future).

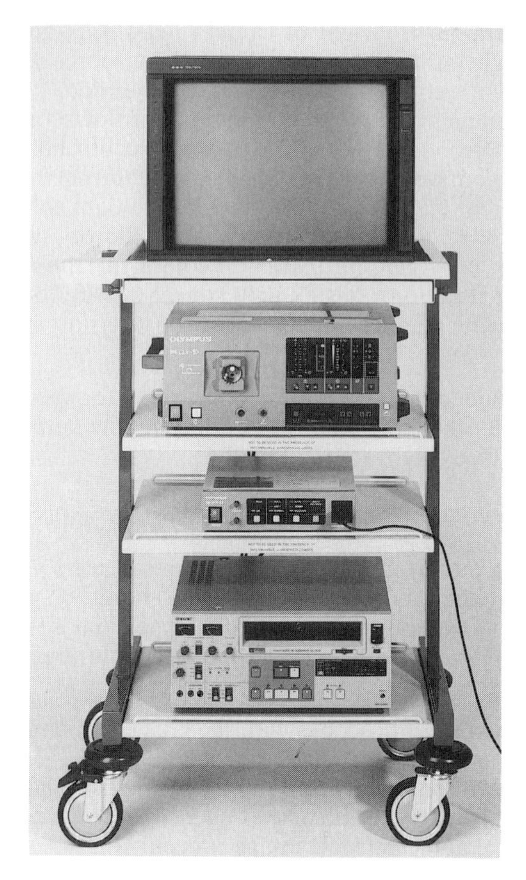

Figure 13. Video unit with (from top to bottom) RGB monitor, integrated light source, video camera control unit and U-matic recorder.

For very high quality recordings 0.75-inch U-matic high-band (BVU) should be used. The most widely used U-matic videorecorders are the Sony VO-5600 (0.75-inch U-matic low-band) and the recently introduced Sony VO-9600P (0.75-inch U-matic high- and low-band, see Figure 8). For routine use any good quality VHS recorder can be applied. Of course the norm-standard again has to match the one used in the video imaging system.

Additional equipment

Text or title generator

Titles, dates, times and sometimes more information can be superimposed on the video image with text generators or keyboards, connected to the camera control unit. The manufacturers of endoscopic video cameras usually have their own versions.

Video printers

A full-colour, hard copy of the video image nears photographic quality and this instant documentation method will become the first choice in instant, hard-copy documentation in endoscopy with video imaging. Video printers available today are manufactured by Hitachi and Mitsubishi. A Sony version is expected to be introduced soon.

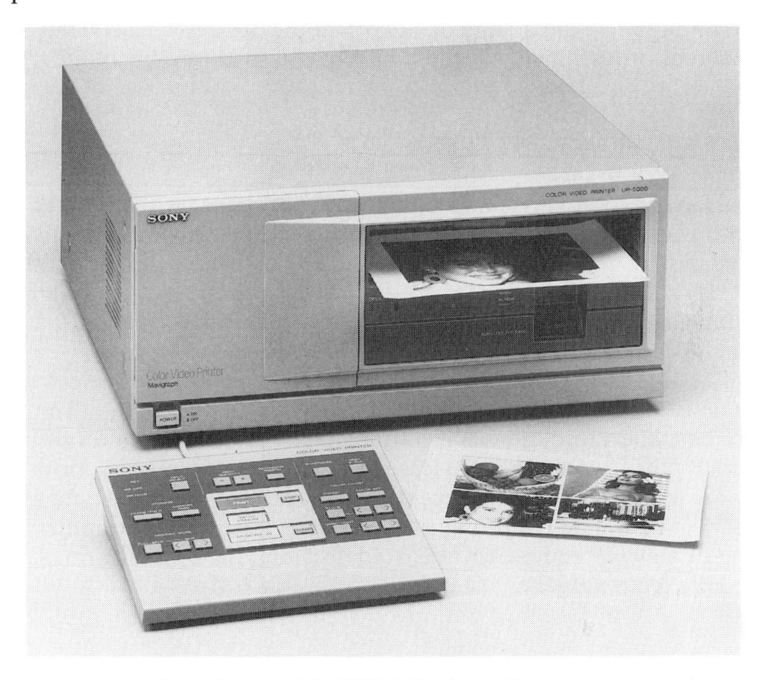

Figure 14. Sony UP-5000P full colour video printer.

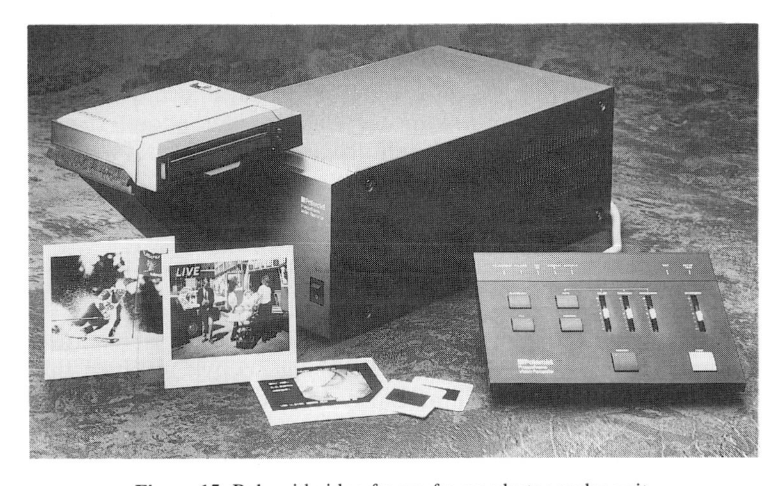

Figure 15. Polaroid video freeze-frame photography unit.

As the quality of a normal photograph is about 15 dots/mm, the new Sony UP-5000P, with about 10–12 dots/mm, will provide the best available quality (Figure 14). The Hitachi and Mitsubishi printers have less dots/mm, but are cheaper than the Sony UP-5000P is likely to be.

A video printing-like system is provided by Polaroid, using a freeze-frame and instant Polaroid photography system. The quality of reproduction of the video image is less than that of the aforementioned video printers (Figure 15). In the coming years the quality of video printing devices will probably rise to 12 dots/mm, providing an excellent alternative to hard-copy photography.

HIGH FREQUENCY INTERFERENCE

Several laparoscopic surgical techniques are performed with high frequency current. The frequency of the current has to exceed a lower frequency limit to avoid muscle and nerve stimulation and is usually in the range of 300 kHz to 2 MHz. As these frequencies are situated within the bandwidth of every video imaging system, this can cause electromagnetic interference to a video imaging system in use during electrosurgery (Flachenecker, 1987).

High frequency (HF) electrosurgery causes complicated electric and magnetic fields, disturbing video equipment in close proximity. The video system has, therefore, to be electromagnetically shielded, or the high-frequency power of the electrosurgical unit must be reduced. Both techniques are applied in the more recently developed equipment. These aspects should be investigated carefully when buying new video equipment with existing or new HF equipment, to avoid discouraging results during laparoscopic HF electrosurgery.

FUTURE DEVELOPMENTS

Image processing

With electronic video signals, image processing will soon be possible in endoscopic video imaging. Several different pictures could be displayed simultaneously on the display and/or other data could be added. In addition, colour-filtering techniques will be able to perform structural analysis of a tissue surface.

Three-dimensional endoscopy

Flexible endoscopes with electronic image transmission and distal CCD chips do not yet seem to provide any advantage for laparoscopy as they cannot compete with the image quality of rigid optical 'lens' laparoscopes. Flexible endoscopes may be useful for salpingoscopy, but even then the electronic video endoscopes will probably be too thick.

The electronic video endoscopes, however, do have the ability to house two CCD chips at the distal end, thus providing the possibility of three-dimensional endoscopic imaging, and opening up new avenues for three-dimensional laparoscopy. Research in the field of endoholography has not so far produced encouraging results.

Video communication networks

Video imaging and documentation, at first seen just as a modern alternative to film, has in fact provided many more possibilities than film, of particular importance in teaching and communication in medical endoscopy. Being an electronic medium, it enables the transmission of pictures and sound, live or recorded, over any distance to any number of locations. These advantages could not be fully utilized in endoscopy until video endocameras were sufficiently small and sensitive to provide high quality images without impeding the surgeon during his endoscopic procedures.

The growing number of hospital departments producing electronic images and using video techniques is creating an enormous potential for interdepartmental and interhospital communication, teaching and exchange of records. Central image databases and image communication networks will become a realistic possibility in the near future. The following main groups of technology are already available for this purpose (Holdoway, 1987):

1. Videotapes. The simplest means of image communication is the distribution and exchange of video tapes. This method is most widely used in scientific communication at present.

2. Cables. High quality coaxial cables can be used for the transmission of video signals. The signal has to be amplified and equalized after 200 m. A central remote control unit can also be added.

3. Slow-scan. Still pictures can be transmitted by telephone lines, after digital conversion.

4. Glass fibreoptics. The modern improvement in traditional cable systems is due entirely to fibreoptics. All signals are converted to light energy by a solid state laser. This light is guided down glass fibres to its destination where it is decoded.

The advantages are that this system has a very low signal attenuation of 0.8 dB/km, it allows a much greater bandwidth for transmission (easy two-way video and sound signal), its transmission capacity is 140 MBits/s and it is free from electromagnetic interference. The diameter of glass fibres is only 125 μm (Williams, 1987). A fibreoptic system therefore has good potential for communication between different departments (LAN, local area network).

5. Lasers. A straight laser beam between two buildings can easily transmit full quality moving colour pictures and sound. Its range is limited to 2 km.

6. Microwave. Microwave transmission is mainly used for broadcast television live on location. It is quite expensive and requires a licence.

7. Satellite video transmission. Satellite video transmission can be used for scientific video-conferencing between different countries. Transmission of analogue signals is expensive as it requires a wide bandwidth. Digital signals require much less bandwidth and hence digital satellite transmission is much cheaper.

Central image databases

Better image and data transmission facilities allow the possibility of setting up central image databases. Storage can be magnetic or optical (laser disc). Every type of data can be entered in powerful central memories and can be retrieved via a computer terminal at any desired location in the hospital. Eventually facilities could be made available for external sources to tap into the system, which would allow communication between hospitals.

For endoscopy the new Sony Laser VideoDisc Recording system (LVR-6000 recorder and LVS-6000P processor) is able to store 24 minutes video (or 36.250 frame pictures in PAL) on each side of an optical video disc.

SUMMARY

Technological developments have increased tremendously the possibilities for the application of image documentation techniques in gynaecological laparoscopy. Increased quality of optical endoscopes, powerful light sources, highly sensitive photographic films and miniature electronic video cameras have largely removed the barriers to efficient documentation. This equipment is no longer considered to be only for 'hobbyists', but has become an essential part of diagnostic and surgical laparoscopy. Future developments can only increase its applications further.

REFERENCES

Cooper D (1987) Advances and applications in high resolution video endoscopy. In Wamsteker K, Jonas U, van der Veen G & van Waes PFGM (eds) *Imaging and Visual Documentation in Medicine*, pp 95–104. Amsterdam: Excerpta Medica.

Flachenecker G (1987) High frequency interference: Basic electrotechnical principles. In Wamsteker K, Jonas U, van der Veen G & van Waes PFGM (eds) *Imaging and Visual Documentation in Medicine*, pp 85–94. Amsterdam: Excerpta Medica.

Gisolf AC (1987) Video systems: Fighting the chaos. In Wamsteker K, Jonas U, van der Veen G & van Waes PFGM (eds) *Imaging and Visual Documentation in Medicine*, pp 77–79. Amsterdam: Excerpta Medica.

Holdoway A (1987) The use of video for intra-hospital training and communication. In Wamsteker K, Jonas U, van der Veen G & van Waes PFGM (eds) *Imaging and Visual Documentation in Medicine*, pp 723–732. Amsterdam: Excerpta Medica.

Marlow JL (1983) Endoscopic Photography. *Clinical Obstetrics and Gynecology* **26:** 359–365.

Marlow JL (1989) Hysteroscopic Photography. In Baggish MS, Barbot J & Valle RF (eds) *Diagnostic and Operative Hysteroscopy*: pp 215–222. Chicago: Year Book Medical Publishers.

Noordveld RB, Algra PR & Wamsteker K (1987) The DOCUMED philosophy: The Imaging Chain in Medicine. In Wamsteker K, Jonas U, van der Veen G & van Waes PFGM (eds) *Imaging and Visual Documentation in Medicine*, pp 5–7. Amsterdam: Excerpta Medica.

Semm K (1987) Photographs, films and television in endoscopy. In Wamsteker K, Jonas U, van der Veen G & van Waes PFGM (eds) *Imaging and Visual Documentation in Medicine*, pp 303–312. Amsterdam: Excerpta Medica.
Sivak MV (1986) Video Endoscopy. *Clinics in Gastroenterology* **15:** 205–234.
Williams AR (1987) A fibre-optic communications network for teaching clinical medicine. In Wamsteker K, Jonas U, van der Veen G & van Waes PFGM (eds) *Imaging and Visual Documentation in Medicine*, pp 599–604. Amsterdam: Excerpta Medica.

12

Assessment of results of laser surgery

MICHAEL P. DIAMOND

In less than two decades, the use of lasers in reproductive pelvic surgery has advanced to the point of routine practice by physicians skilled in their use. Currently, four types of lasers are used in gynaecology: carbon dioxide (CO_2), argon, potassium titanyl phosphate (KTP)-532, and neodymium yttrium-aluminium-garnet (Nd YAG). The first laser available for use was the CO_2 laser. Initially it was used at the time of laparotomy, but with advancements in technology (the ability to pass the laser beam down narrow channels), the laser has also become of use with laparoscopy. The fibre lasers (argon, KTP-532, and Nd YAG), have been used primarily at the time of endoscopic procedures, either laparoscopy or hysteroscopy.

LASER LAPAROTOMY

There has been widespread use of lasers in centres where they are available despite the lack of any evidence demonstrating superiority of lasers over other modalities of therapy. Most animal studies have been unable to demonstrate an advantage of laser over electrocautery at the time of laparotomy, either in terms of subsequent pregnancy outcome or in terms of postoperative adhesion development and tissue damage (Filmar et al, 1986; Luciano et al, 1987). The most eloquent of these studies is that by Luciano et al, comparing injuries to the rabbit uterine horn and ovary. In that report, the same power density was calculated for both CO_2 laser and electrocautery. At the time of the initial injuries as well as at subsequent necropsy, there was no difference in tissue damage. Additionally, there was no difference in adhesion development between these two modalities.

Evaluation of the efficacy of lasers at the time of laparotomy in humans has unfortunately been very limited. Diamond et al (1984) compared adhesion development in women who underwent reproductive pelvic surgery procedures utilizing a continuous-wave CO_2 laser, and compared the results to a previously described report by diZerega et al (Adhesion Study Group, 1983), based on a similar patient protocol. Evaluating adhesions at multiple sites throughout the pelvis (ovaries, fimbria, cul-de-sac, small bowel, large bowel, and omentum), they were unable to demonstrate any consistent difference noted at the time of a subsequent second-look laparoscopy. Furthermore, the pregnancy outcome following neosalpingostomy reported by Daniell et al (1986), is no different than those previously described in the literature for non-laser therapy. Finally, the incidence of adhesions at the time of the second-look procedure was no different than previous reports performed using non-laser techniques (Diamond, 1988).

Thus, at this time there remains no substantiated evidence demonstrating a superiority of laser over other therapeutic modalities at the time of laparotomy. The reasons for use of the laser at the time of laparotomy thus most likely relates to personal preferences. It is felt by many investigators that the use of the CO_2 laser will result in decreased time of the operation and in decreased blood loss during the operative procedure. Also, there may be advantages in performance of certain procedures such as treating endometriosis or adhesions deep in the posterior cul-de-sac, which might be more difficult to reach using other modalities. Another example is in the performance of a neosalpingostomy. After creation of the cruciate incisions, it is often possible to 'flower back' the 'petals' using a defocused laser beam instead of the more traditional method of suturing.

LASER LAPAROSCOPY

Unfortunately, trials describing outcome of the use of lasers at the time of laparoscopy have also been exceedingly limited, mainly being retrospective reviews by individual investigators describing their experience rather than prospective evaluations comparing the different therapeutic parameters.

There are several potential benefits to performing operative procedures at laparoscopy as compared to laparotomy. Foremost would be the decreased patient morbidity following endoscopic procedures as compared to those performed at laparotomy. Even with multiple puncture techniques, it is rare for patients not to be discharged the day of their operative procedure, and to return to normal activities within 3–5 days. In contrast, patients undergoing laparotomy are frequently not discharged until 3–5 days postoperatively and do not return to normal activities until 4–6 weeks later. A corollary to the decreased morbidity is the decreased cost of endoscopic techniques. This is not so much in regard to actual costs of the physician or hospital for the procedure, but for decreased expenses for the total hospital stay and decreased potential loss of time at work. Thus, what remains is to establish the relative efficacy of procedures performed at the time of laparoscopy utilizing the laser as compared to the same procedures performed at the time of laparotomy. If results of laser laparoscopy are superior, or even equivalent to, those obtained at laparotomy, then major benefits will accrue to those performed endoscopically. The final issue, which has been to a great extent ignored in the gynaecology literature is the safety of use of lasers. Complications have been described at the time of intra-abdominal procedures including bowel perforation, bladder damage, ureteral damage, and vascular damage. With regard to laser laparoscopy specifically, the largest report to date is that of the CO_2 Laser Adhesion Study Group (Diamond et al, 1987). In over 671 endoscopic procedures performed utilizing the CO_2 laser, the intraoperative and postoperative complications were very limited, and by and large due to performance of the operative techniques independent of the surgical modality (CO_2 laser) utilized. Thus, in the hands of experienced physicians, it appears that laser procedures, like other endoscopic procedures, can be performed with a fairly large margin of safety.

Reasons for using laser laparoscopy

If reports in the literature do not demonstrate a superiority of laser to other techniques for reproductive pelvic surgery, the question becomes 'Why has the use of the laser become so popular?' It is to be hoped that the answer does not lie in the idea that use of the laser is a promotional gimmick to attract patients. Such a concept has been fostered by the many reports in the lay press describing the laser as a 'magic wand' for the treatment of endometriosis and pelvic adhesions. More likely, for most physicians, the answer relates to the belief that the laser is a therapeutic modality which allows performance of procedures at laparoscopy which otherwise would require laparotomy.

CLINICAL TRIALS

Unanswered questions

There are many unanswered questions in the fields of reproductive pelvic surgery. Some of the issues which are currently most debated are:

1. Efficacy of laparotomy v. operative laparoscopy?
2. Value of laser v. non-laser modalities for surgical procedures (neosalpingostomy, fimbrioplasty, treatment of endometriosis, adhesiolysis)?
3. Relative efficacy of the available lasers (CO_2, argon, KTP-532, Nd YAG with sapphire tips)?
4. Safety of laser surgery, both at laparotomy and laparoscopy, when performed by less experienced surgeons?

Why haven't trials been conducted?

Unfortunately, well-designed comparative clinical trials of the issues described have not been performed. Yet, this is not surprising since even the development of microsurgery, as an alternative to macrosurgery, for tubal anastomosis and other procedures has not been based on well-designed clinical studies. There are several possible reasons for this. First is the issue of the endpoint for the clinical trial. The most important endpoint for our infertile couples is pregnancy, but, as is well known, there are many factors involved in the attainment of pregnancy, such as ovulatory status, semen quality, the morphological and hormonal endometrial milieu, and the exposure frequency. If the surgical endpoint is considered alone, however, only tubal patency can be currently evaluated without performance of a second operative procedure. Second, even the busiest surgeon will have only a limited number of subjects with a particular abnormality treated in a particular way for comparison. Third, is the expense involved in conducting a well-designed trial, particularly if this involves more than one centre.

There are also ethical issues potentially involved in the decision to perform a randomized clinical trial. First is the question of whether it would be ethical to perform a laparotomy on a subject in whom the same procedure could be performed at the time of laparoscopy. Currently, there would probably be a great deal more controversy about whether a primary neosalpingostomy should be performed at laparoscopy, while few experienced surgeons would question the utility of treating an unruptured ectopic pregnancy or moderate endometriosis at laparoscopy. Yet, neither of the latter two conditions have undergone intense scrutiny by a randomized clinical trial. Additionally, would patients agree to subject themselves to laparotomy for the purposes of a clinical trial when their physicians felt they could do an equivalent job at the time of laparoscopy. Of course, the converse ethical question also remains, whether it is appropriate to recommend laparoscopy to a subject when it has not been definitively shown that results are equivalent or better with endoscopic therapy.

Recipe for solutions

The ideal human clinical trial would be a randomized prospective double-blind evaluation, but this is rarely going to be possible in reproductive pelvic surgery. Most human trials have been a summary of outcome with various modalities. Often the choice of therapy was based on availability at the time of the operative procedure, a variation over the time that the report describes, or physician preference for uncertain reasons; bias is inherent in each of these methods of choice. Another variable is retrospective versus prospective data collection. Retrospective evaluation offers the advantage of being able to collect a large amount of data from previous procedures rather than having to await subsequent performance. However, a major disadvantage of a retrospective review is that the parameters of interest are not always available, such as whether primary or secondary infertility was at issue, whether coexisting infertility factors existed. Prospective protocols allow for collection on all pertinent variables, but these must be identified at the outset. They require much more time because of the need to collect patients, and then to monitor their progress over a specified follow-up period.

Accurate recording of data is essential for any evaluation. Ideally this should be done at the time the procedure is performed rather than later when recall may be faulty. Additionally, the data form should be completed by an individual well versed in the procedure performed to avoid any mistakes because of misinterpretations or use of different wording.

A concern of all trials and investigations is how to handle patients lost to follow-up in whom the endpoint is not available. It is probably most appropriate to consider that the endpoint has not been achieved, i.e. in an infertility population to assume that the couple has been unable to conceive.

Most human trials compare outcome of one group of patients with that of a subsequent group. Difficulty in such analysis is based on the assumption that other parameters are equivalent. This bias can potentially be minimized by inclusion of a large number of subjects, thus increasing the likelihood that biases would be equivalent in each of the study groups. A better alternative, when possible, would be to use each subject as her own control. For example, the patient with bilateral hydrosalpinx or adnexal adhesions, could have each side treated by different surgical modalities. Of course, the characteristics of the hydrosalpinx or the adhesions on each side would have to be equivalent for this comparison to be fully justified. Again, differences between the two sides could be minimized by randomly assigning the two sides to the two different therapies and collecting a large number of subjects. Such a design would allow minimization of variation of characteristics and healing between patients. That such a difference does exist is suggested by studies which show that most patients benefit from reproductive pelvic surgical procedures, yet approximately 10% end up with worse adhesions than they had at the time of their initial operative procedure (Diamond et al, 1984; Garcia et al, 1985).

Once results are collected, appropriate methods must also be used for data analysis. Simply to compare pregnancy outcome at a given point in time may introduce bias if the two therapeutic parameters vary in relation to the time of input. This would not only be an issue in sequential protocols but may also be a bias in designed protocols. The bias can be minimized by performance of life table analysis.

For many of these suggested solutions, the point is made that a large number of subjects reduces potential bias in patient selection and assignment to the various groups. The difficulty with this is that of getting a large enough group of patients from any one physician. In multipartner groups, this can be overcome by combining results from different surgeons. A second option would be to combine the results of several physicians who work at the same centre, although not together. This would minimize variation in equipment availability and ancillary support, and would maximize the ability to coordinate protocol monitoring and reporting. Unfortunately, even the largest centres rarely have enough facilities to allow timely collection of data. For this reason, multicentre groups have been formed to evaluate the outcome of reproductive pelvic surgery. In addition to the ability to collect data rapidly, this tends to limit potential bias from individual physicians who may be significantly better or worse than most other physicians performing similar procedures. The disadvantages of such groups are also clear, namely that there is a much greater potential for variations in the patients referred to individual physicians, in the classification and observation of the extent of disease present, in the therapeutic modalities employed, in the techniques employed in the performance of the procedure, in patient follow-up, and subsequently in the reporting.

SUMMARY

The use of lasers in reproductive pelvic surgery has been established, based more on the reports of clinical experience than demonstration of improved efficacy as compared to other therapeutic modalities. Superiority of one type of laser over another has not been demonstrated.

It is the author's opinion that the advantage of using lasers lies in the ability to treat pelvic pathology endoscopically rather than at laparotomy. We have been trained in the use of the laser and find it to be of great use; it is quite possible, however, that other physicians, trained in alternative endoscopic techniques, can achieve similar results. Of course, appropriate clinical trials are needed so that surgical treatments can be based on scientific knowledge rather than clinical impressions. Until such time that this information is available, however, experience gained from clinical observation and reports of clinical outcome do serve as guides for counselling and treating our patients.

REFERENCES

Adhesion Study Group (1983) Reduction of postoperative pelvic adhesions with intraperitoneal 32% Dextran 70: a prospective, randomized clinical trial. *Fertility and Sterility* **40:** 612–619.

Diamond MP, Daniels JF, Martin DC et al (1984) Tubal patency and pelvic adhesions following use of the carbon dioxide laser and early second look laparoscopy: initial report of the Intra-abdominal Laser Study Group. *Fertility and Sterility* **42:** 717–723.

Diamond MP, Feste J, McLaughlin DS, Martin DC & Daniell JF (1986) Pelvic adhesions at early second-look laparoscopy following carbon dioxide laser surgery. *Infertility* **7:** 39–44.

Diamond MP, Daniell JF, Martin DG et al (1987) Safety of CO_2 laser laparoscopy: report of the carbon dioxide (CO_2) laser laparoscopy study group (LLSG). *16th Annual Meeting, American Association of Gynecologic Laparoscopists, San Francisco, California, November.*

Diamond MP (1988) Surgical aspects of infertility. In Sciarra JJ (ed.) *Gynecology and Obstetrics*, vol. 5, pp 1–23. Philadelphia: Harper and Row.

Daniell JF, Diamond MP, McLaughlin DS et al (1986) Clinical results of terminal salpingostomy using the CO_2 laser: report of the intra-abdominal laser study group. *Fertility and Sterility* **45:** 175–178.

Filmar S, Gomel V & McComb P (1986) The effectiveness of CO_2 laser and electromicrosurgery in adhesiolysis: a comparative study. *Fertility and Sterility* **45:** 407–411.

Garcia JE, Jones HW Jr, Acosta AA & Andrews MC (1985) Reconstructive pelvic operations for in vitro fertilization. *American Journal of Obstetrics and Gynecology* **153:** 172–178.

Luciano AA, Whitman G, Maier DB, Randolph J & Maenza R (1987) A comparison of thermal injury, healing patterns, and postoperative adhesion formation following CO_2 laser and electromicrosurgery. *Fertility and Sterility* **48:** 1025–1029.

13

New techniques in advanced laparoscopic surgery

HARRY REICH

Most gynaecological surgery can be performed using laparoscopic visualization (Table 1). Laparoscopy is a method of access and not a method of treatment. While the surgeon's hands are much further from the area being treated than during laparotomy, his eye (or eyes with video) is right on top of it, much like when using the operating microscope for pelvic reconstructive surgery. Instrument development for laparoscopic surgery is just beginning and beckons the innovator. The major advantages of a laparoscopic approach are short hospitalization, rapid recuperation, superior cosmetics, and results at least equivalent to those obtainable by laparotomy.

The operator must replace fear of failure with knowledge of pelvic anatomy and available instrumentation. Every laparoscopic procedure is an anatomy lesson, especially the easy cases, with identification of the ureters, the common iliac vessels and their branches, the liver and gallbladder, the bowel, and the appendix. The location of pelvic retroperitoneal structures should be second nature for surgeons performing advanced gynaecological endoscopy. Laparoscopic surgical procedures can last from 1–4 hours, and operating rooms must prepare their schedules accordingly.

Table 1. Laparoscopic procedures listed according to degree of difficulty.

1.	Ectopic pregnancy
2.	Pelvic abscess
3.	Excision peritoneal endometriosis
4.	Oophorectomy
5.	Cyst excision including dermoids
6.	Excision of ovarian endometrioma
7.	Salpingostomy for hydrosalpinx
8.	Endometrioma excision after danazol
9.	Ureteral dissection
10.	Hysterectomy
11.	Tubal reversal
12.	Salpingo-ovariolysis for thick 'fused' tubo-ovarian complex
13.	Myomectomy for large fibroids
14.	Pelvic lymph node dissection
15.	Cul-de-sac dissection for deep fibrotic endometriosis
16.	Small bowel adhesions

This chapter details several techniques useful in performing the procedures listed in Table 1. A brief introduction and definition of these techniques follows. Useful incisions are described and specific procedures discussed.

TECHNIQUES

Aquadissection (Reich and McGlynn, 1987; Reich, 1987a)

A suction–irrigation–dissection instrument is used to irrigate, suction irrigant fluid and smoke, suction-retract, and to perform blunt dissection with its tip by using the hydraulic effect of the pressurized irrigant delivered through it. The Aquapurator (WISAP USA, Tomball, Texas) is the first and most popular of these devices. Aquadissection is performed by placing the tip of the Aquapurator against the adhesive interface between bowel–adnexa, tubo-ovarian, or adnexa–pelvic sidewall and using the pressurized fluid gushing from it to develop a dissection plane which can be extended either bluntly or with more fluid pressure. Often, adhesions can be 'weakened' with laser and then taken down with the Aquapurator using either the hydraulic effect or suction-traction. The suction–irrigation–dissection device is the single most important instrument for treating acute adhesions including pelvic abscesses.

Aquaexpression

A technique for treating ampullary intraluminal ectopic pregnancy: the tip of a suction–irrigation device is inserted through the open end of the affected tube into the ampulla and fluid under pressure used to dislodge and expel the products of conception.

Laser dissection

Use of the CO_2 laser through a laser laparoscope converts the umbilical incision into a portal for performing surgery. The CO_2 beam, which travels down the 5–8 mm operating channel of an operating laparoscope, has a focal point of approximately 20 mm from the end of the laparoscope and remains in focus for several centimetres beyond this point. This beam is adjusted into a 1 mm spot from which the tissue effect will be slightly greater than 1 mm. A useful technique is to align the beam emanating from the laparoscope into the centre of the operating channel by using transparent tape or the cuff of the surgeon's glove over the scope tip to identify where the beam exits. Tension on the laser laparoscope as it traverses the trocar sleeve will modify the beam-spot as will the extent of hydration of tissue being vaporized, irrigant on the scope tip, and smoke in the peritoneal cavity. Power delivered to tissue is reduced by 30–50% with an 8 mm laparoscopic operating channel and by 70% with a 5 mm operating channel (Table 2). In addition, the passage of CO_2 gas through the lumen of the laparoscope, presently a necessity, results in a reduction in transmitted energy and an increase in spot size at higher power settings. With these limitations in mind,

Table 2. Power at the distal end of the laparoscope.

Power entering laparoscope* (laser setting)	Power leaving laparoscope, i.e. at tissue 8 mm Channel†	5 mm Channel‡
20 W	11 W	5 W
40 W	24 W	14 W
60 W	40 W	20 W
80 W	52 W	27 W
100 W	70 W	32 W

* Sharplan 1100 Laser (Tel-Aviv, Israel).
† Sharplan Laser Laparoscope with 8 mm channel.
‡ Wolf Laser Laparoscope with 5 mm channel (Rosemont, Illinois).

I use a setting of 35 W superpulse on a Sharplan 1100 laser (Tel Aviv, Israel) through a 5 mm operating channel for most procedures (1500 W cm^{-2} at the tissue).

The main effect of the carbon dioxide laser on tissue is vaporization. This can be used for direct vaporization of lesions, but is more often used for dissection or separation of adhesions and for excision of tissue in a manner similar to using scissors. Blood vessels less than 1 mm in diameter are often coagulated in the process but application of the beam to an actively bleeding vessel usually results in 'burnt, black blood'.

I performed most of the procedures listed in Table 1 prior to the addition of laser to my surgical armamentarium. The major advantage of CO_2 laser is its 0.1 mm depth of penetration, allowing a greater margin of safety when working around the bowel, ureter, and major vessels. Yet, it must be emphasized that laser surgery is still associated with a zone of thermal necrosis surrounding treated tissue and, in susceptible patients, adhesions will form. Laser surgery does not result in a reduced rate of adhesion formation when compared to other energy sources. I do not use fibre lasers (potassium titanyl phosphate (KTP), argon, and neodymium-yttrium aluminium garnet (ND-YAG)), as, in my view, they hold no advantage over the cutting and coagulation possible with electrosurgery.

Electrodissection

Electrosurgery is the mainstay of microsurgical laparotomy surgery today. As techniques for laparoscopic surgery are patterned on laparotomy microsurgery, it seems logical that the instruments should match. A 3 mm knife or a 1 mm needle electrode are excellent instruments for lysing adhesions and draining ovarian cysts. The effective power density of the electrode can be modified by applying either the sharp tip or the wider body to the tissue being treated. The electrode is connected to a low-voltage electrosurgical generator (Valleylab SSE2L, Boulder, Colorado) with a low power attenuator control which limits all three generator outputs to less than 100 W and less than 600 V peak. For lysing adhesions or draining cysts, pure cutting current (40–80 W) is used. Cutting or coagulation current through a knife, hook or button electrode is used for coagulating specific blood vessels or haemorrhagic ovarian cysts. If possible, the vessel should be compressed to occlude it prior to coagulation. A quick application of cutting current following coagulation often avoids pulling off the char that results.

Scissors dissection

Microscissors and hooked scissors, both 5 and 3 mm, are used to cut sharply both thin and thick adhesions between tube and ovary. This is the main technique used for adhesiolysis in infertile women to diminish the potential for adhesion formation; electrosurgery and laser are reserved for tubal, ovarian and pelvic sidewall haemostasis. Vasopressin (20 units in 50 ml Ringer's lactate) can be used for adnexal haemostasis without electrosurgery in selected cases.

Bipolar desiccation for large vessel haemostasis (Reich, 1987; Reich and McGlynn, 1986a)

The bipolar forceps use high-frequency, low-voltage current (25–50 W) to desiccate vessels as large as the ovarian and uterine arteries. Bipolar desiccation seals arterial blood vessels immediately so that they can withstand the pulsating arterial pressure until permanent sealing can be accomplished through the healing process.

For large vessel haemostasis using bipolar forceps, electrical current flow must be monitored to ensure total desiccation of the tissue between the tips of the bipolar forceps. The bipolar forceps must be applied so as to completely occlude the vessels between its tips. If the vessels are not occluded, current will continue to flow between the tips of the instrument as heat is carried from the operative site, i.e. the tissue will not become completely desiccated. Only when complete desiccation has occurred will flow of current cease between the tips of the bipolar electrodes. Then, and only then, is it safe to divide the structures involved.

I have had experience only with the Kleppinger bipolar forceps (Richard Wolf, Rosemont, Illinois) for large vessel haemostasis. Specially insulated bipolar forceps are available that allow current to pass only through their tips; with these, precise haemostasis can be obtained. A channel for irrigation is a useful addition to microbipolar forceps. In addition to irrigating bleeding sites to identify vessels prior to their desiccation, irrigation can be used during underwater examination to push away blood products and clots from the bleeding vessel, making its correct identification easier.

Short trocar sleeves (Figure 1) (Reich and McGlynn, 1989)

I use trocar sleeves of a special design: short, self-retaining, secondary to a screw grid on its external surface, and without a trap (Richard Wolf, Rosemont, Illinois). These trocar sleeves facilitate efficient instrument exchanges and eliminate time spent reinserting trocar sleeves removed during these exchanges. Once placed, their portal of exit stays fixed at the level of the anterior abdominal wall parietal peritoneum, permitting more room for instrument manipulation.

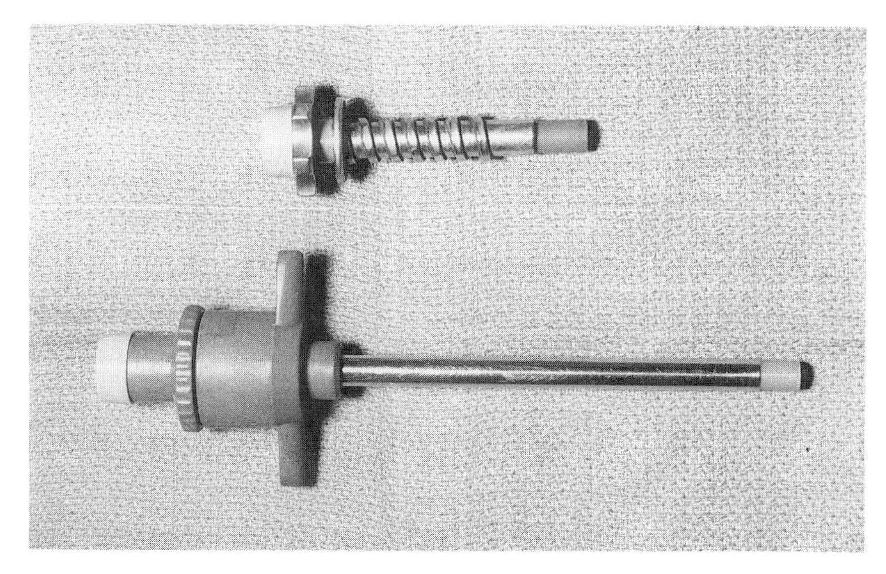

Figure 1. Short self-retaining trochar sleeve without trap adjacent to conventional sleeve.

Suturing

The ability to suture during laparoscopy greatly expands the indications for laparoscopic surgery as well as the confidence of the surgeon performing more difficult procedures. Pioneered by Semm (1978), indications include ovarian repair after excision of the cyst wall of an endometrioma, eversion of tubal ostia following salpingostomy, closure of salpingotomy following removal of a tubal pregnancy, tubal anastomosis and excision of omentum. They are essential in the reperitonealization of the rectosigmoid, and in closure of peritoneal and smooth muscle defects after rectal mobilization during cul-de-sac reconstruction in cases of severe endometriosis. Two lower abdominal puncture sites are necessary and through these, laparoscopic needle holders are introduced to manipulate suture, needle, and involved tissue. The suture, 4-0 polydioxanone (PDS) on a taper ST4 needle (Ethicon Z-420), is tied outside the peritoneal cavity using a half-hitch slip knot. Average operating time for placing and tying a suture is less than 5 minutes.

Staples

Disposable stapling instrumentation for laparoscopic surgery will soon become available. US Surgical Corporation, Norwalk, Connecticut, is introducing an automatic clip applier. The clip itself is of medium to large size and is made of titanium, an inert, non-reactive metal. A second stapler will place six rows of staples, 30 mm in length, and simultaneously divide the desired tissue. This instrument will function similarly to the gastrointestinal anastomosis stapler (GIA) which thoracic and general surgeons have used for the past 25 years. These devices should prove valuable for large vessel haemostasis in the pelvis and make advanced laparoscopic techniques such as oophorectomy and hysterectomy more prevalent.

Preventive haemostasis (vasopressin)

This technique, popularized by Pouly et al (1986), is particularly useful for infiltrating the mesosalpinx prior to surgery for ectopic pregnancy and following tubal surgery in an attempt to avoid the thermal injury which always results from laser- or electrosurgery. Dilute vasopressin solution (Pitressin, Parke Davis, Morris Plains, New Jersey) combines 20 units (1 ampoule) and 50 cm^3 of normal saline. More dilute or more concentrated solutions may be used. Either a 3 mm or 5 mm injection and puncture cannula can be used through the lower quadrant trocar sleeves. Alternately, a 22-gauge spinal needle can be inserted directly through the skin at pubic hairline, usually just lateral to the deep inferior epigastric vessels. Care must be taken at initial insertion into the mesosalpinx to avoid injection of the blood vessels. The solution (approximately 10–20 cm^3) is infiltrated, causing a grossly visible swelling in the mesosalpinx. This effect persists for approximately 2 hours, allowing physiological haemostasis to occur.

Rectal, vaginal and uterine probes (manipulators)

A sponge on a ring forceps is inserted into the posterior vaginal fornix and a no. 81 French rectal probe (Resnik Instruments, Skokie, Illinois or Cheshire Medical, Cheshire, CT) is placed in the rectum. In addition, a no. 3 or 4 Sims curette is placed in the endometrial cavity to markedly antevert the uterus and stretch out the cul-de-sac to aid in its identification. Devices to stabilize or fix the curette in this position are available.

Underwater surgery at the end of each procedure

At the end of each operation, haemostasis is checked in stages using the 10 mm straight laparoscope. First complete haemostasis is established with the patient in the Trendelenberg position. Next, complete haemostasis is obtained by underwater examination with the patient supine using underwater bipolar coagulation. Finally, complete haemostasis is documented with all instruments removed, including the uterine manipulator. To visualize the pelvis with the patient supine, the laparoscope and the Aquapurator are manipulated into the deep cul-de-sac beneath floating bowel and omentum, and this area is alternately irrigated and suctioned until the effluent is clear. An 'underwater' examination is then performed to observe the completely separated tubes and ovaries and to confirm complete haemostasis. Two litres of Ringer's lactate are left in the peritoneal cavity to displace CO_2 and to prevent fibrin adherences forming between surfaces that have been operated upon during the initial stages of reperitonealization. No drains, antibiotic solutions, or heparin are used.

The 'chopstick' manoeuvre refers to the synchronized movement of the actively irrigating Aquapurator tip just in front of the laparoscope tip to maintain a clear underwater view in a bloody field deep in the pelvis. Bloody fluid is diluted, circulated and aspirated. Individual blood clots are isolated, usually in the pararectosigmoid gutters, and aspirated.

Video

A video camera with or without beam-splitter attached to the laparoscope enables the surgeon and his staff to operate while watching a video monitor. Beam-splitters supply 80–90% of available light to the video monitor providing an excellent picture, but operating while viewing the surgical field through the laparoscope produces considerable eye-strain. Recently, beam-splitters have been developed that supply 50% of available light to the operator's eye, thus easing the problem of eye-strain.

ANAESTHESIA CONSIDERATIONS

In our unit, all laparoscopic surgical procedures are performed under general anaesthesia. No preoperative medication is given, but intravenous (i.v.) sedation with midazolam (Versed) is considered if indicated. Prior to the induction of general anaesthesia, bilateral ulnar pads (Zimfoam: laminectomy arm cradle set: Zimmer, Warsaw, Indiana) are applied and both arms are tucked at the side, the right on a padded arm board. Shoulder braces are placed over the acromio-clavicular joint to prevent brachial plexus injury. The legs are placed in knee stirrups.

Approximately 10 minutes preinduction, droperidol (Inapsine) 1.25 mg is given i.v. General anaesthesia is induced using 100% oxygen, followed by a bolus of a narcotic, alfentanil (Alfenta), 50–75 μg/kg. Thirty seconds later a bolus of a muscle relaxant, vecuronium bromide (Norcuron) 0.1 mg/kg is given i.v. Within 30 s, thiopentone (Pentothal) 1–2 mg/kg, is administered as a bolus. Intubation is achieved with a 7.0 mm oral endotracheal tube and controlled respiration is established. At this point an end-tidal CO_2 monitor is placed, and an oral gastric tube is inserted to empty the stomach contents.

General anaesthesia is maintained with 100% oxygen, an inhalational anaesthetic, isoflurane (Forane), alfentanil infused at a rate of 1 μg/kg/min and vecuronium bromide infused at a rate of 1 μg/kg/min. Awakening usually occurs in 5–10 minutes following the completion of the operation. The administration of droperidol preinduction, the avoidance of nitrous oxide, and placing an oral gastric tube may help decrease postoperative nausea. With the rapid recovery from anaesthesia and decreased amount of postlaparoscopic nausea in procedures lasting more than 3 hours, time from end of procedure to hospital discharge is usually 2–4 hours.

GENERAL CONSIDERATIONS

The patient is supine (0°) until after the umbilical trocar sleeve has been placed. Hysteroscopy with CO_2 is performed during the initial peritoneal insufflation to assess the endometrial cavity. Thereafter, a Cohen cannula or a curette is inserted into the uterus (if present) for manipulation and tubal lavage. The resectoscope is used to treat intrauterine fibroids, septa, and endometrial ablation, using sorbitol (Travenol Labs, Deerfield, Illinois) as the distension medium. A Foley catheter is inserted only if the bladder is distended.

Initial laparoscopic examination is performed with a straight 10 mm laparoscope. First the upper abdomen is assessed. The patient is then placed in steep Trendelenburg position (20–30°) and the pelvis examined. The laparoscope is manoeuvred into the pelvic side-wall tunnels lateral to the lateral surface of the ovaries in search of endometriosis and adhesions. Lower quadrant incisions are placed if pelvic pathology is present.

Four laparoscopes are available: a 10 mm straight viewing laparoscope, a 10 mm laser laparoscope with 5 mm laser channel, a 10 mm operating laparoscope with 5 mm operating channel, and a 5 mm straight viewing laparoscope for introduction through the lower quadrant 5 mm trocar sleeve. I use my right foot to activate the laser and my left foot for the electrosurgical pedals. An average of 10 litres of Ringer's lactate irrigant is used per case; over 30 litres have been used on occasion. CO_2 insufflation up to 5 l/min is used to compensate for the rapid loss of CO_2 during suctioning.

INCISIONS (Reich, 1989b)

The intraumbilical incision

A vertical intraumbilical incision to accommodate an 11 mm trocar sleeve takes advantage of the scar resulting from the sloughing of the umbilical cord. It overlies the area where skin, deep fascia, and parietal peritoneum of the anterior abdominal wall meet; thus, little opportunity exists for the parietal peritoneum to tent away from the Veress needle.

The description that follows is for a right-handed surgeon. With the surgeon standing on the patient's left side and the patient supine, the left thumb (with or without sponge) is inserted into the umbilicus as deep as possible, after which the thumb and surrounding umbilicus are rolled over the lower left forefinger, stretching and widening the umbilical fossa, which is further enlarged with the blunt back end of the scalpel. A no. 15 blade (never a no. 11) should be used to make a vertical midline incision on the inferior wall of the umbilical fossa extending to and just beyond its lowest point. In thin patients, this incision frequently traverses the deep fascia, but intraperitoneal injury is avoided by pulling the umbilicus onto the surgeon's forefinger, a manoeuvre which controls the incision's depth.

The Veress needle (or Auto Suture Surgineedle, US Surgical, Norwalk, Connecticut) is grasped near its tip, like a dart, between thumb and forefinger. The lower anterior abdominal wall is stabilized, not elevated, by grasping its full thickness in the operator's fist and holding it there. The Veress needle tip is then inserted at right angles to the anterior abdominal wall for a distance of approximately 1 cm. Insertion of the Veress needle should be an anatomical exercise with the surgeon cognizant of the anatomical structures traversed. Individual layers can be felt, i.e. deep fascia and peritoneum, or occasionally, peritoneum alone. If the Veress needle is inserted according to these principles, there is little need to test for proper positioning of the needle. After complete insertion, the needle is connected to a CO_2 insufflator flowing at 1 l/min with a pressure of approximately 10 mmHg.

The umbilical or 'first-puncture' trocar, with its surrounding trumpet-valved trocar sleeve, is placed within the umbilicus. It is not necessary to lift the anterior abdominal wall during insertion of the trocar after establishment of a 4 litre pneumoperitoneum. The trocar should be 'palmed' so that only 1 cm of the sharp tip protrudes beyond the operator's fingers. Holding the trocar sleeve higher unsheathes a lethal weapon. Following shallow penetration of the peritoneum at a 60–90° angle, the trocar is upturned to approximately 30°. This continuous motion is almost straight down at first, and then becomes almost horizontal, with the wrist rotating nearly 45°. The result is a parietal peritoneal puncture directly beneath the umbilicus.

When this intraumbilical approach is used, the trocar leaves the undersurface of the umbilicus closer to the aortic bifurcation than is encountered with the more common transverse infraumbilical incision with trocar inserted at 30°. Accordingly, an important prerequisite to performing an intraumbilical puncture is the ability of the surgeon to palm the trocar. Some trocars are too long and some hands too small. If palming is neither feasible nor possible, the trocar should be aimed at the hollow of the sacrum to avoid the aortic bifurcation, or because elevation of the lower abdominal wall is not necessary with adequate pneumoperitoneum, the trocar can be controlled with two hands to avoid a sudden thrust, i.e. the thumb and forefinger of one hand provide resistance to the insertional pressure exerted by the other.

Lower quadrant incisions

Laparoscopic puncture sites should be kept to a minimum, because deep fascia never fully regains its previous strength after division. Three puncture sites in the anterior abdominal wall are sufficient for 99% of laparoscopic procedures. Large puncture sites or incisions bordering on minilaparotomy should be replaced by an umbilical extension or a laparoscopic culdotomy approach (see below).

Two lower quadrant incisions are made in a uniform manner regardless of the pathology involved. Consistency with incisions results in a spatially reproducible procedure with less need to make time-consuming intraoperative decisions.

Lower quadrant incisions are made with a no. 11 blade near the top of the pubic hairline, adjacent to the deep inferior epigastric vessels. These vessels—an artery flanked by two veins (venae comitantes)—are located by direct vision of the inner abdominal wall, lateral to the umbilical ligaments (obliterated umbilical artery), as they generally cannot be consistently found by traditional transillumination.

A 3 mm trocar sleeve is inserted on the right side, and through this, atraumatic grasping forceps are used to retract tissues as needed. Larger instruments for retraction may result in laceration or avulsion of tube, ovary, or bowel, especially if they are held by a scrub nurse whose other duties are keeping the uterus elevated and passing the surgeon the instruments he needs before he realizes he needs them. Grasping instruments, the knife and the hook electrode for electrosurgery, and microscissors all fit through the 3 mm puncture site. A 3 mm ratchet handle grasping forcep in a spread-open position holds the ovary or bowel out of the operative field during most cases.

The 5 mm lower quadrant puncture is always made on the patient's left to avoid mechanical malfunctions from the Aquapurator, which is draped over the patient's left leg and connected by tubing to wall suction and to a pressurized source of Ringer's lactate irrigant. The tubing of the Aquapurator, normally manipulated with the surgeon's left hand, is more likely to become kinked when stretched across the abdomen to a right-sided abdominal puncture site. Other instruments used through the 5 mm puncture site include bipolar forceps, biopsy forceps, grasping forceps, hook and microscissors, and laparoscopic needle holders. (Alternatively two 5 mm lower quadrant trocar sleeves can be used with a sleeve reducer for 3 mm instrumentation.)

Closure

The umbilical incision is closed with a 4-0 Vicryl suture opposing deep fascia and skin dermis. The knot is buried beneath the fascia. The lower quadrant 5 mm and 3 mm incisions are loosely approximated with a Javid vascular clamp (V. Mueller, McGaw Park, Illinois) and covered with Collodion (AMEND, Irvington, New Jersey) to allow drainage of excess Ringer's lactate solution should increased intra-abdominal pressure be present.

MORE INCISIONS: FOR OVARIAN AND MYOMA EXTRACTION (Reich, 1989b)

Many surgeons dilate 5 mm lower-quadrant puncture sites to 11 mm so that larger instruments including morcellators can be used to extract ovaries, tubes, and fibroids. Surgeons should be aware that incisional hernias can occur from 11 mm lower-quadrant incisions. Morcellation is rarely necessary for removal of an ovary from the peritoneal cavity.

Because of my bias against large lower-quadrant incisions, techniques for umbilical incision enlargement and laparoscopic culdotomy were developed to remove ovaries from the peritoneal cavity. Postmenopausal cystic ovaries should always be removed intact through the cul-de-sac, as should perimenopausal cystic ovaries that do not drain chocolate-like material upon mobilization from their respective pelvic side-wall or utero-sacral ligament. Large endometriomas in women not desiring future fertility are usually sufficiently cystic and pliable so that, once separated from the pelvic side-wall, they can be removed through the umbilical incision.

For small ovaries or ruptured cysts without any solid components, an operating laparoscope is used. Biopsy forceps in the operating channel grasp the tissue which is then partially delivered into the tip of the umbilical trocar sleeve. The trocar sleeve and laparoscope are popped out of the umbilicus in one motion, after which the protruding tissue is grasped with haemostats or Kocher clamps and gently teased out of the peritoneal cavity. Alternatively a 5 mm laparoscope can be used for visualization through the 5 mm lower trocar sleeve and the tissue to be removed grasped with 11 mm grasping forceps inserted through the umbilicus and extracted.

Umbilical extension

With large ovaries (benign pathology) and small fibroids, the umbilical incision can be enlarged, especially if the initial skin incision was vertical intraumbilical as described above. The operating laparoscope is used with a scissors in the operating channel. The tip of the laparoscope is placed 1 cm above the tip of the trocar sleeve which is then carefully removed from the peritoneal cavity. Peritoneum first is visualized and incised downward in the midline with the scissors in the operating channel of the operating laparoscope. Next, deep fascia is identified and incised to add another 1 cm or more to the incision. Finally, the skin incision inside the umbilicus can be extended upwards to incorporate the superior wall of the umbilical fossa. Most ovaries can be removed through this incision.

Laparoscopic culdotomy

Ovarian cysts of unknown pathology separated intact from the pelvic side-wall are best removed through the cul-de-sac. The anatomical relationship between the rectum and the posterior vagina must be confirmed to avoid cutting the rectum while making the laparoscopic culdotomy incision. A curette is placed in the uterus for elevation; a sponge at the end of ring forceps is placed just behind the cervix to identify the posterior vaginal fornix; and a rectal probe assures that the rectum is out of the way. Before the rectal probe is removed it may be necessary to reflect the rectum off the posterior vaginal fornix. This is performed using either cutting current through a knife electrode or the laparoscopic laser at 35 W superpulse. The peritoneum at the junction of the rectum and vagina is incised and using the Aquapurator, the plane between rectum and vagina is developed and the rectum pushed downward.

Following these manoeuvres, and when it is clear that the rectum has been separated off the posterior wall of the vagina (regardless of the presence or absence of the uterus) the posterior fornix is distended by the wet sponge on ring forceps. The transverse laparoscopic culdotomy incision is made with the knife electrode at 80 W or the CO_2 laser with 1 mm spot size and power set at 80 W continuous. This incision is usually bloodless and the sponge in the posterior vagina rapidly comes into view. Some difficulty may be encountered in maintaining adequate pneumoperitoneum once the vagina is entered, but the sponge in contact with the incision is usually adequate for this purpose. Laparoscopic biopsy forceps can then be inserted through the vagina and used to grasp the ovary and pull it out through the culdotomy incision. Alternately, the 3 or 5 mm lower-quadrant grasping forceps can be used to push the mass through the culdotomy incision. On occasion, the operator's fingers can be inserted into the peritoneal cavity and used to grasp the ovary.

For large cystic masses an 18-gauge needle directed through the vagina is used for decompression or, if a dermoid is present, the mass can be incised so that the thick cyst contents drain into the vagina until the mass is small enough to be pulled through the incision. Following removal of the mass, the incision is closed with a figure-of-eight 0-Vicryl suture or laparoscopic sutures (4-0 PDS: Ethicon, Somerville, New Jersey).

LAPAROSCOPIC OOPHORECTOMY WITHOUT ENDOLOOPS OR MORCELLATION (Reich et al, 1986a; 1987b)

In 1980 Semm and Mettler reported 37 laparoscopic oophorectomies using a loop ligature and a tissue punch morcellator. I modified their technique to feature bipolar electrosurgery for oophorectomy and to eliminate the need to morcellate by using the incisions just described. Comparison between the two techniques is not possible as I have never used endoloops for oophorectomy.

Indications

The indications for laparoscopic oophorectomy (or salpingo-oophorectomy) include: pelvic pain secondary to ovarian adhesions from previous hysterectomy, pain from ovarian adhesions unresponsive to laparoscopic lysis, pelvic mass secondary to hydrosalpinx from pelvic inflammatory disease (PID) or previous surgery, postmenopausal palpable ovary (PMPO), and pain or mass arising from ovarian endometrioma, haemorrhagic corpus luteum cyst, or dermoid cyst in women not desiring future fertility. The acronym PMPO is used for the palpation of an ovary which, in a premenopausal woman, would be interpreted as normal size, i.e. 3–4 cm in its largest dimension (Barber and Graber, 1971). Such ovaries can almost always be removed intact through a culdotomy incision.

Ureteral dissection

Before starting oophorectomy it is imperative that the surgeon visualizes the course of the ureter. It usually crosses the external iliac artery near the bifurcation of the common iliac artery at the pelvic brim. The peritoneum above the ureter can be opened with laser, sharp-scissors dissection, or cutting-current electrosurgery. Thereafter, the space can be further developed by flushing irrigant (Ringer's lactate) under pressure from an Aquapurator into the space. Smooth grasping forceps are then opened parallel and perpendicular to the retroperitoneal structures until the ureter is identified and grasped. Scissors, laser, or Aquapurator can then be used to further dissect the ureter throughout much of its course along the pelvic side-wall. On the left side, the ureter can be harder to find as its entrance into the pelvis is covered by the inverted V-shaped root of the sigmoid mesocolon.

Oophorectomy

Prior to removal, the ovary must be released from all pelvic side-wall and bowel adhesions using a combination of aquadissection, electrodissection, and laser dissection. After lysis of adhesions and drainage of ovarian endometriomas, if present, Kleppinger bipolar forceps and laparoscopic scissors are used to desiccate and divide the infundibulopelvic ligament, the broad ligament (mesovarium and mesosalpinx), the fallopian tube isthmus, and the utero-ovarian ligament. In some cases the mesovarium alone can be desiccated and divided. Medial retraction with grasping forceps is helpful while the adnexa is being freed from the pelvic sidewall. The free ovary is then removed through the umbilicus or culdotomy as previously described.

Results

I have performed 116 laparoscopic oophorectomies in 100 women using bipolar desiccation of the infundibulopelvic and utero-ovarian ligaments without complication. The average age of these women was 44 with a range from 26 to 74. Thirty-six of the 100 women (36%) had previously undergone hysterectomy. The right ovary was removed in 35% of cases, the left in 49% and both in 16%. The ovary (or ovaries) was removed through the umbilicus in 61 cases, the cul-de-sac in 24, and by morcellation in 11. Pathology included 28 endometriomas, 20 benign ovarian neoplasms including 6 dermoid cysts, one papillary serous cystadenoma of borderline malignancy, and one bilateral serous cystadenocarcinoma. Of the 100 women, 66 were discharged on the day of the procedure.

LAPAROSCOPIC TREATMENT OF TUBO-OVARIAN AND PELVIC ABSCESS

The goals in management of acute tubo-ovarian abscess (TOA) are prevention of the chronic sequelae of infection, including infertility and pelvic pain, both of which often lead to further surgical intervention. Laparoscopic treatment is effective and economical. It offers the gynaecologist 100% accuracy in diagnosis while simultaneously accomplishing definitive treatment with a low complication rate (Henry-Suchet et al, 1984; Reich and McGlynn, 1987; Reich, 1988a).

The commonly accepted belief that surgical intervention during acute pelvic infection would result in greater injury than waiting for the infection to subside began with a New York City study by Simpson (1909) suggesting increased surgical technical difficulty. This opinion prevailed until recently, even though the risks associated with surgical interventions had changed drastically since the early part of this century.

In reality, it is much easier to operate on acute adhesions than it is to deal with dense adherences between structures that obliterate normal anatomic relationships and have, by their chronicity, developed neovascularization. For example, second-look laparoscopic adhesiolysis soon after infertility surgical procedures is much easier than the original procedure. Electrosurgery, laser surgery, and sharp-scissors dissection, all of which are useful during surgery for chronic pelvic inflammatory disease, have no place in the treatment of acute adhesions. Simply stated, the laparoscopic treatment of acute pelvic inflammatory disease with or without abscess does not require the high level of technical skill necessary to excise an endometrioma, open a hydrosalpinx, or remove an ectopic pregnancy under laparoscopic control. It is essentially an exercise in careful blunt dissection using a probe or aquadissection with an Aquapurator and can be performed by gynaecologists experienced in operative laparoscopy using equipment available in most hospitals.

Preoperative considerations

Women presenting with lower abdominal pain in association with a palpable or questionable pelvic mass should undergo laparoscopy to determine the true diagnosis as endometriomas, haemorrhagic corpus luteum cysts, or appendix abscesses can all mimic a tubo-ovarian abscess.

The diagnosis of TOA should be suspected in women with a recent or past history of pelvic inflammatory disease who have persistent pain and pelvic tenderness on examination. Fever and leukocytosis may or may not be present. Following a presumptive diagnosis of TOA, the patient should be admitted to hospital so that laparoscopy can be performed soon thereafter.

Antibiotics

In patients suspected of having TOA, intravenous antibiotics should be initiated on admission to the hospital, usually 2–24 hours prior to laparoscopy. Adequate and sustained blood concentrations of antibiotics are required to combat transperitoneal absorption of bacteria during the operative procedure. This author prefers cefoxitin, 2 g i.v., every 4 hours from admission until discharge, usually on postoperative day two or three. Oral doxycycline is started on the first postoperative day and continued for 10 days following discharge. Although clindamycin and metronidazole have both demonstrated greater ability to enter abscess cavities and reduce bacterial counts therein, cefoxitin is used to simplify therapy to a single i.v. agent and further assess the efficacy of the laparoscopic surgical procedure; in other words the intravenous antibiotic alone should not be considered the reason for successful therapy.

Operative technique

The upper abdomen is examined and the patient is placed in 20° Trendelenburg position before focusing attention to the pelvis. Through the 3 mm right-sided trocar sleeve, either a blunt probe or grasping forceps is inserted and used for traction and retraction. Through the 5 mm left-sided trocar sleeve, a suction–irrigation–dissection instrument or a suction probe attached to a 50 cm^3 syringe is inserted and used to mobilize omentum, small bowel, rectosigmoid, and tubo-ovarian adhesions until the abscess cavity is entered. Purulent fluid is aspirated while the operating table is being returned to a 10° Trendelenburg position. Separate cultures should be taken from the aspirated fluid, inflammatory exudate excised with biopsy forceps, and exudate near the tubal ostium using a bronchoscope cytology brush.

Following aspiration of the abscess cavity, the Aquapurator is used to completely separate the bowel and omentum from the reproductive organs and to lyse completely tubo-ovarian adhesions (aquadissection). Grasping forceps (3 mm) are used to place the tissue to be dissected under tension so that the surgeon can identify the distorted tissue plane accurately before aquadissection. Upon completion of the dissection, the abscess cavity (necrotic inflammatory exudate) is excised in pieces using 5 mm biopsy forceps.

It is important to remember that following ovulation, purulent material from acute salpingitis may gain entrance to the inner ovary by inoculation of the corpus luteum, which may then become part of the abscess wall. Thus, following drainage of the abscess cavity and mobilization of the entire ovary, a gaping hole of varying size may be noted in the ovary which heretofore had been intimately involved in the abscess cavity. This area should be well irrigated; it will heal spontaneously, and significant bleeding is rarely encountered.

The next step is to insert grasping forceps into the fimbrial ostia and spread them in order to free agglutinating fimbria. Retrograde irrigation of the tube should be performed with the Aquapurator to remove infected debris and diminish chances of recurrence. The fimbrial mucosa can also be visualized at this time and its mucosal quality assessed for future prognosis.

Tubal lavage with indigo-carmine dye through a Cohen cannula in the uterus should be attempted. With early acute abscesses, tubal lavage rarely demonstrates tubal patency because of interstitial tubal oedema. In contrast, when the abscess process has been present for longer than 1 week and/or the patient has been previously treated with an antibiotic, tubal lavage frequently documents tubal patency. Rarely, inspissated necrotic material can be pushed from the tube during the tubal lavage procedure.

The last step has been characterized by Dr Gerry Hulka as 'Reich's solution to pollution is dilution'. The peritoneal cavity is extensively irrigated with Ringer's lactate solution until the effluent is clear. The total volume of irrigant often exceeds 15 litres. As part of this procedure, 2 litres of Ringer's lactate solution are flushed through the Aquapurator into the upper abdomen (one on each side of the falciform ligament) to dilute any purulent material which may have gained access to these areas during the 20°

Trendelenburg positioning. Reverse Trendelenburg position is then used for the 'underwater' examination and at least 2 litres of Ringer's lactate is left in the abdomen.

Laparoscopic adhesiolysis using the Aquapurator is rarely bloody. Capillary oozing does occur, but it ceases spontaneously as the procedure progresses. Blood loss is rarely greater than 100 cm^3.

Without question, the more acute the abscess, the easier the dissection. Delay often makes the laparoscopic procedure more difficult than it need be. However, even chronic abscesses can be successfully treated by careful blunt aquadissection.

Postoperative care

Postoperatively, the patient is usually ambulatory and on a 'diet as tolerated' regimen following recovery from anaesthesia. Temperature elevations rarely persist past the first postoperative day. The patient is examined 1 week after discharge after which all restrictions are removed.

Results

Forty pelvic abscesses were treated using laparoscopic surgical techniques from 1976 to 1989. One patient required TAH, BSO in 1977 for recurrence 1 month postoperatively. All others demonstrated long-term resolution of their TOA. Fourteen second-look laparoscopies documented minimal filmy adhesions.

Why laparoscopic treatment works

Peritoneal defence mechanisms that protect the host from invading bacteria include absorption of the microbes from the peritoneal cavity via the lymphatic system, phagocytosis by macrophages and polymorphonuclear leukocytes, complement effects, and fibrin trapping (Skau et al, 1986). Fibrin trapping and sequestration of the bacterial inoculum by the omentum and intestine and the formation of a tubo-ovarian complex act to contain the infection initially, although eventual abscess formation may occur. Although the deposition of fibrin does trap bacteria and decreases the incidence of septicaemic death, thick fibrin deposits ultimately represent a barrier to in situ killing by neutrophils, with resultant abscess formation. Once formed, the abscess walls inhibit the effectiveness of antibiotics and the ability of the host to resolve the infection naturally.

Ahrenholz and Simmons (1980) studied the role of purified fibrin in the pathogenesis of experimental intraperitoneal infection. Their conclusion was that fibrin delays the onset of systemic sepsis, but the entrapped bacteria cannot be easily eliminated by normal intraperitoneal bactericidal mechanisms and, as a result, abscess formation occurs. They also felt that radical peritoneal debridement or anticoagulation may reduce the septic complications of peritonitis. Stated another way, procedures which decrease fibrin deposition and/or facilitate fibrin removal, either enzymatically or surgically, decrease the incidence of intraperitoneal abscess formation, and thus the rational for extensive peritoneal lavage and radical excision of inflammatory exudate in patients with TOA. Success with laparoscopic and laparotomy treatment of TOA by this author (Reich and McGlynn, 1987) and others (Hudspeth, 1975; Henry-Suchet et al, 1984; Rivlin and Hunt, 1986) substantiates the laboratory work of Ahrenholz and Simmons (1980). Laparoscopic drainage of a pelvic abscess followed by lysis of all peritoneal cavity adhesions and excision of necrotic inflammatory exudate allows host defences to control the infection effectively.

ENDOMETRIOSIS

Extensive stage IV endometriosis can be controlled laparoscopically if the surgeon is willing to spend the time. If endometriosis is the sole cause of infertility, laparoscopic removal will often result in a pregnant patient, regardless of the severity of the endometriosis. Danazol rarely relieves infertility or pain when ovarian endometriomas and/or deep fibrotic endometriosis exist. Surgical skill and tenacity are the keys to successful treatment of cul-de-sac obliteration.

Peritoneal implants

To treat superficial peritoneal endometriosis, the endometriosis implant and its adjacent peritoneum is excised, using either a CO_2 laser beam at 35–40 W superpulse, a knife or a needle electrode at 80 W cutting current, or scissors. An elliptical incision is made around the lesion, its edge lifted upward, and the lesion undermined using the hydraulic effect of pressurized irrigant from an Aquapurator. This pushes pelvic side-wall structures or the rectum away and makes undercutting of the lesion with laser, electrosurgery or scissors easier and safer. Following excision with the laser, the ureter, the anterior rectal wall, and upper posterior vagina are checked and superficial endometriosis in these areas excised or vaporized.

Small pinpoint lesions can be vaporized or fulgurated using the CO_2 laser or electrosurgery with resultant drainage of haemosiderin filled fluid in cases where deposits have infiltrated beneath the peritoneum. The base of the lesion must also be vaporized until normal tissue is seen. Cutting current with a knife or needle electrode may give better results due to its greater depth of penetration.

Endometriomas

An Aquapurator is used to lift up the ovaries if they are attached by adhesions to their respective utero-sacral ligament and/or pelvic side-wall. Often this manoeuvre will result in drainage of an endometrioma from the undersurface of the ovary. If no endometrioma is readily identified, and the patient has 'unexplained infertility' or pre- or postmenstrual spotting, a 3 mm knife electrode connected to unmodulated unipolar cutting current (80 W) is used to incise and drain areas on the ovary with superficial endometriosis and cysts suspicious for endometrioma. If an endometrioma is discovered by either of these two methods, the cyst cavity is rinsed with Ringer's lactate solution and then excised using 3 mm and 5 mm biopsy forceps, grasping forceps, and/or scissors. To help delineate the initial plane between normal ovarian cortex and endometrioma cyst wall, cutting current through the knife electrode tip applied at the cyst wall–cortex junction results in the development of a dissection plane. This step is particularly useful near the utero-ovarian ligament as rough avulsion can lead to excessive bleeding. Grasping forceps are then used to stabilize ovarian cortex while the endometrioma cyst wall is avulsed. Excision can be performed with minimal bleeding from the cyst wall bed and the ovarian wall edges usually re-approximate quite well, though occasionally extracorporeal suturing is required (Reich and McGlynn, 1986b).

Results (endometriomas)

Fertility outcome was 65% (28 of 43) for those women without male factor infertility. Twenty-two of the 28 women (80%) conceived within 6 months of laparoscopic treatment. There were no intraoperative or postoperative complications. There were no selection criteria in this series as a primary laparoscopic procedure was performed in all endometriosis cases, whether diagnosed at initial laparoscopy or from a previous surgeon's operative report. Danazol was not used, and if conception did not occur within 6 months of laparoscopy, a second laparoscopy was encouraged to treat any adhesions, if present, and search for occult ovarian endometriomas.

Partial and complete cul-de-sac obliteration (Reich, 1988b,d)

Cul-de-sac obliteration implies the presence of deep fibrotic endometriosis. Partial cul-de-sac obliteration means that deep fibrotic endometriosis, i.e. endometriosis beneath the peritoneum, is present and is severe enough to alter the course of the rectum. The deep fibrotic endometriosis is usually located on the rectum, in the rectovaginal space, on the upper vagina, in the space between the upper vagina and the cervix (cervical vaginal angle), or in one or both utero-sacral ligaments (Table 3). With deep cul-de-sac obliteration, fibrotic endometriosis and/or adhesions involve the entire area between the cervico-vaginal junction (and sometimes above) and the recto-vaginal septum; often one area predominates.

Careful inspection of the cul-de-sac is necessary to evaluate the extent of upward tenting of the rectum. To determine if cul-de-sac obliteration is partial or complete, a sponge on a ring forceps is inserted into the posterior vaginal fornix. Complete cul-de-sac obliteration implies that the outline of the posterior fornix cannot be visualized initially through the laparoscope, i.e. the rectum or fibrotic endometriosis nodules completely obscure the identification of the deep cul-de-sac. Partial cul-de-sac obliteration occurs where rectal tenting is visible but a protrusion from the sponge in the

Table 3. Location of deep fibrotic endometriosis in cul-de-sac obliteration.

Low:	in recto-vaginal septum or on rectum beneath cul-de-sac reflection
Medium:	on posterior vaginal wall (posterior fornix)
High:	at cervico-vaginal junction (inverted 'U' of utero-sacral ligaments)
Lateral:	in utero-sacral ligament

posterior vaginal fornix is noted between the rectum and the inverted 'U' of the utero-sacral ligaments.

When extensive cul-de-sac involvement with endometriosis is suspected, either clinically or from another doctor's operative record, a mechanical bowel preparation should be considered. Polyethylene glycol-based iso-osmotic solution (GoLYTELY or Colyte) works well. Following dissolution in water to a volume of 4 litres, oral administration induces a diarrhoea that rapidly cleanses the bowel, usually within 4 hours. GoLYTELY is usually taken the afternoon before surgery so as not to interfere with sleep later. Reglan, 10 mg *per os*, 30 minutes earlier helps promote gastric emptying and thus reduce abdominal bloating and distension.

In contrast to the procedure performed for superficial peritoneal endometriosis, deep fibrotic nodular endometriosis involving the cul-de-sac, often with invasion into posterior vagina, rectum, or posterior cervix, is a much more difficult problem and should be attempted only by the most expert laparoscopist. Rather than concentrating on excision of the nodular mass, attention is first directed to complete dissection of the anterior rectum throughout its area of involvement. Following placement of rectal, vaginal, and uterine probes, the rectal serosa is opened at its junction with the cul-de-sac lesion using CO_2 laser or scissors. Careful dissection then ensues using the Aquapurator for blunt dissection and laser surgery, electrosurgery, or scissors for sharp dissection until the rectum, with or without fibrotic endometriosis, is separated from the posterior uterus and upper vagina. Loose areolar tissue of the recto-vaginal space should be reached. Only after the rectum is mobilized should excision of the fibrotic endometriosis be attempted from the rectum, posterior vagina, and utero-sacral ligaments.

Should a ureter be close to the lesion, its course should be traced starting at the pelvic brim, and on occasion, the peritoneum overlying the ureter should be opened to confirm ureteral position deep in the pelvis. The rectum, with or without a fibrotic lesion must be separated from the posterior uterus and upper vagina, especially when operating close to the uterine vessels, as entry into these vessels can produce life-threatening haemorrhage requiring immediate application of the bipolar forceps.

Following separation of the rectum from the back of uterus and the upper posterior vagina, the dissection continues on top of the posterior vagina, the position of which is confirmed by the sponge in the posterior fornix. This dissection on the outside of the vaginal wall uses laser, aquadissection, electrosurgery or scissors. On occasion, the lesion may extend deep into or completely through the vaginal wall. Dissection should be performed accordingly with removal of all visible fibrotic endometriosis. Lesions extending totally through the vagina demand an *en bloc* resection from cul-de-sac to posterior vaginal wall; the posterior vaginal wall can then be closed either vaginally or laparoscopically depending on the surgeon's preference (Martin, 1988).

Endometriosis nodules infiltrating the rectal muscularis are excised, partially or totally, usually with the operator's or the assistant's finger, in the rectum just beneath the lesion. In some cases, the anterior rectum is reperitonealized by plicating the utero-sacral ligaments and lateral rectal peritoneum across the midline using 4-0 PDS (Ethicon Z-420) or Vicryl. The suture is tied either outside the peritoneal cavity and then slipped downward, or inside, if Vicryl is available.

Results

One hundred women with cul-de-sac obliteration secondary to endometriosis (48 partial, 52 complete) were treated laparoscopically. The goal of laparoscopic surgery was to excise all macroscopic fibrotic endometriosis and restore normal anatomic relationships. Indications were pain (46 cases), infertility (46), hypermenorrhoea (7), and mass (1). Cases were staged according to the AFS Classification: 6% stage II; 30% stage III; and 64% stage IV. A total of 148 laparoscopies were performed including second- and third-look procedures. Average age was 32 years (range 22–54). Fifty-two women had a prior history of medical or surgical therapy for endometriosis. Surgical techniques included aquadissection, electrosurgery (44 cases), and a combination of laser surgery, electrosurgery, and/or scissors dissection (56). Average operating time was 178 minutes (partial cases, 126 minutes; complete cases, 227 minutes). Eighty nine per cent (41/46) had pain relief and 86% (6/7) had relief of hypermenorrhoea; no hysterectomies were necessary. Overall fertility outcome was 74% (34/46); excluding male factor the pregnancy rate was 85% (34/40). Three women had spontaneous abortions; there were no ectopic pregnancies. No laparotomies were required. Seventy-two women were discharged on the operative day; 28 the next morning. Results for partial and complete obliteration were similar in all categories confirming our impression that we were dealing with the same disease process, i.e. deep fibrotic endometriosis.

ECTOPIC PREGNANCY (CONTROVERSIAL CONCEPTS)

This author has used laparoscopic techniques exclusively for the treatment of 60 cases of ectopic pregnancy since 1982. Laparoscopic salpingectomy and salpingotomy have been well described in the medical literature (Bruhat et al, 1980) and are discussed in detail in Chapter 8. Thus only controversial techniques are discussed here (Reich et al, 1987; Reich, 1988c).

Fimbrial evacuation of tubal pregnancy

Fimbrial evacuation, tubal aspiration without salpingotomy, and tubal abortion without salpingotomy all refer to the technique of removing products of conception at or near the fimbrial end of the tube using either suction or grasping forceps, and on occasion, using grasping forceps to gently push the products of conception towards the fimbrial end. In some cases, tubal abortion is already in progress.

Concern about the incomplete removal of trophoblast and increased tubal damage has resulted in fimbrial evacuation of tubal pregnancy using either laparoscopic or laparotomy techniques being condemned, especially following Budowick et al's study (1980) that implied most tubal pregnancies occur in the extraluminal space. The recent findings of Sherman et al (1987) may encourage the laparoscopic surgeon to reconsider this method.

If the vast majority of ampullary tubal pregnancies rapidly invade the tubal wall and grow in the loose connective tissue between mucosa and serosa, milking the ectopic pregnancy out of the fimbria would cause further tubal destruction. We have not seen a high incidence of extraluminal tubal pregnancies and have treated eight of our last 18 tubal pregnancies by 'aquaexpression'. With this technique the tip of a suction–irrigation device is inserted through the open end of the affected tube into the ampulla and fluid under pressure used to dislodge and expel the intraluminal products of conception, which can then be aspirated from the peritoneal cavity. There were no intraoperative or postoperative complications. β-HCG titres were in the non-pregnant range in all cases 2 weeks postsurgery.

Interstitial ectopic pregnancy

Interstitial ectopic pregnancies are rare. This author has treated a ruptured interstitial pregnancy laparoscopically by electrosurgical wedge resection resulting in preservation of most of the distal portion of the tube but destruction of much interstitium, making a future anastomosis unlikely to succeed. Bipolar desiccation of both the ascending uterine and utero-ovarian arteries was necessary to gain haemostasis. Vasopressin was not used.

The same techniques employed during laparotomy can be applied to laparoscopic resection of an interstitial pregnancy, i.e. segmental resection of the cornua using cutting current electrosurgery. The principles involved are very similar to those gained from removing fibroids from the myometrium during laparoscopic surgery: large vessel haemostasis can be achieved with bipolar forceps and dissection planes developed with the Aquapurator. Alternatively, following vasopressin infiltration, an incision can be made with the knife electrode or laser down to the gestational sac which can then be aspirated with an Aquapurator.

Methotrexate may prove to be a useful adjuvant for interstitial pregnancy. Tanaka et al (1982) and Brandes et al (1986) have documented its successful use.

Extraluminal tubal pregnancy

Budowick et al (1980) from a series of 20 dissections of tubal pregnancies, concluded that the growing product of fertilization rapidly penetrates the wall of the tube and subsequently most of its growth occurs in an extratubal location between the tubal serosa and its muscularis. Stock (1985) reviewed the histopathology of 110 cases of tubal gestation and concluded that the developing tubal pregnancy was intraluminal, within the muscularis of the tube, in all but one case. Pauerstein et al (1986), following a systematic gross and histopathological study of 25 consecutive ectopic pregnancies concluded that an intraluminal location was present in 67%. This evolving understanding of the pathophysiology of ectopic tubal pregnancy has significant clinical implications regarding management decisions.

In most cases of extraluminal ectopic pregnancy, upon opening the tubal serosa over the most distended portion of the tube, products of conception will be evident and often extrude themselves. Thereafter, irrigation with the Aquapurator will produce distention of the tube without any flow of irrigant out of the fimbrial end. Should bleeding be present, the operator can err by trying to open the tube further.

In my experience with these cases, rarely will the surgeon enter the true tubal lumen. Occasionally the blood clot and/or products of conception will envelop the space between serosa and muscularis through 360°. After removal of the bulk of the products of conception and obtaining haemostasis with pressure, coagulation electrosurgery, or laser, the surgeon should end the procedure and follow the patient carefully with β-HCG titres. Adjuvant therapy with methotrexate may have to be considered.

Ruptured tubal pregnancy

Ruptured tubal pregnancy has been considered a contraindication to a laparoscopic approach. However, most ruptured tubes can be easily and safely removed with bipolar desiccation.

In the series of 109 consecutive tubal pregnancies compiled by Reich et al (1988), there were 16 cases of ruptured tubal pregnancy. Salpingectomy or partial salpingectomy was performed in 13 of these cases and salpingotomy in three. Subsequently two women have had intrauterine pregnancies. Another woman in this group, who underwent salpingectomy, has since had two pregnancies in her remaining tube, both treated by laparoscopic salpingotomy.

Of 118 women reported by Pouly et al (1986), who had tubal pregnancies treated by laparoscopic salpingotomy while still desiring fertility, a ruptured tube was present in 47. Intrauterine pregnancies were later recorded in 27 of these women (57.4%) and recurrent ectopic pregnancy in nine (19%). A ruptured tube was present in 32 of the 100 cases of laparoscopic salpingectomy recently reported by Dubuisson (1987).

OTHER PROCEDURES

Dermoid cysts

Oophorectomy with culdotomy extraction can be considered for previously diagnosed or intraoperatively discovered dermoid cysts in women not desiring future fertility. Spillage is rare and can be directed through the culdotomy incision (Reich and McGlynn, 1986a,b; Reich, 1989).

Should laparoscopic cyst excision with associated intentional spillage be considered? Kistner (1952) described the aftermath of intraperitoneal rupture of benign cystic teratomas. The intraperitoneal spill of dermoid contents sets up a granulomatous reaction in the peritoneum which, when viewed grossly, may be confused with tuberculosis or carcinomatosis.

In 1986, at a national meeting, Kurt Semm described the treatment of over 70 dermoid cysts using laparoscopic surgical techniques. The cysts were drained into the cul-de-sac and then stripped from surrounding normal ovarian tissue. No adverse effects occurred. Bruhat's group in France and this author have had a similar experience. Shelling out a dermoid from inside an ovary following drainage is usually much easier than endometrioma cyst wall excision. Vigorous peritoneal cavity irrigation with at least 10 litres of Ringer's lactate and underwater examination with direct suctioning of fatty and epidermal elements per underwater examination is recommended to prevent a future chronic granulomatous reaction.

Alternatively, it is possible to remove dermoid cysts intact and still preserve the ovary. The laser is used to drill a superficial hole in the ovarian cortex, avoiding rupture of the delicate cyst wall. After locating the cleavage plane between the cyst wall and the ovarian cortex, microscissors are inserted and the opening extended. Aquadissection is very useful to separate the dermoid cyst from surrounding ovarian tissue. Laser and scissors are used to separate fibrous adhesions and vessels near the hilum. Caution is constantly exercised to prevent puncturing the cyst wall. Following complete excision of the intact cyst from inside the ovary, it is removed through the cul-de-sac using the previously described laparoscopic culdotomy incision.

Myomectomy

Enucleation of myomas can be a frustrating, time-consuming experience when attempted laparoscopically. Bleeding problems are common and difficult to resolve. An instrument capable of holding an intramural fibroid on tension during its dissection from surrounding myometrium is essential; the 5 mm corkscrew (WISAP, Tomball, Texas) is such an instrument.

The serosa and surrounding myometrial shell are entered with a knife electrode at 80 W cutting current. Thereafter, the corkscrew is screwed into the myoma, which is pulled outward so that the tip of the Aquapurator can be inserted between the fibroid and surrounding myometrium to aquadissect tissue planes. The exposed portion of the fibroid can then be bivalved using cutting current electrosurgery. Small fibrous adhesions between the fibroid and its myometrial shell can be divided with laser and larger pedicles separately desiccated with bipolar forceps. Little blood loss occurs. Vasopressin is not administered preoperatively.

Hydrosalpinx (Reich, 1987a)

Chronic pelvic inflammatory disease with hydrosalpinx can almost always be treated laparoscopically. Scissors dissection should be attempted on the most favourable side, with laser or electrosurgery reserved for the other. With hydrosalpinx, the distal end of the tube is often fused to the ovary and is opened by dividing all adhesions between distal tube and ovarian surface. Difficult surgical decisions must be made when dissecting the distal tube from the ovary as bleeding often ensues in the tubo-ovarian ligament or fimbria ovarica which can compromise fimbrio-ostial blood supply.

Following mobilization of the distal tube, microscissors are inserted into the phimotic ostium and spread. Avascular areas are divided. Then 3 mm grasping forceps are inserted, spread, and the ostium stretched. Finally, 5 mm smooth grasping forceps are inserted, spread, and again avascular areas divided, usually resulting in a wide-open ostium with fimbrial mucosa protruding from it. Laser eversion is avoided if possible, as the thermal effect of laser eversion frequently causes phimosis or adhesions. More physiological eversion can often be obtained by cutting bands of fibrous tissue surrounding the tubal ostium, and on occasion, performing a suture eversion with 4-0 PDS. With a large sactosalpinx, laser eversion at power setting of 1–3 W is followed by a suture approximating ostial mucosa to tube serosa, effectively covering most of the thermally-damaged serosa.

Tubal anastomosis

I have performed 25 laparoscopic tubal anastomoses for reversal of tubal ligation using the two-stitch technique of Swolin (1988). This procedure was performed on one tube only during screening laparoscopy for evaluation prior to laparotomy tubal ligation reversal. Thus far there have been two intrauterine pregnancies and two ectopic pregnancies, both in the contralateral untreated tube.

The problem with laparoscopic tubal ligation reversal lies not in the magnification, but in the available suture needles and needle holders. The needles available for laparoscopic procedures today are large, without curve, and with taper tips. The needle holders hold the needle loosely at right angles. I have performed many procedures with many different types of stents passed through the uterus by hysteroscopy and through distal and proximal tube segments. Stents are not the answer.

The proximal tube is easily opened with hook scissors. Bleeding usually stops spontaneously. The orifice can be identified by intrauterine lavage with indigo carmine dye. It is very difficult to open the distal tube segment at its proximal end. Often there are adhesions in the area and the ampullary lumen is without circumferential support characteristic of isthmic musculature. After using distal tubal stints in over 20 cases, this author feels that a much better approach is to insert a double-lumen balloon catheter into the peritoneal cavity through the umbilical incision adjacent to and beneath the laparoscopic trocar sleeve. It is then inserted just inside the fimbrial end to occlude and irrigate the distal tube retrograde with indigo-carmine dye to identify the proximal end of the lumen which is then opened with hook scissors. Sutures are then placed at the mesenteric and anti-mesenteric borders with 4-0 PDS.

Laparoscopic hysterectomy (Reich, 1989a)

Laparoscopic hysterectomy has been performed by this author using laparoscopic surgical techniques including aquadissection to develop appropriate tissue planes and bipolar electrosurgery for large vessel haemostasis, including uterine vessels. Laparoscopic staples should facilitate this procedure in the future.

Lymphadenectomy

Lymphadenectomy has been performed retroperitoneally by Dargent and Salvat (1988) and transperitoneally by Querleu (1989) in Roubaix, France, and by this author. The ovarian vessel pedicle and surrounding peritoneum is stripped back to the level of the aortic bifurcation. Adipose and lymph tissue lateral to the common and external iliac vessels is excised using laser dissection close to the vessels. Following mobilization of the medial and undersurface of the external iliac vein, the obturator internis fascia of the pelvic side-wall and the obturator nerve are identified and surrounding nodal tissue removed, taking great care while operating close to the hypogastric vein.

CONCLUSION

The techniques described in this chapter should prove useful to both the novice and the expert laparoscopic surgeon. The practical limit to laparoscopic surgery has yet to be defined, despite the widespread use of this operation for two decades (Reich, 1987c). It is becoming increasingly clear that complex gynaecological procedures can be performed using laparoscopic surgical techniques.

Acknowledgements

Len Romanowski, CRNA was the technical advisor for the 'Anesthesia Considerations' section. Fran McGlynn, CRNP, MS, Ronald Batt, MD, FACOG, and Jerry Hulka, MD, FACOG assisted with the preparation of this manuscript. Bridget Evans, provided secretarial assistance.

REFERENCES

Ahrenholz DH & Simmons RL (1980) Fibrin in peritonitis. I. Beneficial and adverse effects of fibrin in experimental *E. coli* peritonitis. *Surgery* **88:** 41–47.

Barber HRK & Graber EA (1971) The PMPO syndrome (postmenopausal palpable ovary syndrome). *Obstetrics and Gynecology* **38:** 921–923.

Brandes MC, Youngs DD, Goldstein DP et al (1986) Treatment of cornual pregnancy with methotrexate: case report. *American Journal of Obstetrics and Gynecology* **155:** 655–657.

Bruhat MA, Manhes H, Mage G et al (1980) Treatment of ectopic pregnancy by means of laparoscopy. *Fertility and Sterility* **33:** 411–414.

Budowick M, Johnson TRB, Genadry R et al (1980) The histopathology of the developing tubal ectopic pregnancy. *Fertility and Sterility* **34:** 169–171.

Dargent D & Salvat J (1988) *Envahissement Ganglionnaire Pelvien*. Paris: Medsi/McGraw-Hill.

Dubuisson JB, Aubroit FX & Cardone V (1987) Laparoscopic salpingectomy for tubal pregnancy. *Fertility and Sterility* **47:** 225–228.

Henry-Suchet J, Soler A & Loffredo V (1984) Laparoscopic treatment of tuboovarian abscesses. *Journal of Reproductive Medicine* **29:** 579–582.

Hudspeth AS (1975) Radical surgical debridement in the treatment of advanced generalized bacterial peritonitis. *Archives of Surgery* **110:** 1233–1236.

Kistner RW (1952) Intraperitoneal rupture of benign cystic teratomas: review of the literature with a report of two cases. *Obstetrical and Gynecological Survey* **7:** 603–617.

Martin DC (1988) Laparoscopic and vaginal colpotomy for the excision of infiltrating cul-de-sac endometriosis. *Journal of Reproductive Medicine* **33:** 806–808.

Pauerstein CJ, Croxatto HB, Eddy CA et al (1986) Anatomy and pathology of tubal pregnancy. *Obstetrics and Gynecology* **67:** 301–308.

Pouly JL, Mahnes H, Mage G et al (1986) Conservative laparoscopic treatment of 321 ectopic pregnancies. *Fertility and Sterility* **46:** 1093–1097.

Querleu D (1989) Laparoscopic pelvic lymphadenectomy. Second World Congress of Gynecologic Endoscopy. Clermont-Ferrand, France.

Reich H (1987a) Laparoscopic treatment of extensive pelvic adhesions, including hydrosalpinx. *Journal of Reproductive Medicine* **32:** 736–742.

Reich H (1987b) Laparoscopic oophorectomy and salpingo-oophorectomy in the treatment of benign tuboovarian disease. *International Journal of Fertility* **32:** 233–236.

Reich H (1988a) Endoscopic management of tubo-ovarian abscess and pelvic inflammatory disease. In Levine RL & Sanfilippo JS (eds) *Gynecologic Endoscopy: Pelviscopic Surgery and Laser Laparoscopy*. Springer-Verlag.

Reich H (1988b) Laparoscopic treatment of cul-de-sac obliteration secondary to endometriosis. American Fertility Society, 44th Annual Meeting. Atlanta, Georgia.

Reich H (1988c) Ectopic pregnancy. In Levine RL & Sanfilippo JS (eds) *Gynecologic Endoscopy: Pelviscopic Surgery and Laser Laparoscopy*. Springer-Verlag.

Reich H (1989a) Laparoscopic hysterectomy. *Journal of Gynecologic Surgery* **5**(2).

Reich H (1989b) Laparoscopic oophorectomy. *Contemporary OB/GYN* (in press).

Reich H & McGlynn F (1986a) Laparoscopic oophorectomy and salpingo-oophorectomy in the treatment of benign tuboovarian disease. *Journal of Reproductive Medicine* **31:** 609.

Reich H & McGlynn F (1986b) Treatment of ovarian endometriomas using laparoscopic surgical techniques. *Journal of Reproductive Medicine* **31:** 577–584.

Reich H & McGlynn F (1987) Laparoscopic treatment of tuboovarian and pelvic abscess. *Journal of Reproductive Medicine* **32:** 747.

Reich H, Friefeld ML, McGlynn F et al (1987) Laparoscopic treatment of tubal pregnancy. *Obstetrics and Gynecology* **69:** 275–279.

Reich H, Johns D, DeCaprio J et al (1988) Laparoscopic treatment of 109 consecutive ectopic pregnancies. *Journal of Reproductive Medicine* **32:** 885–890.

Rivlin ME & Hunt JA (1986) Surgical management of diffuse peritonitis complicating obstetric/gynecologic infections. *Obstetrics and Gynecology* **67:** 652–656.

Semm K (1978) Tissue-puncher and loop-ligation—new aids for surgical therapeutic pelviscopy (laparoscopy) endoscopic intraabdominal surgery. *Endoscopy* **10:** 119–124.

Semm K & Mettler L (1980) Technical progress in pelvic surgery via operative laparoscopy. *American Journal of Obstetrics and Gynecology* **138:** 121–127.

Sherman D, Langer R, Herman A et al (1987) Reproductive outcome after fimbrial evacuation of tubal pregnancy. *Fertility and Sterility* **47:** 420–424.

Simpson FF (1909) The choice of time for operation for pelvic inflammation of tubal origin. *Surgery and Gynecology and Obstetrics* **9:** 45–62.

Skau T, Nystrom PO, Ohman L et al (1986) The kinetics of peritoneal clearance of *Escherichia coli* and *Bacteroides fragilis* and participating defense mechanisms. *Archives of Surgery* **121:** 1033–1039.
Stock RJ (1985) Histopathologic changes in tubal pregnancy. *Journal of Reproductive Medicine* **30:** 923–928.
Swolin K (1988) Tubal anastomosis. *Human Reproduction* **3:** 177–178.
Tanaka T, Hayashi H, Kutsuzawa T et al (1982) Treatment of interstitial ectopic pregnancy with methotrexate. *Fertility and Sterility* **37**(6): 851–852.

Index

Note: Page numbers of article titles are in **bold** type.